Medical Assisting
Administrative *and* Clinical Competencies

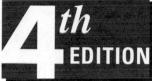
4th EDITION

Lucille Keir, CMA-A
Barbara A. Wise, BSN, RN, MA(Ed)
Connie Krebs, CMA-C, BGS

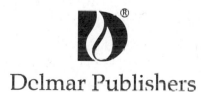

Delmar Publishers

an International Thomson Publishing company I(T)P®

Albany • Bonn • Boston • Cincinnati • Detroit • London • Madrid
Melbourne • Mexico City • New York • Pacific Grove • Paris • San Francisco
Singapore • Tokyo • Toronto • Washington

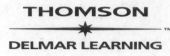

Medical Assisting: Administrative and Clinical Competencies
by Lucille Keir, Barbara A. Wise, Connie Krebs

Publisher:
Susan Simpfenderfer

Acquisitions Editor:
Marlene McHugh Pratt

Development Editor:
Helen Yackel

Project Editor:
William Trudell

Art/Design Coordinator:
Rich Killar

Production Coordinator:
Cathleen Berry

Marketing Manager:
Daryl L. Caron

Editorial Assistant:
Sarah Holle

Cover Design:
Charles Cummings Advertising/Art, Inc.

Library of Congress Cataloging-in-Publication Data
Keir, Lucille.
    Medical assisting: administrative and clinical competencies / Lucille Keir, Barbara A. Wise, Connie Krebs—4th ed.
        p.   cm.
    Includes bibliographical references and index.
    ISBN 0-8273-7712-6 (alk. paper)
    1. Medical assistants. I. Wise, Barbara A. II. Krebs, Connie. III. Title.
    [DNLM: 1. Physician Assistants. 2. Clinical Competence. 3. Practice Management, Medical. 4. Vocational Guidance.
    W 21.5 K27m 1998]
    R728.8K44   1998
    610.73'7—dc21
    DNLM/DLC   97-16219
    for Library of Congress   CIP

NOTICE TO THE READER

Publisher does not warrant or guarantee any of the products described herein or perform any independent analysis in connection with any of the product information contained herein. Publisher does not assume, and expressly disclaims, any obligation to obtain and include information other than that provided to it by the manufacturer.

The reader is expressly warned to consider and adopt all safety precautions that might be indicated by the activities herein and to avoid all potential hazards. By following the instructions contained herein, the reader willingly assumes all risks in connection with such instructions.

The Publisher makes no representation or warranties of any kind, including but not limited to, the warranties of fitness for particular purpose or merchantability, nor are any such representations implied with respect to the material set forth herein, and the publisher takes no responsibility with respect to such material. The publisher shall not be liable for any special, consequential, or exemplary damages resulting, in whole or part, from the readers' use of, or reliance upon, this material.

TABLE OF CONTENTS

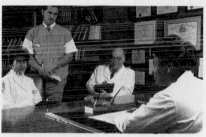

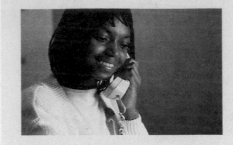

SECTION 2
THE ADMINISTRATIVE ASSISTANT   99

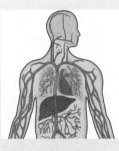

SECTION 3
STRUCTURE AND FUNCTION OF THE BODY   205

■ CHAPTER 11
Anatomy and Physiology of the Human Body   207

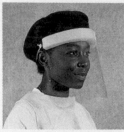

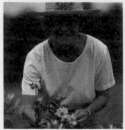

SECTION 5
BEHAVIORS AND HEALTH 717

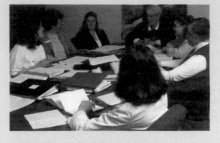

SECTION 6
EMPLOYABILITY SKILLS 751

INDEX OF TABLES

INDEX OF PROCEDURES

■ INDEX OF PROCEDURES cont.

PREFACE

Medical Assisting: Administrative and Clinical Competencies, 4th Edition is a proven competency-based learning system with a twelve year history of success. The text is full-color throughout and written in an interesting, easy to understand format. The content covers the knowledge, skills, attitudes, and values necessary to prepare you to become a successful, multiskilled medical assistant. Information is presented in six major sections which are divided into 21 chapters with a total of 81 units of instruction. There are hundreds of color photos, illustrations, charts, and tables to visually supplement and reinforce the written material. A student workbook, student practice software, instructor's manual, computerized testbank and instructor's resource kit complete this learning system.

The text, workbook and practice software are comprehensive, covering the administrative, clinical and general areas identified as necessary for entry level employment by the current Role Delineation Study for Medical Assisting issued by the American Association of Medical Assistants (AAMA) and the National Board of Medical Examiners. The cognitive and performance competencies are identified by Learning Objectives which are stated at the beginning of each unit of instruction or as Terminal Performance Objectives with each written administrative or clinical procedure.

A clear and concise presentation of human anatomy and physiology is included in the text. The structure and function of each system is followed by a discussion of the common diagnostic examinations and the diseases and disorders of that system. To facilitate learning, a new expanded outline format organizes the description, signs and symptoms, causes, and treatments for each disease.

The text, workbook and practice software are designed as instructive guides to learning the attitudes, behaviors and skills necessary for a successful career as a multiskilled medical assistant in today's dynamic health care environment. It can be used in a variety of settings:

- a structured classroom setting, with the expertise of a qualified instructor
- for individualized instruction of learners in programs of diversified training, because much of the content and format are appropriate for self-study
- for on-the-job training in a physician's office, where the learning package serves as a supplement to employee instruction and as a resource manual
- for review by medical assistants who wish to prepare for the certification examination

Completion of the learning materials, including an understanding of the learning and performance objectives and application of the standard competencies during externship or employment, prepare the learner to successfully complete the CMA or RMA certification examination.

Student Practice Software is now packaged with this text is an easy-to-use Windows® (3.1 or higher) program consisting of over 800 exercises and activities that make individual or group study effective and fun. For each exercise, the learner has two attempts to answer each question correctly and then receives immediate feedback on all answers. For additional information, refer to the "How to Use the Student Practice Software" section on the pages immediately before Chapter 1.

Together the authors have over 50 years of medical and academic educational preparation and employment experience. In addition, many medical assistants, educators, nurses, and physicians from general and specialty practices have reviewed and contributed to this 4th Edition.

WHAT'S NEW IN THE FOURTH EDITION?

Many changes were made to reflect the impact of technology, recent legislation, medical advances and revised accreditation standards. Limitations on clinical laboratory procedures and the impact of this and other legislation on the operation of a medical office are explained. Other changes involve third-party payments, the shift to managed care, and the communication revolution. The anatomy and physiology content reflects advances in cellular biology applications and the ever changing diagnostic and treatment methods.

The major content changes are as follows:

Administrative and General

- *New*–chapter on the role of the medical assistant which covers training, career opportunities, personal characteristics, and professionalism
- *New*–discussions on career opportunities and career laddering
- *New and Expanded*–certification requirements and eligibility; employment opportunities and continuing education
- *Expanded*–information on time management.
- *Expanded*–information on acquiring, maintaining, and advancing your career
- *New*–Fundamentals of Managed Care Unit explains various changes and types of health care coverage and the purpose of each including HMO's. Managed Care is also covered throughout the text where appropriate, eg scheduling and billing

- *New*–advances in communication technology including voice mail, e-mail, pagers, cellular phones, conference calls, teleconference, and telemedicine
- *New*–office environment content including office design, Americans with Disabilities Act implications, and expanded information on ergonomics

Insurance and Coding

- *New*–historical beginnings of CPT and ICD coding methods and discussion of the development and impact of managed care
- *Expanded*–third-party reimbursement

Anatomy & Physiology Content

- *New*–all diseases and conditions are organized in a format outlining the description, signs and symptoms, cause, and treatment
- *New*–most diseases and disorders include phonetic pronunciations to facilitate learning
- *New*–categories of HIV infection and the determining factors which classify the disease as AIDS
- *New*–information on fingerprinting, genetics, the Human Genome Project, gene therapy, and genetic engineering along with the legal, ethical, and moral issues involved
- *New*–completely new computer-generated full-color illustrations which match those found in the workbook exercises

Clinical

- *Revised*–discussion of Clinical Laboratory Improvement Amendments (CLIA), Occupational Safety and Health Administration (OSHA), and Physicians Office Laboratory (POL) regulations including new Standard Precautions
- *Revised*–blood glucose equipment and computer link capabilities
- *Revised*–information on cardiopulmonary diagnostic equipment and illustrations
- *Expanded and revised*–immunization content
- *New*–nomogram for calculating medication dosages
- *Expanded*–telephone and on-site triage
- *Revised*–chapter on emergency care, including office readiness, acute illness, injuries, and first aid applications
- *Expanded*–information on exercise, nutrition and habit-forming drugs
- *Revised and Reorganized*–unit on mobility and range of motion exercises, including canes, crutches and wheelchairs

Additional Changes:

- *New*–all procedures are numbered along with corresponding Performance Evaluation Checklists in the workbook
- *New*–rationales have been added to procedures
- *Expanded*–medical-legal ethical highlights throughout text with critical-thinking discussion scenarios

COMPREHENSIVE LEARNING PACKAGE

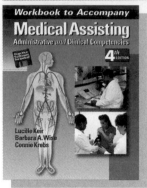

Student Workbook (0-8273-7713-4) contains unit specific assignment sheets with a variety of review questions, vocabulary and skill exercises, forms to complete, puzzles, and other activities that reinforce the text content. New to this edition, *the anatomy and physiology section will now be full-color*. The workbook also includes new Performance Evaluation Checklists for determining student competency of administrative, clinical and general competencies of the text and *includes a point rating for each step*. The checklists correlate with the steps in the textbook procedures and reflect the terminal performance objectives. The organization of the workbook has been revised to include the assignment sheets, in the same order as the text content, within the front section. The Performance Evaluation Checklists are numbered as they are in the textbook and are in one complete section in the back of the workbook to make them easier to locate and use. Evaluation Checklists include a documentation section for students to practice charting after appropriate procedures.

A Certificate of Completion, to be completed and signed by the instructor, is included at the back of each workbook.

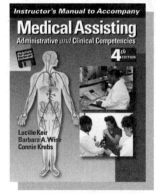

Instructor's Manual (0-8273-7715-0) has been improved to make it easier for instructors to identify answers to student workbook questions and exercises. The questions as well as the answers have now been included to facilitate evaluating the workbook assignment sheets. The Instructor's Manual includes:

- Correlation guide from the third to the fourth edition, identifying what features are new, expanded, or revised and where they can be found
- Instructional strategies and suggestions for presenting the course content, including integrating technology into the curriculum
- Instructional suggestions, organizational tips, and sample lesson plan format
- Section on establishing an externship program along with suggested tracking forms
- Chapter by chapter workbook questions with correct answer plus additional suggested activities for each chapter

- Documentation record of student scores for assignment sheets and performance evaluation sheets which may be used in lieu of a gradebook, if so desired.
- Student Practice Software Program instructions, including system requirements, installation, a description of the program, and technical support

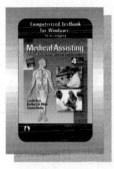

Computerized Testbank (0-8273-7716-9) includes over 1,800 questions and answers. The Testbank is available in a new easy-to-use Windows® (3.1 or higher) format to allow easy creation of testing materials.

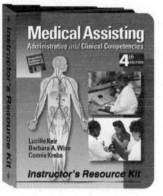

Instructor's Resource Kit (0-8273-7714-2) is a comprehensive 3-ring binder packed with instructional support for instructors at any level of educational program. It includes sections on:

- **Concepts and Principles of Teaching and Learning** - discusses what teaching is, how students learn, basic learning principles and steps in the learning process
- **From Objectives to Evaluation** - discusses the purpose and benefits of identifying objectives, how to evaluate student competence, and how objectives and evaluation provide a solid framework for a competency-based education.
- **Instructional Strategies** - identifies ideas and methods of planning that make up the media of content presentation; describes a variety of methods for delivering instruction.
- **Lesson Plans** - discusses four-step lesson planing and design along with complete presentation outlines for each of the textbook units.
- **Class Activities** - provides additional ideas, activities and materials to reinforce lessons, to make learning more relevant, and to help students apply concepts from theory to practice.
- **Transparency Masters** - includes individualized sheets that can be photocopied into overhead transparencies, aiding in the visual presentation of material.

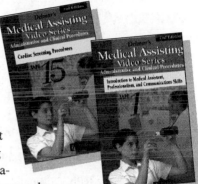

Delmar's Medical Assisting Video Series: Administrative and Clinical Procedures, 2nd Edition (0-8273-8304-5) is a collection of 15 tapes with over nine hours of instruction to complement Delmar's medical assisting texts. They cover administrative, clinical and laboratory procedures as well as interpersonal skills and characteristics.

Delmar's Medical Assisting CD-ROM (0-8273-8404-1) is a multimedia interactive program developed specifically for the field of medical assisting. The CD-ROM's menu structure is based on AAMA's new Role Delineation Study plus an add-on Managed Care Segment. The CD-ROM can be used as a standalone program or as an integrated enhancement to any medical assisting textbook.

The use of the textbook, reinforced by the Student Practice Software, Student Workbook, and the instructional assistance in the Instructor's Manual, Computerized Testbank, and Instructor's Resource Kit provides a complete, multiskilled competency-based learning system, that is innovating, easy to comprehend, and provides the necessary competencies for a career in medical assisting.

ACKNOWLEDGMENTS

A textbook of this nature requires the input and assistance of many friends, professional colleagues and acquaintances, and subject matter experts as well as the publishing team and the group of reviewers. We owe them all a great deal of appreciation and recognition for their willingness to contribute of their time and expertise to assist with this revision.

Special recognition is due to the following:

- **Anne Burns**, RPh, Clinical Assistant Professor and manager of the Proficiency Practice Laboratory, The Ohio State University College of Pharmacy, for assistance with Chapter 18 on medications.

- **Kim Knueven**, RN, BS medical office manager, for her insights and assistance with Chapter 21, Employability Skills.

- **Holly Herron Meader**, RN, MS, Life Flight trauma nurse for reviewing and making recommendations for emergency care and first aid in Chapter 19.

- **Lee A. Speck**, MT (AMT), LMLT (ASCP), Smith, Kline, Beecham Laboratories, for review and recommendations for Chapter 15, Laboratory Procedures.

- **James B. Soldano**, MD for reviewing the content regarding physical examination in Chapter 14.

- **Warner M. Thomas**, Jr. Attorney at Law, for his review and recommendations of Chapter 3 on Medical Ethics and Liability.

- **Kent Vedder**, BSME, engineer in medical disposables research and computer-aided design, who provided information pertaining to electronic networking by voice and E-mail, and demonstrated data retrieval from the Internet.

- **Carol Watts**, CMA, a practicing medical assistant manager, who provided assistance to revise Chapters 8, 9, and 10.

Invaluable contributions from physicians, nurses, and educators were truly outstanding. Their involvement took hours of reviewing, identifying and recommending content to be deleted, added or technically updated in the 13 units of the anatomy and physiology chapter. Words are inadequate to express our appreciation.

Very special acknowledgment to the following:

- **Stephen D'Ambrosio**, PhD, Professor of Radiobiology and Pharmacology, The Ohio State University, College of Medicine, for resources and assistance with cellular structure and genetics in Unit 1.

- **Phil Diaz**, MD, The Ohio State University researcher and practicing physician specializing in pulmonary diseases, for review and assistance with The Respiratory System, Unit 7.

- **Ann Eaton**, MD, pediatrician in community practice, for answers to inquires in various areas as they related to infants or children.

- **James English**, MD, family practice physician and former anatomy and physiology instructor in The Ohio State University College of Medicine, for his contribution to this revision, (his third time). His remarkable investment of time to review Units 2, 3, 4, 8, 10, and 12 is truly outstanding.

- **Elaine Glass**, RN, MS, OCN, a clinical nurse specialist at the Arthur G James Cancer Hospital and Research Institute, for sharing her materials on the Immune System in Unit 9.

- **Diane Hohwald**, RN, CNN, Grant/Riverside Methodist Hospital, Dialysis Educational Coordinator for her information on dialysis in Unit 11, the Urinary System.

- **Peter Pema**, MD, Neurologist and Radiologist, for assistance to understand some radiological procedures.

- **Michael Staub**, MD, surgical resident in Orthopedics for his in-depth review and recommendations for Units 5 and 6, the Skeletal and Muscular Systems.

- **Nancy Wise Vedder**, RN, BSN, OCN, Grant/Riverside Cancer Institute, Oncology Research Nurse, who reviewed and provided information relating to the diagnosis and treatment of cancer and Unit 9, the Immune System.

- **Henry A Wise**, MD, Urologist, who reviewed and provided extensive comments on the Urinary System, Unit 11 and male reproductive content in The Reproductive System, Unit 13.

REVIEWERS

The authors are particularly grateful to the reviewers who continue to be a valuable resource in guiding this book as it evolves. Their insights, comments, suggestions, and attention to detail were very important in guiding the development of this textbook.

- **Emma Anderson**, CMA/LPT
  Ogden Webster Applied Technology College
  Ogden, UT

- **Alisa Bowhay**, BSN
  Topeka Technical College
  Netawaka, KS

- **Kevin Brown**, BA, RMA, (AMT)
  Formerly of Apollo College
  Tucson, AZ

- **Adrienne Carter-Ward**, CMA, BA,
  Corinthian Schools
  San Bernadino, CA

- **Laura Durham**, BS, CMA,
  Forsyth Technical Community College
  Winston-Salem, NC

- **Julie Orloff**, RMA, CMA, CPT
  National School of Technology
  North Miami Beach, FL

- **Ursula Pennell**
  Hesser College
  Epping, NH

- **Vicki Prater**, CMA
  Concorde Career Institute
  San Bernadino, CA

- **Kimberly Shinall**, R.N.
  Tidewater Tech Institute
  Norfolk, VA

- **Mary Wahl**, RN, BSN, MEPD, CMA,
  Mid-Sate Technical College
  Marshfield, WI

DEDICATION

We gratefully acknowledge the support and encouragement of our families, loved ones, and friends throughout the preparation of this edition. We especially recognize the wonderful friendship and strong commitment we share, which goes far beyond the pages of this book. Because of our experiences in employment and education, we felt a need for this text and we therefore wish to dedicate it to you, the reader, for you are the reason it was written.

APPRECIATION TO DELMAR PUBLISHERS

The authors especially wish to acknowledge and commend the editors and staff of Delmar Publishers for their guidance and expertise during the preparation of this edition. We especially thank Sarah Holle for responding to all our calls and requests. A special thanks goes to Helen Yackel who patiently encouraged and pleaded for manuscript until we finally got it finished. The assistance and dedication of the total staff during the development of the text was greatly appreciated.

Administrative Editor - **Marlene Pratt**
Developmental Editor - **Helen Yackel**
Editorial Assistant - **Sarah Holle**
Project Editor - **William Trudell**
Art and Design Coordinator - **Rich Killar**
Production Coordinator - **Cathleen Berry**
Marketing Manager - **Darryl L. Caron**

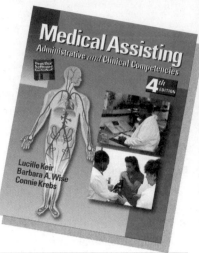

HOW TO USE THIS TEXT

Medical assisting is an ever-evolving health care profession full of opportunity and challenge. This complete learning system is designed to help you acquire the knowledge and skills necessary to become a successful multiskilled medical assistant. The text is organized into six main sections which reflect the broad areas of medical assisting responsibility. The sections are then divided into a total of 21 chapters of related information. Chapters are further divided into 81 units of specific content. The text has many unique features which will make it easier for you to learn and integrate theory and practice, including:

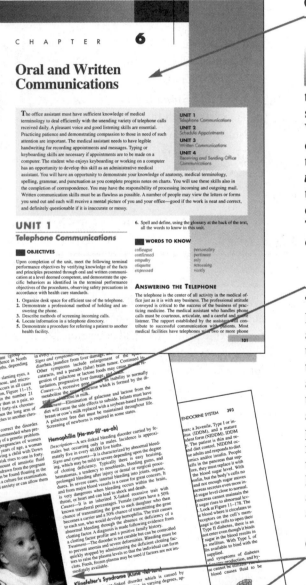

Chapter Openers

1 At the beginning of each chapter is a brief overview of the content presented within the chapter. Each chapter opener lists the **Units** of study within the chapter and the **Objectives** of the chapter, which can be used to self-test your understanding of the chapter content. When you're finished reading the chapter, review the objectives and re-read the necessary portions of the text until you can accomplish all objectives. The **Words to Know** identify the medical- and general-related terminology used in the unit. These are listed alphabetically and appear in blue the first time they are used. These terms are all defined in the glossary at the back of the book.

Anatomy and Physiology Section

2 This comprehensive anatomy and physiology section is organized into 13 general and body system units. Each body system unit includes the structure and function of the system, and the common diagnostic examinations and tests used to determine pathological conditions in that particular body system. Each body system unit also includes **Common Diseases and Disorders** with phonetic pronunciations to assist in building your medical vocabulary. Pathology is presented consistently throughout, and has been completely reorganized to highlight the description, cause, signs and symptoms, and treatment of the disease or condition where appropriate.

Color Photographs, Illustrations, Forms and Tables

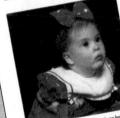

FIGURE 11-15 Child with Down Syndrome features.

3 Throughout the text, there are visual images to aid in the explanation and understanding of the subject matter. Full-color anatomy **illustrations** help differentiate human structures and organs, and explain physiological processes. **Color photos** throughout provide realistic examples of the material described. Actual medical **forms** duplicate those used in today's medical facilities. **Tables** summarize important facts or concepts presented in the text.

Procedures

Administrative and clinical competencies are presented in complete step-by-step procedures with distinct components. The *Title* identifies the procedure competency. Icons indicate whether the procedure is administrative 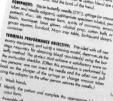 or clinical . The *Purpose* states the reason for performing the procedure. The *Equipment* lists the materials and supplies needed to perform the task. The *Terminal Performance Objective* states the competence (or task), the conditions for its performance, and the standard by which it will be evaluated. Throughout the steps, *Notes* identify specific instructions or cautions, and *Rationales* explain why a step in the procedure is required.

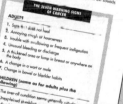

Patient Education Boxes

These purple-shaded boxes alert the student to issues and information that may be discussed with patients regarding tests and examinations, providing information to assist patients or their families in actively participating in their own health care. These education boxes can be found throughout the clinical content of the text, where appropriate.

Medical-Legal Ethical Highlights

At the close of most chapters, you will find Medical-Legal Ethical Highlights. These summarize the concepts within the chapter or include critical-thinking situations. This feature is included to provide "food for thought" and topics for learner discussion.

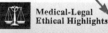

References

References are listed at the end of each chapter. These articles, pamphlets, periodicals, and books identify related sources of information.

Appendix

The appendice include sections on: Converting Measurements, Common Household Measures and Weights, Medical Symbols and Abbreviations, Medical Terminology Derivatives, and Prefixes and Suffixes. An extensive Glossary provides the definitions for all the Words to Know from each unit.

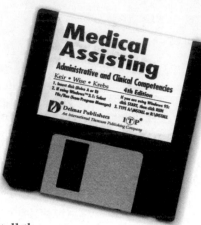

HOW TO USE THE PRACTICE SOFTWARE

The Student Practice Software has been designed to accompany *Medical Assisting: Administrative and Clinical Competencies, 4th Edition.* By using these exercises and games, you'll challenge yourself and other students, make your study of medical assisting more effective, and have fun!

Getting started is easy. Follow the simple directions on the disk label to install the program on your computer. Then take advantage of the following features:

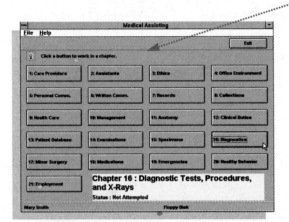

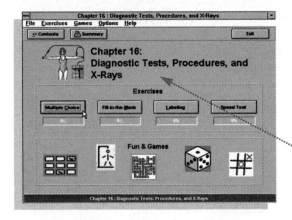

Minimum System Requirements:
Operating System: Windows 3.1 or higher
Computer: 386 or higher
Memory: 4 MB
Graphics: 16 bit color VGA
Hard Drive Space: 2 MB

Main Menu

The main menu follows the chapter organization of the text exactly—which makes it easy for you to find your way around. Just click on the button for the chapter you want, and you'll arrive at the chapter opening screen.

Toolbar

The button at the top left of every screen allows you to retrace your steps, while the Exit button gets you out of the program quickly and easily. As you navigate through the software, check the toolbar for other features that help you use individual exercises or games.

On-Line Help

If you get stuck, just press F1 or click on the *Help* menu for assistance. The on-line help includes instructions for all parts of the Student Practice Software.

The Chapter Screen

Here you have the opportunity to choose how you want to learn the material. Select one of the exercises for additional practice, review, or self-testing. Or click on a game to practice the content for that chapter in a fun format.

Exercises

The Student Practice Software acts as your own private tutor. For each exercise, it chooses from a bank of over 800 questions covering all 21 chapters. Putting these exercises to work for you is simple:

• Choose an exercise from those displayed, eg. multiple choice, true or false, fill-in-the-blank, or labeling exercise.

• You'll encounter a series of 8-10 questions for each exercise format; each question gives you two chances to answer correctly.

• Instant feedback tells you whether you're right or wrong—and helps you learn more quickly by explaining why an answer was correct or incorrect.

• The Practice Software displays the percentage of correct answers on the chapter screen. An on-screen score sheet (which you can print) lets you track correct and incorrect answers.

• Review your previous questions and answers in an exercise for more in-depth understanding. Or start an exercise over with a new, random set of questions that gives you a realistic study environment.

• When you're ready for an additional challenge, try the timed Speed Test. Once you've finished, it displays your score and the time you took to complete the test, so you can see how much you've learned.

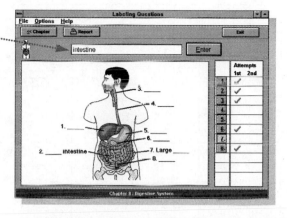

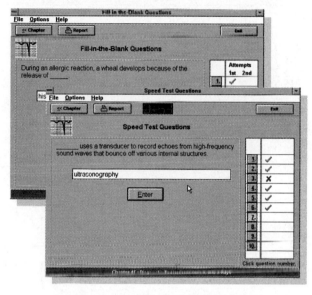

Fun & Games

To have fun while reinforcing your knowledge, enjoy each of the five simple games on the software. You can play alone, with a partner, or on teams.

• **Concentration:** match terms to their corresponding definitions under the cards as the timer runs.

• **Hangman:** review your spelling and vocabulary by choosing the correct letters to spell medical words appropriate to the chapter before you're "hanged."

• **Crossword Puzzles:** using the definition clues provided, fill in the medical words to complete each puzzle. A click of the Check button highlights incorrect answers in blue.

• **Board Game:** challenge your classmates and increase your knowledge by playing this question-and-answer game.

• **Tic-Tac-Toe:** you or your team must correctly answer a medical question before placing an X or an O.

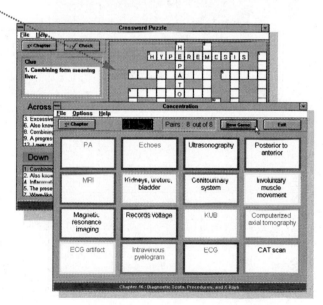

CORRELATION CHART TO ROLE DELINEATION STUDY

CH	TEXT	Administrative Procedures	Practice Finances	Fundamental Principles	Diagnostic Orders	Patient Care	Professionalism	Communication Skills	Legal Concepts	Instruction	Operational Functions
		Administrative		Clinical			General (Transdisciplinary)				
1.	Health Care Providers						X				
2.	The Medical Assistant						X		X		
3.	Medical Ethics and Liability	X		X	X	X	X	X	X	X	
4.	The Office Environment	X									X
5.	Interpersonal Communications	X					X	X	X	X	
6.	Oral and Written Communications	X		X	X	X	X	X	X	X	X
7.	Records Management	X	X				X	X	X		
8.	Collecting Fees	X	X				X	X	X		
9.	Health Care Coverage	X	X				X	X	X	X	
10.	Medical Office Management	X	X				X	X	X	X	X
11.	Anatomy and Physiology of the Human Body				X	X				X	
12.	Preparing for Clinical Duties			X	X	X	X		X	X	
13.	Beginning the Database			X	X	X	X	X	X	X	
14.	Preparing Patients for Examination				X	X	X	X	X	X	
15.	Specimen Collection & Laboratory Procedures			X	X	X	X	X	X	X	
16.	Diagnostic Test Procedures & X-rays			X	X	X			X	X	
17.	Minor Surgical Procedures			X	X	X		X	X	X	
18.	Assisting with Medications			X		X	X	X	X	X	
19.	Emergencies, Acute Illness, and Accidents			X		X	X	X	X	X	
20.	Behaviors Influencing Health				X	X	X	X	X	X	
21.	Achieving Satisfaction in Employment	X		X	X	X	X	X	X	X	X
	Appendix	X			X		X	X		X	
	Glossary	X			X			X			
	Workbook	X	X	X	X	X	X	X	X	X	X
	Instructor's Guide	X	X	X	X	X			X	X	X

Medical Health Care Roles and Responsibilities

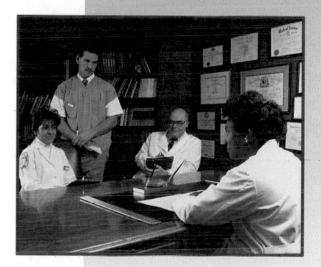

1

Health Care Providers

Health care providers have held prominent positions in society since the beginning of time. A look into the history of medicine reveals that for thousands of years, disease was thought to be the result of evil spirits and demons, brought on by disobedience to the gods. Therefore, early medical practitioners were primarily religious leaders. Eventually, scientific interest led to the discovery of microorganisms and understanding of the human body. Unit 1 of this chapter highlights ancient, medieval, and modern health care practitioners.

UNIT 1
A Brief History of Medicine

UNIT 2
The Health Care Team

UNIT 3
Medical Practice Specialties

Current medical practice has become very technical and is constantly undergoing change due to clinical research and development. Because of the vast amounts of accumulated knowledge and clinical procedures, it is impossible for a physician to provide competent care in all areas of medicine. In order to meet the needs of patients, some physicians become medical specialists, spending additional years in the study of one particular field of medicine. Unit 2 lists many specialties, the practitioner's titles, the areas of practice, and the types of patients treated.

Due to the complexity of health care, many other health care practitioners and specialists are needed in order to provide complete patient care. These professionals are also members of the health care team. They work in a variety of settings providing specialized care or services related to their education or training. A listing and brief discussion of various team members is included in Unit 3.

Because of the great technological advances in health care which have controlled plagues, increased survival rates, and extended the years of life, another major problem has developed: overpopulation. Unless controlled very soon, the masses of people will outstrip the world's capacity to support their existence. The current presence of air, water, and land pollution and the destruction of vital resources is evidence of impending problems. Once again disease, famine, and epidemics of viruses yet unknown and uncontrolled, may affect the people of the world.

UNIT 1

A Brief History of Medicine

■ OBJECTIVES

Upon completion of the unit, meet the following terminal performance objectives by verifying knowledge of the facts and principles presented through oral and written communication at a level deemed competent.

1. Explain how the caduceus may have been acquired as the medical symbol.
2. Discuss the reason Hippocrates is known as the Father of Medicine.
3. Tell why many of Galen's findings were invalid.
4. Explain the differences in the role of the physician, the surgeon, and the barber-surgeon.
5. Identify the contributions of Jenner, Pasteur, Lister, Roentgen, Reed, Barton, Blackwell, Nightingale, Curie, Papanicolaou, Domagk, Banting, Fleming, Salk, and Bernard.
6. Spell and define, using the glossary at the back of the text, all the words to know in this unit.

■ WORDS TO KNOW

acupuncture
anesthesia
apothecaries
apprenticeship
asepsis
caduceus
cautery
chloroform
disease
epidemics
ether
exorcism
guilds

Hippocratic oath
infectious
pandemic
physicians
plague
practitioners
Roentgen rays
scientific
surgeons
surgery
trephining
vaccination

ANCIENT HISTORY

To fully understand the high technical level of current health care and the responsibilities of those who provide it, we must look back at its history and learn how it has developed. Ancient times were filled with **infectious disease** and **epidemics** as well as illnesses and injuries caused by dietary deficiencies and unhealthy or hostile environments. Eighty percent of primitive man died by the age of thirty, as a result of a hunting accident or violence. He lived primarily alone so there was little risk of widespread diseases or **plagues**. However, when he began settling in communities, farming, and domesticating animals, overcrowding, filth, and the natural presence of microorganisms caused epidemic diseases. Initially, tuberculosis, tetanus, malaria, smallpox, typhus, typhoid, and later leprosy ravaged early civilizations.

Because these ancient people did not understand the concept of microorganisms or the function of the human body, the presence of disease was credited to evil spirits and demons brought on as punishment for disobedience to the gods. Therefore, medical practice became the role of priests or medicine men. "Treatments" involved rituals to drive out demons. At times, a surgical procedure called **trephining** was performed. This remarkable operation involved cutting a hole in the skull with a flint knife presumably to treat migraines, epilepsy, paralysis, or insanity. Later, it was used to treat head injuries incurred in battle or from accidents. Archaeologists have examined hundreds of skulls and determined that some trephining ended in death, but surprisingly, the majority showed healing and several years of survival.

Evidence has been found in Egyptian tombs and on papyri which indicates that the people of the area around the Nile River had developed a level of medical practice as early as 3000 BC. Egyptian **physicians** were priests who studied medicine and **surgery** in the temple medical schools. They too tried to drive out evil spirits with spells. If this failed, they used concocted repellents to fight the demons. These were made from the excretions of the lion, panther, gazelle, and ostrich. Insects, either crushed or alive, were swallowed along with the backbones of ravens and fat from black snakes. In addition to the "black magic," they also used about one-third of the medicinal plants still used in pharmacies today.

Egyptians believed that blood in the body flowed through canals like those constructed along the Nile for irrigation. When it was thought that the body's canals were "clogged," they were opened by bloodletting or the application of leeches. The leech not only removed blood and disease toxins but also produced hirudin in the process, which prevented coagulation. The use of leeches continued until the 19th century and is being reintroduced today in specific traumas where a large amount of blood is present within the tissues. Egyptian physicians (priests) were very conservative in treating patients. They adhered to rules of the Sacred Books so they would be free from blame if a patient died. If the physician tried a different treatment and the patient did not survive, the physician was executed; therefore, medical progress was impossible. The physicians became famous and were in high demand. An Egyptian named Imhotep was considered outstanding and became the physician for the royal family. As a reward, he was given deity and named the Egyptian God of Medicine.

People from surrounding regions had medical problems similar to the Egyptians. The average person lived in squalor, drank filthy water, and had very poor personal hygiene. By the year 2000 BC, the ruler of Babylon established a legal code for medical practice that set fees for services and established rules of conduct. It provided that the physician's hands be cut off if he killed a patient or destroyed his sight. It is worth noting that these stiff penalties applied only to patients from nobility—a slave just had to be replaced.

The Sacred Books tell of priest-doctors in India around 1500 BC and listed their deadly diseases as malaria, dysentery, typhoid, cholera, the plague, leprosy, and smallpox. The Hindus had the world's first nurses and hospitals. There was extensive use of drugs, including those for **anesthesia** which undoubtedly assisted with the main Hindu contribution to the art of healing: surgery. Their knowledge of anatomy was limited but their **surgeons** performed a fairly technical form of cataract and plastic surgery. Early writings reveal that they used approximately 120 surgical instruments in many different operations. The Hindu environment was greatly improved with walled sewer drains and underground water pipes. Their level of medical knowledge and drugs spread to other lands through trade, migration, and by conquerors.

The Chinese, India's neighbor, had a highly developed center of early medical learning. Their belief in evil spirits as the cause of illness gradually changed; they began searching for medical reasons for illness. About 3000 BC, the emperor, who was known as the Father of Chinese Medicine, had a document called Great Herbal (a translation) which contained over a thousand drugs; some are still in use today. The art of **acupuncture** was originally used as a means to drive out demons. Today, the ancient procedure has become a respected alternative form of treatment. Acupuncture consists of the insertion of needles of various metals, shapes, and sizes into one or several of the 365 specified spots on the head, trunk, and extremities. It is believed to relieve internal congestion and restore the equilibrium of the bodily functions.

The Greeks also played a large role in the development of medicine. Beginning about 2000 BC, they invaded many lands and established a remarkable civilization. They ac-

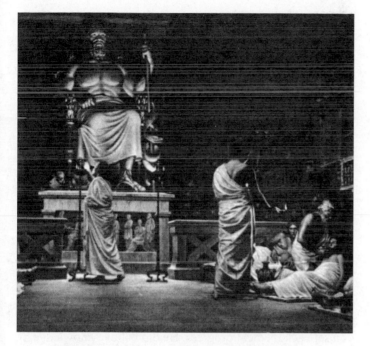

Figure 1-1 The temples and cult of Aesculapius.

quired knowledge from their conquered, but still practiced the religious/healing rituals. They believed Apollo, the Sun God, taught the art of medicine to a centaur who in turn taught others including Asklepios, the Greek God of Healing, who lived about 1250 BC. The priests in the temples of Asklepios (also called Aesculapius) used massage, bathing, and exercise in treating patients. They also depended on the magical power of large, yellow, nonpoisonous snakes. After the patient purified himself by bathing and made an offering to the god, he was given tablets to read that described cures of former patients. Then he was put into a drug-induced sleep in the temple. During the night, the snakes licked the wounds, and Asklepios applied salves. The god was usually depicted holding a staff with a serpent coiled around its shaft, Figure 1-1. This is probably the origin of the medical symbol known as a **caduceus**,

Figure 1-2, even though it shows two instead of one coiled serpent as did the staff of Aesculapius. Both are accepted as symbols of medical practice.

The Greeks absorbed ideas, drugs, and earlier methods of treatment from their predecessors. Their great interest in the unknown led them to question the accepted knowledge and seek information themselves. They began to investigate the causes of and reasons for illness in nature, which started the tradition of medical inquiry. About 500 BC, Alcmaeon dissected animals to study sight and hearing. Another Greek named Empedocles believed that blood gave life and the heart distributed it around the body. Medical schools began to observe what happened in illness rather than accept the teachings of the past. Upon the island of Cos, in about 460 BC, Hippocrates, the founder of **scientific** medicine, was born. During his 99 years of life, he took medicine out of the realm of priests and philosophers and produced an organized method of gaining knowledge through the means of observation, Figure 1-3. He taught that illness was the result of natural causes and not punishment for sin. He advocated examining a patient's environment, his home and place of work. He stressed the importance of diet and cleanliness. He felt medical knowledge could only be acquired through accurate clinical observation of the sick. He discovered that the course of certain diseases could be traced by listening to the chest of a patient. Over 2000 years passed before a French physician named Laennec invented the stethoscope to improve this method of observation, Figure 1-4. Hippocrates studied with the most distinguished teachers of the day. He practiced in many parts of the Greek world and was admired for his cures. He wrote many detailed studies among which are ones on prognostics, fractures, and surgery. He is best known for his code of behavior known as the **Hippocratic oath**, which medical schools still teach and physicians repeat as they enter practice. For all his accomplishments, Hippocrates became known as the Father of Medicine.

Aristotle, a contemporary of Hippocrates, was a philosopher and scientific genius, and became the tutor of Alexander the Great. He brought together medicine, biology, botany, and anatomy. His findings were based upon

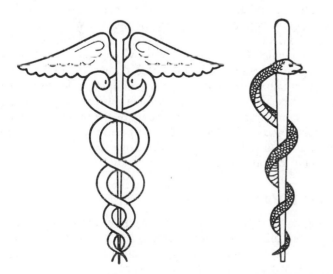

Figure 1-2 (Left) Caduceus (Right) Staff of Aesculapius.

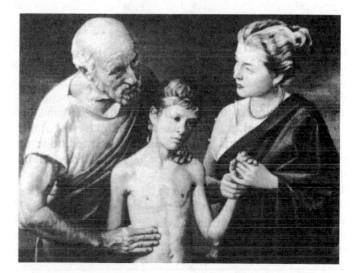

Figure 1-3 Hippocrates: medicine becomes a science.

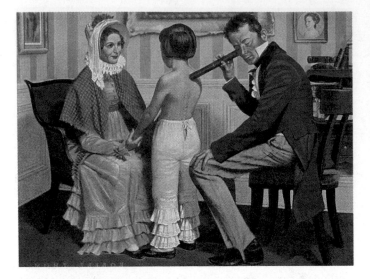

Figure 1-4 Laennec and the stethoscope (Courtesy Parke-Davis & Company, copyright 1957).

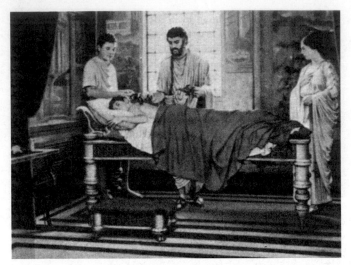

Figure 1-5 Galen: influence for forty-five generations.

animal dissection because human dissection was illegal where he lived. However, in Alexandria, Egypt, human dissection was legal. Students throughout the ancient world went there to study and use its library of 700,000 books. Alexandria became the center of learning and the home of a famous medical school. However, it declined with the rise of the Roman Empire and medicine reverted to supernatural theories of disease.

Medicine was held in very low esteem in the Roman Empire. The Romans distrusted and despised the wandering Greek physicians who came to Italy about 200 BC, many as slaves. Roman men treated their own families with early, primitive methods. In 46 BC, Julius Caesar gave physicians citizenship rights and they began to achieve status. But the great demand for physicians opened medicine to anyone and little clinical teaching took place. The teachings of Hippocrates were largely ignored and rival schools of medicine argued about his ideas.

About this time Claudius Galen, a physician from Asia Minor emerged, professing to following the teachings of Hippocrates. He was born in 129 AD and became a surgeon to a gladiatorial school after minimal medical training. He received much experience treating the severe wounds the gladiators received in the arenas. He later went to Rome and quickly became famous, but his arrogance caused hostility from other physicians and he was forced to return home. He was called back to Rome by Marcus Aurelius, the emperor. He successfully cured his stomach ache and remained in Rome until his death in 199 AD. He produced over 500 books during this time. His theories were accepted for the next 1300 years because he claimed they had the authority of Hippocrates, Figure 1–5. However, he had ignored observation and explained diseases as unbalanced "humors." The body was believed to be composed of and regulated by the four fluids (humors) of life, namely the blood, phlegm, black bile, and yellow bile. An imbalance or disturbance of the humors was thought to result in illness. He prescribed diets, massage, exercise, and drugs to cool, heat, dry, or moisten the body as needed. His beliefs regarding blood and circula-

tion set back medical progress. He did believe knowledge of anatomy was necessary so he dissected pigs and apes, since human dissection was still illegal, and related his findings. His viewpoints went unchallenged until the 16th century. The Romans made almost no contribution to medicine but established superior methods of sanitation and water supply. They realized disease was connected to filth and overcrowding. They drained the marshes to reduce the incidence of malaria. There were laws to maintain public health and clean streets. They built an extensive underground sewer system and pure water aqueducts capable of bringing an estimated 300 million gallons of drinking water a day into the city. The emperor provided for teachers of medicine to maintain a supply. Medical officers and surgeons, usually Greek, served in the Army. A private hospital system was also developed, first for the wealthy and slaves, then for the campaign armies. Later, public hospitals were founded and the hospital movement expanded with the growth of Christianity and its tradition of caring for the sick.

Despite Rome's advances, the empire began to fall as political, social, and economic factors collapsed. The real cause, however, was the spread of disease which resulted from the disuse of the drainage system and the return of the swamps which followed invasions by other empires. The resulting malaria and smallpox killed thousands. In 542 AD, the remnants of the eastern Roman Empire were destroyed by the first major historically known **pandemic** (occurring at the same time in different places) of the bubonic plague. It had come from China, spread through trade routes to Egypt, along the coast of North Africa to Palestine, Syria, and into Europe. It affected all the known world.

MEDIEVAL HISTORY

The great Roman Empire was overrun by barbarians. Europe was controlled by Teutonic tribal groups. The people were agricultural and established health standards vanished. The centers of learning and medicine decayed. From the 5th to the 16th centuries, there was no progress in medical knowledge or practice. There was a blend of pagan magic, superstition, and herbalism. According to Hastings in *Medicine, An International History*, the Anglo-Saxon settlers in Britain believed illness was caused by "nine venoms, the nine diseases, or of 'worms', elves, and witches." It was treated with charms and incantations or with herbs, some of which were effective. However, they lived in filth and had a total absence of sanitation and personal hygiene. Writings from the 6th to the 10th centuries tell of epidemics of smallpox, dysentery, typhus, and plague. In addition, there was widespread famine. Eventually, medicine passed into the hands of the Christian Church and Arab scholars. The church did not foster medical science. They recommended prayer and fasting since they believed that illness was a punishment for sin. In 391 AD, a religious fanatic mob burned the great library at Alexandria. Christianity forbade human dissection, so anatomy and physiology died except for the erroneous pages of Galen. Priests again became healers, using exorcism and holy relics to cure the sick. Parts of the body were assigned a patron saint who could cure and inflict disease. The church did care for the sick and established religious orders that provided care. Most monasteries had rooms and herb gardens to care for their own sick and members of the general public. The monasteries also took on the task of translation and transcription of the ancient manuscripts of the classical physicians, a task which preserved and circulated information before the invention of the printing press.

A second storehouse of medical knowledge was in the Moslem Arab Empire which, by 1000 AD, extended from Spain to India. The Arabs were eager for knowledge and the classical learning was translated into Arabic. Medicine began a revival. Arab physicians learned much about epidemics, but their great knowledge of chemistry resulted in their major medical contribution in pharmacology. They also continued the Roman system of hospitals, including at least four major teaching centers. One had specialized wards for specific conditions. All patients were admitted regardless of race, creed, or social status. Upon departure, patients were given sufficient money to cover their convalescence.

One of the greatest physicians was known as Rhazes, the Arab Hippocrates. He was forty before beginning medical study and was responsible for the construction of a hospital. He produced about 150 books including a medical encyclopedia weighing 22 pounds. He based his diagnosis upon observation of disease and his major contribution was distinguishing smallpox and measles. Anatomy was still based upon Galen. Since it was considered unclean to touch the human body with the hands, the Arabs were not good surgeons. This was left to inferior practitioners; however, Rhazes is credited with the use of animal gut sutures to sew wounds. The major surgical instrument was the cautery (a red hot iron) applied to wounds and infected ulcers to "burn out the poison," always very painful and disfiguring and often fatal.

The union of medical knowledge from both the East and West produced an outstanding medical school at Salerno around 850 AD. It was believed to be founded by a Jew, a Roman, a Greek, and an Arab and was open to both men and women of all nationalities. Since it was not a church school, it could teach medicine using a sound basis. It became the

convalescent center for wounded Crusaders. By the 12th century it had a highly organized curriculum upon which students were examined and issued degrees to become the first "true" doctors. Both anatomy and surgery were taught, but it was still based upon animal dissection. Other medical centers followed, including ones in Paris, Oxford, and Cambridge. Despite earlier beliefs, however, religious and scholarly factions prohibited advancement. Hippocrates and Galen remained the unquestioned authorities. Medical teaching was predominately oral since books were scarce (for example, the medical school in Paris had only twelve books at the end of the 14th century). Dissection was rare. One university did secure the right to dissect one executed criminal every three years, but it allowed only a superficial examination of the chest and abdomen.

Medieval European surgeon's practice was limited to nobility, the high clergy, and wealthy merchants. Other patients and minor surgeries were treated by ignorant barber-surgeons. Their trademark became the white poles around which they wrapped their blood-stained bandages. The red and white pole has descended to barbers today. They cut hair, practiced blood-letting, opened abscesses, pulled teeth, and occasionally did amputations—all with the same razor.

The Roman tradition of hospitals continued but public health and personal hygiene was gone. The environment was overrun with disease. Famine and population movement due to wars increased the problems. Typhus was flourishing due to the custom of wearing the same underclothing, which was often infested with fleas. Tuberculosis was endemic due to poverty and food shortage. Tuberculosis of the neck was common and its principal remedy was "the king's touch." In one month in 1277 AD, Edward I touched 543 persons attempting to affect a cure. Smallpox was returned to Europe by the Crusaders in the 13th century causing at least twenty epidemics. Danish ships even spread the disease to Iceland.

Two of the greatest medieval diseases, however, were leprosy and the bubonic plague. Leprosy was present in the early centuries, brought perhaps by the Roman soldiers. It was one of the few diseases recognized as being contagious, but was believed to be a result of sins against God. The afflicted were herded into leper houses outside the towns, forbidden to marry, proclaimed dead citizens, and ordered to wear a black cloak with white patches. In 1313, King Philip the Fair wanted to burn them all but was forbidden by the church. Incidences of leprosy decreased with the coming of the "Black Death" (or, the bubonic plague) which killed many lepers. Black Death was a term used to describe the dark, mottled appearance of the corpse due to hemorrhages beneath the skin. (In 1905, it was determined that this disease was caused by a bacillus which grew in fleas of infected black rats.) The disease was devastating. Symptoms included sudden shivering, headache, vomiting, and pains in the abdomen and limbs, followed by delirium. Large, painful boils appeared at the body joints and unless treated, proved fatal in five days. Other variations included the pneumonic plague which affected the lungs, causing death in three days and the septicemic plague, caused by direct bacillus injection into the blood by the flea, which caused death within twenty-four hours.

The plagues probably began after flooding drove rodents inflicted with fleas from their habitats. China reported 13 million deaths. The plague traveled to India, Asia Minor, Egypt, and North Africa. An army fighting for a trading port realized they were becoming infected, catapulted their infested corpses into the port, and fled homeward to Sicily. This same sequence occurred in other areas, thereby carrying the plague into other ports. By 1352, all Europe, Iceland, Greenland, and Russia were infected. The plague was blamed on a corrupt atmosphere: foul vapors created by Jupiter, infection from decomposing bodies of a plague of locusts, and the most favored, invisible arrows shot by Christ. All were attributed to the wrath of God. Finally, the Jews were blamed. All Jews living in Switzerland and Germany, approximately 28,000 people, were put in wooden buildings and burned alive. Before it subsided, it is estimated that thirty percent of the total European population died. There were four additional outbreaks before the end of the 14th century. In *Medicine, An International History*, Hastings states, "infectious disease has been a more deadly enemy to man than war—hence the ghastliness of the modern concept of bacteriological warfare." The Black Death was not forgotten and fear of the plague was an important motivation to stimulate a return to medical learning.

EARLY MEDICAL PIONEERS

Beginning in Italy in the 14th century, there was a revival of culture and concern for life. Gradually, they began to escape the limitations of the church. There was a new attitude toward the human body. The classical artists, Michelangelo, Durer, and da Vinci, began to practice dissection in order to draw the human body—especially the bones, muscles, and internal organs—accurately.

An anatomist named Vesalius was from a medical family in Brussels. He was the student of a strong believer in Galen. The teacher thought the new anatomical discoveries were merely changes that had occurred naturally since Galen's time. Vesalius was not convinced and did his own dissections on corpses that he took from the gallows or bought from grave robbers. He determined that the structures he dissected were all the same and not as Galen had described. In 1537 he became a professor of Surgery and Anatomy and four years later, while dissecting a monkey, discovered Galen's descriptions had been the result of animal dissection, not human. He published a book on the human body which contained over 300 illustrations proving Galen's errors; however, he made little attempt to discuss physiology, or, the function of organisms.

It was in 1578 when an Englishman named William Harvey observed that blood in the arteries always flowed away from the heart while blood in the veins flowed toward it, with valves that prevented it from changing direction. He also calculated that two ounces of blood passed with each heartbeat; therefore, with seventy-two beats per minute, the body would require 270 pounds of blood for just half an hour. He also realized that the same blood had to be pumped repeatedly. He knew blood passed through the lungs to be purified, but he died without discovering the capillaries between the arteries and veins.

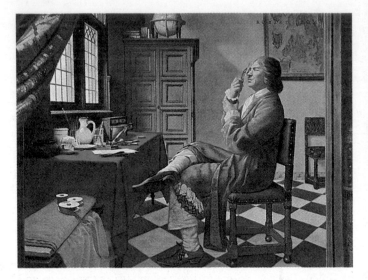

Figure 1–6 Leeuwenhoek and his microscope (Courtesy Parke-Davis & Company, copyright 1957).

The microscope was the invention of an Italian named Malpighi and a Dutchman named van Leeuwenhoek, Figure 1–6. Malpighi first saw capillaries in 1661. Van Leeuwenhoek was a wealthy merchant and in his leisure built over 200 microscopes, some which magnified up to 270 times, allowing him to see, for the first time, red blood cells.

An outstanding surgeon of this era was a Frenchman named Pare. He studied four years at the Paris hospital and earned his Diploma of Barber-Surgeon. For the next 30 years, he accompanied the army in its many battles, making discoveries first-hand. He accidentally discovered a dressing of egg-yolk, oil of roses, and turpentine; this was the only thing he had after his traditional boiling oil used to cauterize wounds, ran out. He also discovered it was possible and much more successful to tie bleeding vessels with a ligature, rather than to burn them. He invented special forceps to grasp arteries and developed new techniques for treating fractures and dislocations. He was not well recognized by his peers because he could not use the Latin or Greek language of the formally educated physicians; however, he became Europe's greatest surgeon and served four French kings.

Intensive intellectual activity toward the end of the 17th century resulted in the development of scientific societies in different countries. The most famous was the Royal Society of London, established by Charles II in 1662. It was there that the mystery of circulation was solved and the recognition that oxygen was responsible for the change in the color of blood in the lungs was made. Soon after, pipes were inserted into veins and arteries of animals to measure blood pressure and attempts at transfusions were made.

The practice of medicine in the beginning of the 17th century was divided among the members of three **guilds** (an association of persons engaged in a common trade or calling, for mutual advantage and protection): the physicians, the surgeons, and the **apothecaries**. The physicians were the most prestigious because they usually possessed a university degree. They preferred studying, teaching, and debating the theories of disease to actually dealing directly with the sick. They limited their practice to the upper classes. The surgeons were considered inferior to the physicians. They were divided into two classifications: Surgeons of the Long Robe or, the more humble, barber-surgeons. Only a few surgeons held university degrees. They were trained largely in hospitals or through **apprenticeships** (a period of time when one is bound by agreement to learn some trade or craft). Barber-surgeons used their razors for opening veins as well as barbering. The apothecaries were tradesmen and were permitted to treat people with the drugs they made, prescribed, and sold. They were the general **practitioners** for the masses and also learned through apprenticeships.

MODERN MEDICAL PIONEERS

The discovery and conquest of the Americas had far-reaching medical impact. Colonists from Spain, Portugal, Holland, and France who landed in Southern, North and Central America, brought the diseases from the Old World and infected the Native Indians who had no built-up resistance. Entire tribes were destroyed, making it easy to occupy their lands. However, the Indians were infected with syphilis and "sent" it back to Europe with sailors. It flourished and spread throughout Europe. Reportedly, one-third of all the people in Paris alone were infected.

In the first settlement at Jamestown in 1607 there were only six medical men among the 208 settlers. Within three years, the population was reduced by half. This state of health continued for the next century, caused mainly by the fear of eating unknown fruits and vegetables. In addition, some settlers returned to Europe and there was a shortage of female settlers. There were only three or four trained physicians in all of Virginia before 1700. The Virginia Company offered free passage to apothecaries and their families to increase medical immigration. It was necessary for the settlers to practice self-medication using herbs and old practices. Bleeding was still practiced for fevers, infections, and even toothache. One French surgeon reportedly bled his patient sixty-four times in eight months. To aid in digestion, some physicians recommended swallowing grit. Queen Anne's physician, the President of the Royal Society, prescribed drinking fifty live millipedes in water twice daily. The preparations in the medicines still contained ingredients recommended in ancient Egypt.

Man had been "practicing" medicine for thousands of years, but only in the last 250 years, since the development of the microscope and the discovery of microbes, has it progressed. In the 18th century, medical science developed rapidly because of advances in the modern sciences of physics and chemistry which gave the physicians new tools and new methods. Brothers William and John Hunter were born in Scotland and they both studied medicine. William became a surgeon in London and John became a surgeon in the army. After leaving the service, John devoted himself to practicing surgery and to the teaching and studying of anatomy. He was especially interested in comparing the bodies of animals with one another and with man. John Hunter has been called the Founder of Scientific Surgery because his surgical procedures were based upon sound pathological findings. In 1778, he introduced artificial feeding by inserting a flexible tube into the stomach of his patient. His great collection of anatomic and animal specimens is in the museum of the Royal College of Surgeons in London, England.

With the emphasis on scientific inquiry, medicine changed rapidly. Many people made contributions that changed medical practice. Following is a list of the more familiar men and their contributions.

Edward Jenner (1749–1823) was an Englishman who studied under John Hunter. In May 1796, he gave the first **vaccination** to an eight-year-old boy using the pus from a cowpox lesion on the hand of a dairymaiden. After two months, he injected the child with smallpox but the disease did not develop. The Royal Society rejected his discovery so he published it himself.

Gabriel Fahrenheit (1688–1736) was a German physicist devoted to the study of physics. He improved the construction of the thermometer, introduced the thermometric scale which is known by his name, and developed the first mercury thermometer. It became available in England in the 1740s.

Rene Laennec (1781–1826), a Frenchman, invented the stethoscope in 1816, out of necessity. He had an obese patient and could not hear the heart and lungs with just his ear. Originally, it was a piece of rolled paper but was later refined into a wooden tube that fit the doctor's ear. Nineteenth century physicians carried it in their top hats.

Dr. Phillipe Pinel (1755–1826), a Frenchman, was the first physician to call for the humanitary treatment of mental patients. He thought mental illness should be treated as a disease and not a crime. In medieval and early modern times, mentally ill persons were burned as witches or kept in chains. Some had been manacled for forty years. It was a popular 18th century pasttime to watch the antics of the chained inmates of Bedlam, the Bethlehem Hospital in London.

Dr. W.T.G. Morton (1819–1868) was practicing medicine in Massachusetts in the mid-1800s when he introduced the use of an anesthetic in the form of **ether** to make his patients more comfortable during surgery. After he died, the city of Boston erected a monument in recognition of his contribution. The use of ether stimulated research into other safer methods of relieving pain.

Dr. James Simpson (1811–1870) of Edinburgh University in Scotland began to use **chloroform** as an anesthetic. It was sprinkled on a towel held over the patient's face. Oliver Wendell Holmes, a writer and physician, suggested the word anesthesia to describe ether and chloroform. The word comes from two Greek words meaning "not feeling."

Louis Pasteur (1822–1895) was born in a small town in France and studied to become a chemist, Figure 1–7. He was working for some wineries trying to discover why their wine often became sour. With the aid of a microscope, he discovered that microorganisms were the cause and that they could be destroyed by heating and sealing the wine. His name is well known because it has been used to name the process that eliminates dangerous microbes from milk: pasteurization. Almost as important was his discovery of a vaccine for the treatment and prevention of deadly rabies. It was first given to a bitten, critically ill child in 1885. The child recovered and the occurrence of death from rabies, which was common, dropped to below 1% worldwide with its extended use.

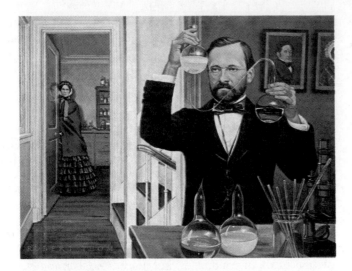

Figure 1-7 Pasteur: the chemist who transformed medicine (Courtesy Parke-Davis & Company, copyright 1957).

Joseph Lister (1827–1912) was born near London, England, Figure 1–8. He was respected as a surgeon but despite his skill, many patients died of wound infections. In 1865, he was reading Pasteur's research articles and thought infections might be caused by microbes in the air. At first, he used carbolic acid as a skin disinfectant, but it was too strong and he severely burned the patient's skin. By adjusting the strength of the solution used on wounds, his hands, the instruments, and the surgical dressings, the wounds healed without becoming infected. He also devised a carbolic spray to pump into the air in the operating room to kill organisms in the air. He laid the foundation for later techniques of medical **asepsis**.

Wilhelm von Roentgen (1845–1923), a German professor of physics, discovered x-rays, perhaps the greatest technical aid to the field of medicine. The name was chosen because he was uncertain about the nature of the invisible rays. Later, they were called **Roentgen rays** in his honor. For the first time, physicians were able to see into the body without operating. At first, Roentgen rays were used to diagnose fractures and the presence of foreign bodies. Later, it was learned

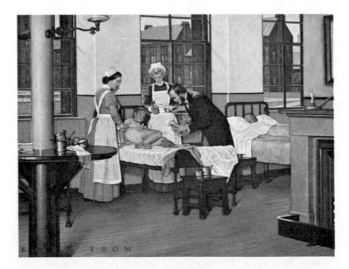

Figure 1-8 Lister introduces antisepsis (Courtesy Parke-Davis & Company, copyright 1957).

that instillation of opaque liquids, either by mouth or injection, allowed viewing of the stomach, brain, kidneys, and bronchial tubes.

Dr. Elias Metchnikoff (1845–1916) was a Russian Jew who devoted much of his life to studying ways to prolong life. Louis Pasteur invited him to work at the Pasteur Institute. He became the director after Pasteur's death. In 1908, Metchnikoff was awarded the Nobel Prize in medicine for his study of the way white blood cells protect us from disease.

Frederick Banting (1891–1941), a young Canadian surgeon, discovered and isolated insulin in 1921. This breakthrough enabled diabetics to lead near normal lives.

Gerhard Domagk (1895–1964), a German bacteriologist, began experimenting with a red dye called prontosil in 1932. By experimenting on mice, he discovered it killed or weakened many germs among the coccus family. This discovery led to the development of sulfa drugs which cured nine out of ten patients with coccal infections.

Sir Alexander Fleming (1881–1955), in 1932, noticed that a mold which accidentally got on his culture plate had prevented the growth of the bacteria around it. He cultured the mold but did not realize its potential. This was the beginning of the development of penicillin. Nothing further was done until 1939 when doctors Howard Florey and Ernst Chain reinvestigated its properties. After months, Florey isolated the chemical substance and proved it effective as a germ killer in humans.

After World War II, surgeons were looking for ways to transfer tissues and organs from one person to another. Heart surgery was performed in the 1940s to repair defects. By 1960, surgeons had successfully placed artificial heart valves, plastic arteries, and pacemakers in the heart. In 1961 kidneys were transplanted. The surgery was successful but the body often rejected the organ and the kidney failed after a year or two.

In 1968, Dr. Christian Barnard performed the first successful heart transplant in South Africa. His first attempt failed but in his second attempt, the patient survived for nineteen months.

EARLY LEADERS IN AMERICAN MEDICINE

Thomas Bond was born in Maryland. Since there were no domestic schools or hospitals in which to serve an internship, he studied in France, England, and Scotland at medical schools affiliated with hospitals. These experiences taught him the value of hospital care for the sick. When he returned to Philadelphia to practice, he tried to secure money from friends to support building a hospital. He made no real progress until he enlisted the help of Benjamin Franklin. Franklin believed in his project and wrote about the proposal in the newspapers. When it was clear the money offerings would not be sufficient, he proposed a bill before the Assembly; the bill passed in May 1751, and the first patients were admitted in 1756. A distinguished Frenchman, M. deWarville, visited the hospital around 1788 and reported it superior to most hospitals he had visited in France. The hospital was clean, and black and white patients were being cared for in the same wards. It was not the first hospital in the American colonies, but it is recognized as the oldest surviving institution for the care of the sick in the United States.

In 1762, William Shippen, Jr., returned to Philadelphia from his study of anatomy under John Hunter in England. He placed an announcement in the *Pennsylvania Gazette* offering a course of anatomical lectures. He had only ten students for the first course, but following years enrollment climbed as high as 200. During this period in our history it was not unusual for bodies to be stolen from graves so that they could be dissected and studied.

William Beaumont (1785–1853) was a surgeon in the U.S. Army during the War of 1812. In 1822, he treated a young man who was in serious condition because of a bullet wound in his stomach. The treatment was successful and the man regained his health, but the flesh never healed completely. As a result, Dr. Beaumont was able to use the open area as a laboratory to study the action of the stomach. These studies added to our understanding of the digestive process.

Ephraim McDowell (1771–1830) was an American physician who studied at the then most famous medical school in the world, the University of Edinburgh. He practiced medicine in Kentucky and was a skilled surgeon. In the early 1800s Dr. McDowell performed an operation never before recorded. He removed a large ovarian tumor that would otherwise have killed his patient. When neighbors and friends found out he was going to perform the operation they called him a murderer. However, the surgery was successful and the patient lived many more years. McDowell was not recognized for his achievement until years later after he had performed other similar operations. Present day surgeons still use many of his techniques for this surgery.

At the time Beaumont and McDowell were practicing medicine, the causes of infection were not understood. Many patients developed blood poisoning or gangrene and died from these complications.

Walter Reed (1851–1902) was a Major serving in the U.S. Army in Cuba when he realized the need to find the cause of yellow fever. He was forced to seek out volunteers who were willing to be given the disease. Certainly these people, some of whom died, also made a great contribution to medicine although their names are not remembered. Dr. Reed's work in stamping out yellow fever made it possible to build the Panama Canal.

Theobald Smith (1859–1934), born in Albany, New York, was a professor of bacteriology. He was responsible for the establishment of a department of animal pathology in 1916 near Princeton University. His research laid the foundation for the prevention of diseases like typhoid, diphtheria, and meningitis, which are now prevented by use of vaccines.

Alexis Carrel was born in 1872 in France. He came to the United States after he received his medical degree and became a staff member of the Rockefeller Institute. He discovered, in his study of body tissues, that severed arteries could be joined and again carry on their function. His research work, which was carried out on animals, showed that it is possible to transplant bones and blood vessels and various organs of the body. He was awarded the Nobel Prize in medicine in 1912 for his work in joining blood vessels.

In 1949 there were 43,000 cases of polio in the United States alone. Dr. Jonas Salk and a group of researchers at the Harvard Medical School successfully isolated the polio virus after discovering it grew in human intestines and was carried in water and food to other contacts. In April of 1954, Dr. Salk began massive trials of a vaccine. By the end of that summer, 1,830,000 children in America had been successfully protected.

WOMEN IN MEDICINE

The earliest known women in the field of medicine were at the famous medical school in Salerno, Italy from 1099 to 1179. The most famous was Trotula Platearius (1100 AD). Her specialty was obstetrics and gynecology. Her textbook, *Diseases of Women,* was a major publication for seven centuries. She married a physician and had two sons, both of whom were physicians.

In England in the 16th century, women were allowed to practice medicine. Then, attitudes changed and they were often persecuted as witches if they tried to cure sickness. In the mid-19th century, even though there was still much opposition, women once again won the right to be trained and qualified as doctors.

Dr. Elizabeth Garrett Anderson (1836–1917) was the first woman to qualify as a doctor in Britain. A hospital is named after her. In 1872 she opened the New Hospital for Women. It was staffed entirely by women.

Clara Barton (1821–1912) cared for the wounded in the Civil War. In the course of this work she not only nursed the wounded but recognized the need for support services to meet the emotional and spiritual needs of the soldiers. After the war she worked at locating missing soldiers. She learned of the Red Cross in 1869 when she visited friends in Geneva, Switzerland. In 1881 she formed the American Red Cross and served as its first president.

Elizabeth Blackwell (1821–1910) was the first woman in the United States to qualify as a doctor, Figure 1–9. She was turned down in 1844 by medical schools in Philadelphia and New York but enrolled in a school in Geneva, New York, and

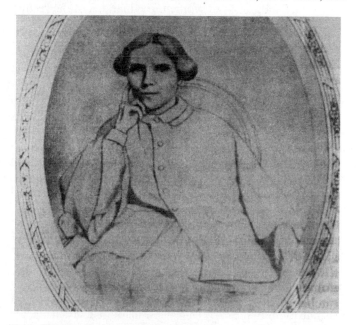

Figure 1–9 Elizabeth Blackwell, first woman in United States to qualify as doctor (Courtesy Elizabeth Blackwell Center, Riverside Methodist Hospital, Columbus, Ohio).

was awarded a degree in 1849. In 1853, Dr. Blackwell, with the help of two other women, who were also doctors, her sister Emily and Marie Zackrzewska, opened a dispensary and medical college for women in New York. They opened a hospital exclusively for women in 1857 despite great opposition.

Florence Nightingale (1820–1910) was the founder of modern nursing. She was born into a wealthy family who were of the opinion that ladies found a suitable husband, were married, and raised children, period. She was greatly influenced by Elizabeth Blackwell, who was a close personal friend. Nightingale studied nursing in Europe and used her knowledge in the Crimean War to care for the wounded and sick. She established a school for nurses in 1860 at St. Thomas Hospital in London.

Dr. Aletta Jacobs (1854–1929) was Holland's first woman physician and opened the world's first birth control clinic in Amsterdam in 1882.

Marie Curie (1867–1934), born Mary A. Sklodowska in Warsaw, Poland, was the first world-famous woman scientist. She discovered the element radium. She won the Nobel Prize in physics with her husband, Pierre, and Henri Becquerel and later won the Nobel Prize herself in the field of chemistry. Her work led directly to the treatment of cancer with radium.

Elsie Strang L'Esperance (1878?–1959) was born in Yorktown, New York. She graduated from Woman's Medical College of the New York Infirmary for Women and Children established by Elizabeth Blackwell. Her concern for the early treatment of cancer led her to establish the Strang Clinic. Her effort represented the first organized attempt to detect cancer in its early stages. The clinic offered complete physical examinations to apparently healthy women to determine the presence of cancer. Major advances were made in the Strang Clinic, including the work of Dr. George Papanicolaou in the diagnosis of cervical cancer. His discovery, the Pap test (using a shortened version of his name) has become a routine screening examination and has saved the lives of thousands of women. Evaluations of the rectum were also studied through use of proctoscopy.

Gerty Theresa Radnitz Cori (1896–1957) was the first American woman to win the Nobel Prize for medicine and physiology. Dr. Cori worked with her husband on the overall process of carbohydrate metabolism in the body.

Dorothy Hansine Anderson (1901–1963) was born in Asheville, North Carolina. She was denied a residency in surgery and an appointment in pathology at the University of Rochester because she was a woman. She was accepted as an assistant in pathology at Columbia and in 1930 was appointed to the teaching staff. Her research into celiac disease of the pancreas led to the discovery of a previously unrecognized disease entity which she called cystic fibrosis. She ultimately developed a simple method of diagnosing this disease. She wrote major publications in the 1940s on chemotherapy for respiratory tract infections in cystic fibrosis.

Grace Arabell Goldsmith (1904–1975) was born in St. Paul, Minnesota, and received her medical training at Tulane University School of Medicine. Her main interest was nutrition. In the early 1940s she instituted, at Tulane, the first nutrition training for medical students anywhere in the world.

Dorothy Hodgkins was born in 1910 in Egypt of British parents. Her work in analyzing the structure of vitamin B12 as a vital substance in the fight against pernicious anemia won her the Nobel Prize for chemistry in 1964.

In 1983, *Ebony* magazine reported that only two black women in the United States, Drs. Alexa Canady and M. Deborah Hyde-Rowan, participated in the field of neurosurgery. They were excellent students and experienced discouraging remarks from faculty members in medical school. Remarks such as "you don't fully understand all that is involved in neurosurgery" and it is "too difficult a field for a woman" did not stop them from realizing their goals. The women are proud of their accomplishments and say "it shows that black women have the determination, discipline, and dedication to succeed in an area such as neurosurgery."

Today, women continue to struggle with determination to achieve positions of leadership in the medical field. Many specialty areas are still dominated and controlled by men. Access to medical schools and opportunities to practice have improved, though. Extensive education and medical practice commitments do present a challenge to female physicians who also want to have and raise children. However, these challenges are being managed and women are making their mark as health care providers.

UNIT 2
The Health Care Team

■ OBJECTIVES

Upon completion of the unit, meet the following terminal performance objectives by verifying knowledge of the facts and principles presented through oral and written communication at a level deemed competent.

1. List and discuss the allied health care professionals described in this unit.
2. Explain why it is necessary to have a basic understanding of other health care team members.
3. Spell and define, using the glossary at the back of the text, all of the words to know in this unit.

■ WORDS TO KNOW

admissions clerk
certified nurse assistant (CNA)
certified ophthalmic technician (COT)
chiropractor
dental assistant
dental hygienist
dietitian
electrocardiogram technician (ECG tech)

emergency medical technician (EMT)
histologist
laboratory technician
licensed practical nurse (LPN)
multi-skilled health care assistants
nurse practitioner
nutritionist
occupational therapist

occupational therapy
assistant (OTA)
office manager/business
office manager
paramedic
patient care technician
(PCT)
pharmacist
pharmacy technician
phlebotomist (accessioning
tech)
physical therapist
physician assistant (PA)

podiatrist/chiropodist
prophylaxis
psychologist
radiologic technologist
radiology technician
registered nurse (RN)
respiratory therapy
technician
ultrasound
unit clerk
ventilatory
x-ray technician

ALLIED HEALTH PROFESSIONALS

In addition to the physicians you will work with, there are many other health care team professionals for whom you should have a basic understanding and respect for their parts in patient care. Each one performs a specific set of duties for which they were trained. Defined hereafter are the many skilled areas, educational requirements, and primary duties of the most frequently encountered health professionals who cross paths in daily patient care. Many of these members you may not work with directly, but you may have contact with them by telephone or by written communication. Often patients can have several health problems at the same time and cooperation with other members of the health care team to accommodate the patient is vital. Knowing the role each plays in the total health care of patients will enable you to speak more intelligently with others in the medical field and become more efficient at what your role is as the medical assistant.

Admissions Clerk

An **admissions clerk** in the hospital or medical center has basic medical terminology and administrative medical office skills. Obtaining a basic medical history and other important information from patients when they are admitted is the primary duty of this person. A college degree is desirable, but not essential.

Certified Ophthalmic Technician (COT)

Certified ophthalmic technicians are valuable members in the field of ophthalmology. Often they are initially medical assistants with a versatile background in both administrative and clinical office procedures as well as a basic understanding of medical terminology. Additional training is necessary and certification is required to perform delicate ophthalmic tests and procedures for patients. COTs must also keep current with the latest treatments, medications, and equipment in assisting patients and physicians.

Certified Nurse Assistant (CNA)

The **certified nurse assistant** provides basic nursing skills and patient care to those in nursing homes, retirement and adult day care facilities under the supervision of the regis-

tered or licensed nurse, Figure 1–10. CNAs are also referred to as nurse aides, nurse technicians, and orderlies.

Chiropractor

A **chiropractor** is highly trained and skilled in the mechanical manipulation of the spinal column. The degree of Doctor of Chiropractic, DC, is awarded after the individual completes two years of premedical studies followed by four years of training in an approved chiropractic school.

Dental Assistant

A **dental assistant** helps a dentist in the performance of generalized tasks, including chairside assistance, clerical work, reception, and some radiography and dental laboratory work. The person learns duties in school or on-the-job and becomes certified by taking the national certification examination to become a CDA, Certified Dental Assistant.

Dental Hygienist

A **dental hygienist** is a person with special training to provide dental services under the supervision of the dentist. Services supplied by a dental hygienist include dental *prophylaxis*, radiography, application of medications, and provision of dental education at chairside and in the community.

Electrocardiogram Technician (ECG Tech)

ECG technicians are skilled in performing electrocardiograms and may be employed in medical clinics and hospitals.

Emergency Medical Technician (EMT)

Emergency medical technicians are trained in and responsible for the administration of specialized emergency care and the transportation to a medical facility of victims of acute illness or injury. EMTs have ongoing training following certification and must be recertified every two years.

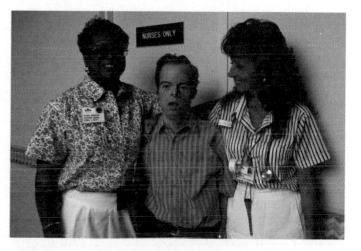

Figure 1–10 The certified nurse assistant is an important member of the health care team in a long-term care facility.

Histologist

A **histologist** is a medical scientist who specializes in the study of histology, which is the science dealing with the microscopic identification of cells and tissues. Histologists are employed in private laboratories, clinics, and hospitals.

Laboratory Technician

A medical technologist or **laboratory technician** is one who, under the direction of a pathologist or other physician or medical scientist, performs specialized chemical, microscopic, and bacteriologic tests of blood, tissue, and bodily fluids. Those who have successfully completed the examination by the Board of Registry of the American Society of Clinical Pathologists, or a similar professional body, are designated as Certified Medical Technologists.

Multi-Skilled Health Care Assistants

Multi-skilled health care assistants are coming of age as a result of health care reform. In the efforts to hold down the cost of health care, many medical facilities have become more and more interested in the health care worker who offers a variety of skills in the area of patient care. There is a vast array of titles for this multi-skilled person which seem to vary from one facility to another as do the expectations of the job. Some medical centers refer to this employee as a patient care technician (PCT). A background in medical assisting and/or nurse assisting is most helpful, and most often required. Additional training is provided by the nursing staff with certification exams that follow. Under the supervision of registered nurses, the duties of this position range from performing vital signs and EKGs, to turning patients, drawing blood, and changing dressings, as well as many other responsibilities.

Nursing

Nursing is the practice in which a nurse assists in the performance of those activities contributing to the health or recovery from illness. The following are specialized areas of nursing:

Nurse Practitioner   A **nurse practitioner** is a **registered nurse (RN)** who, by advanced training and clinical experience in a branch of nursing (they usually hold a Master's degree), has acquired expert knowledge in that special branch of practice. They are employed by physicians in private practice or in clinics.

Registered Nurse   In the United States a registered nurse is defined as a professional nurse who has completed a course of study at a state-approved school of nursing and passed the National Council Licensure Examination (NCLEX-RN). RNs are licensed to practice by individual states. Employment settings for RNs include hospitals, convalescent homes, clinics, and home health care, to name a few.

Licensed Practical Nurse (LPN)   Sometimes referred to as licensed vocational nurses, **licensed practical nurses** are trained in basic nursing techniques and direct patient care.

They practice under the direct supervision of an RN or a physician and are employed in hospitals and convalescent centers.

Nutritionist

A **nutritionist** studies and applies the principles and science of nutrition (which is the study of food and drink as related to the growth and maintenance of living organisms).

Dietitian   A **dietitian** has specialized training in the nutritional care of groups and individuals and has successfully completed an examination and maintains continuing education requirements of the Commission on Dietetic Registration. This member of the health care team assists patients in regulating their diets. Dietitians are employed in hospitals and clinics.

Occupational Therapist

An **occupational therapist** practices skills of occupational therapy most often in the hospital setting. They may be licensed, registered, certified, or otherwise regulated by law. Occupational therapy is "the use of purposeful activity with individuals who are limited by physical injury or illness, psychosocial dysfunction, developmental or learning disabilities, poverty and cultural differences, or the aging process to maximize independence, prevent disability, and maintain health. The practice encompasses evaluation, treatment, and consultation." (American Occupational Therapy Association)

Occupational Therapy Assistant (OTA)

The **occupational therapy assistant** is an important member of the health care team. The certified occupational therapy assistant, or COTA, generally has achieved an associate's degree in Applied Sciences, and works under the direction of a Registered Occupational Therapist. The duties include assisting patients in learning (or relearning) self-care, functional duties of their employment, and recreational activities according to their individual needs.

Office Manager/Business Office Manager

An **office manager** or **business office manager** has managerial skills in the business operations of the medical office or clinic (or hospital). A degree in business administration is most desirable.

Paramedic

Paramedics are also called paramedical personnel and allied health personnel. They act as assistants to physicians or in place of a physician, especially in the military. They are trained in emergency medical procedures and supportive health care tasks.

Pharmacist

A **pharmacist** is a specialist in formulating and dispensing medications. They are licensed by individual states to practice pharmacy, which is the study of preparing and dispensing drugs. Pharmacists are employed in hospitals, medical centers, and pharmacies. Training consists of two years of postgraduate study in pharmacology.

Pharmacy Technician

Pharmacy technicians assist licensed pharmacists in preparing medications for patients and, in certain cases, administering the medicine. They also assist in clerical duties such as telephone communication, typing, filing, and often in patient education regarding medicines. Requirements and duties may vary in different states; however, professional certification can be obtained through individual state pharmacy boards.

Phlebotomist

In some areas, the skilled **phlebotomists** are referred to as **accessioning technicians** because they are extensively trained in the art of drawing blood for diagnostic laboratory testing. Most often they are lab technicians. They must be nationally certified and are employed in medical clinics, hospitals, and laboratories. (Under the supervision of a physician, the medical assistant who has had instruction, practice on a training arm, and evaluation proving competency in this skill may perform this procedure to obtain blood specimens for analysis.)

Physical Therapist

One licensed to assist in the examination, testing, and treatment of physically disabled or handicapped people and those patients who are going through a physical rehabilitation program following accident, injury, or serious illness through the use of special exercise, application of heat or cold, use of **ultrasound** therapy, and other techniques is a **physical therapist**, Figure 1–11. They qualify by having a B.S. in physical therapy or getting a special 12-month certificate course after obtaining a B.S. in a related field.

Physician Assistant (PA)

A **physician assistant**, also called physician associate, is a person trained in certain aspects of the practice of medicine or osteopathy to provide assistance to the physician. These individuals are trained by physicians and practice under their direct supervision and within the legal license of a physician according to the laws of each state. Training programs vary in length from a few months to two years. They may be nationally certified.

Podiatrist/Chiropodist

Podiatrists and **chiropodists** are trained to diagnose and treat diseases and disorders of the feet. They may be awarded these degrees: DSC—Doctor of Surgical Chiropody; PodD—Doctor of Podiatry; and with further training, DPM—Doctor of Podiatric Medicine.

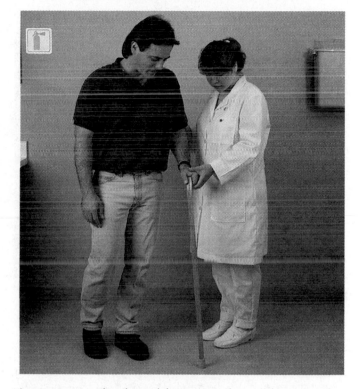

Figure 1–11 The physical therapist explains to the patient the correct way to use ambulatory equipment.

Psychologist

Psychologists specialize in the study of the structure and function of the brain and related mental processes. They have a graduate degree in psychology and training in clinical psychology. They provide testing and counseling services to patients with mental and emotional disorders. Psychologists have private practices or may be a part of a group family practice.

Radiology Technician, Radiologic Technologist, X-Ray Technician

An **x-ray technician**, **radiology technician**, or **radiologic technologist**, Figure 1–12, is one who has had specialized training in the various techniques of visualization of the tissues and organs of the body and who under the supervision of a physician radiologist, operates radiologic equipment and assists radiologists and other health professionals. Competence must be proved by the American Registry of Radiologic Technologists.

Respiratory Therapy Technician

Respiratory therapy technicians are graduates of an AMA-approved school designed to qualify persons for the technician certification examination of the National Board for Respiratory Care. These members of the health care team perform procedures of treatment that maintain or improve the **ventilatory** function of the respiratory tract in patients. The training period for this field is usually a one-year program in a hospital setting.

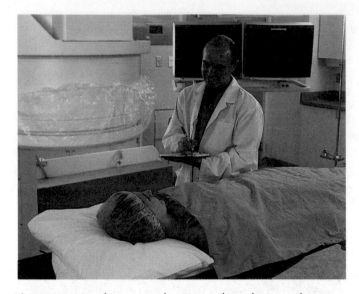

Figure 1-12 The x-ray technician explains the procedure to the patient.

Unit Clerk

A **unit clerk** performs routine clerical and reception tasks in a patient care unit of a hospital. This position requires a self-motivated, mature individual to handle the stress of the hectic pace of coordinating personnel and their duties at the nurses' station. Also called unit coordinator, unit secretary, administrative specialist, ward clerk, or ward secretary. Training is on-the-job or possibly included in a health care program such as medical assisting.

Because medical assistants are the most versatile of all health care workers, it is reasonable for them to seek employment in any of the previously mentioned areas of the medical field. Once these persons have gained basic entry-level skills in medical assisting, they are able to adapt easily to a specialty practice with additional training (the amount of which would obviously depend on the type of practice).

Complete Chapter 1, Unit 2 in the workbook to help you meet the objectives at the beginning of this unit and therefore achieve competency of this subject matter.

UNIT 3
Medical Practice Specialties

▮ OBJECTIVES

Upon completion of the unit, meet the following terminal performance objectives by verifying knowledge of the facts and principles presented through oral and written communication at a level deemed competent.

1. Identify the primary medical specialties and give the abbreviations for those that have them.
2. List eight health care professionals with doctoral degrees. Explain who should be called doctor.

3. Name employment possibilities for medical assistants other than with MDs and DOs.
4. Identify and spell correctly the title of each practitioner in each of the specialties.
5. Discuss the educational process of becoming a physician.
6. Spell and define, using the glossary at the back of the text, all the words to know in this unit.

▮ WORDS TO KNOW

allergy	nuclear medicine
anesthesiologist	obstetrician
cardiologist	occupational medicine
chiropractic	oncology
competency	ophthalmologist
dentist	optometrist
deprivation	orthopedist
dermatologist	osteopathy
diplomate	otorhinolaryngologist
doctorates	pathologist
endocrinologist	pediatrician
gastroenterologist	perception
gerontologist	podiatrist
gynecologist	practitioner
hematologist	preventive
immunology	proprietorship
infertility	psychiatrist
internist	psychologist
internship	psychotherapy
licensure	pulmonary
maintenance	radiologist
manifestation	radionuclides
manipulation therapy	residency
misalignment	surgeon
nephrologist	traumatic
neurologist	urology

HEALTH CARE PROFESSIONS

Ideally, all physicians dedicate their lives to acquiring skills in the art and science of diagnosing and treating disease and maintaining health. Each physician has this same goal. It is, however, impossible for a physician to study in detail every field of medicine. Because of this fact, some physicians become medical specialists. This means that they have chosen to gain expertise in one particular area of medicine. Some doctors additionally have a particular interest that is not a specialty, but is an area they feel worthy of their time and effort and effective in helping their patients toward better health. These areas are viewed as subspecialties or areas of special interest.

Because medical assistants generally are employed by physicians in their offices, they need a basic understanding of the various medical specialties and special interests. The medical assistant who works for a general practitioner may need to initiate contacts with specialists through referrals.

The medical assistant must then be knowledgeable about these areas to help reinforce or clarify the physician's directions to the patient. Moreover, knowing about these various practices will also help the medical assistant to decide in which area to seek employment. Most specialists maintain office practices and have need of medical assistants as general and family practitioners do. Adapting to these special areas after acquiring basic skills and knowledge should be relatively easy. A medical assistant interested in advancement must be willing to put forth the necessary effort.

To help you get familiar with these specialties, Table 1–1 contains basic information concerning each area. You should note that a few specialty practices are not listed in the table. One of those practices is the specialty practice of emergency medicine or traumatic medicine. In this case, the referral may be initiated by the family or general practitioner's office if, when the patient phones in for advice concerning a condition, the patient's symptoms suggest a true emergency or urgency, then referring the patient to an urgent or emergency care center is certainly the procedure. And too, physicians who practice in the specialties of anesthesiology and pathology are usually hospital-based; rarely do they have private practice offices where patients are seen. These specialists work as members of the health care team contributing their expert skills and knowledge in serving patients. More precise knowledge of all these practices will come with experience and further study.

The field of general practice covers perhaps the broadest spectrum. The general practitioner sees all kinds of patients with all kinds of problems. Most can be handled by the general practitioner. If, however, the symptoms of a case suggest a serious or perhaps unknown cause, the patient may be referred to a specialist for further diagnosis and/or treatment, Figure 1–13. When the patient's specific need or problem has been remedied or the recovery plan has been established, the patient returns to the "family doctor" for continued care.

The following pages will introduce you to many fields of medical practice and allied health professions. Because treating patients is a team effort, gaining a basic knowledge of the duties involved in each type of practice will help you better serve the patient. Better communication between colleagues who understand each other leads to more efficient patient care.

Physician Education

All physicians invest a minimum of nine years in learning how to practice medicine, which is the art and science of the diagnosis, treatment, and prevention of disease, and the **maintenance** of good health. Until recently, their training, education, and practical experience included a four-year college degree in premed, four years in medical school, and one year of **internship**. Following this and successful completion of the state board examination for **licensure**, the person was then considered a general **practitioner** and was ready to begin a private practice. This license to practice medicine is renewed periodically throughout the physician's life. Today the phrase Postgraduate year following medical school (PGY-1) denotes the **internship** stage of training. Specialty areas require additional years of study in the particular area of choice. It is usually between two and six years and is commonly known as **residency** or PGY-2, 3, 4, and so on. After satisfactorily accomplishing all requirements, the physician is awarded a certificate of

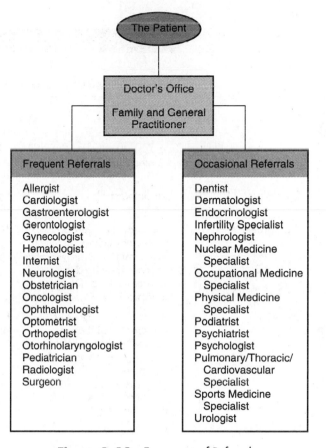

Figure 1-13 Frequency of Referrals.

competency in the specialty area and is recognized as a **diplomate** of that specialty.

Types of Practices

The actual business of practicing medicine may be conducted in several ways. Many physicians prefer to have a solo practice, or sole **proprietorship**, meaning that the individual alone makes all decisions regarding the practice. Being employed as a medical assistant in this type of office requires that you have both administrative and clinical skills essential for the smooth operation of that practice, especially if you are the only employee.

In a partnership, two or more physicians have a legal agreement to share in the total business operation of the practice. In this case, usually two to several medical assistants (or other members of the health care team) are employed to care for patients and conduct business.

A group practice consists of three or more physicians who share a facility for the purpose of practicing medicine. In this legal contract the doctors share expenses, income, equipment, records, and personnel. Many times these practices are a health maintenance organization (HMO) or an independent practice association (IPA) type of practice. You will learn more about these in Chapter 9. Usually several professionals make up the health care team in this setting. Medical assistants, lab technicians, radiology technicians, nurses, physician assistants, and the physicians work together in providing health care.

TABLE 1-1

MEDICAL SPECIALTIES			
SPECIALTY	**TITLE OF PRACTITIONER**	**AREA OF SPECIALIZATION**	**TYPES OF PATIENTS SEEN**
Allergy	Allergist	Diagnosing and treating conditions of altered immunological reactivity (allergic reactions)	Adults of all ages, children, both sexes
Anesthesiology	Anesthesiologist	Administering anesthetic agents before and during surgery	Adults of all ages, children, both sexes
Cardiology	Cardiologist	Diagnosing and treating abnormalities, diseases, and disorders of the heart	Adults of all ages, children, both sexes
Chiropractic	Chiropractor. (Chiropractors are not physicians, but they are licensed in their field of practice. They hold the degree of DC, or Doctor of Chiropractic.)	Manipulative treatment of disorders originating from misalignment of the spinal vertebrae	Adults of all ages, children, both sexes
Dentistry	Dentist (Dentists are not physicians, but they are licensed in their field of practice, which can range from general to highly specialized. They hold the degree of DDS, or Doctor of Dental Surgery.)	Diagnosing and treating diseases and disorders of the teeth and gums	Adults of all ages, children, both sexes
Dermatology	Dermatologist	Diagnosing and treating disorders of the skin	Adults of all ages, children, both sexes
Endocrinology	Endocrinologist	Diagnosing and treating diseases and malfunctions of the glands of internal secretion	Adults of all ages, children, both sexes
Family Practice	Family Practitioner	Similar to general practice in nature, but centering around the family unit	Adults of all ages, infants and children of all ages, both sexes
Gastroenterology	Gastroenterologist	Diagnosing and treating diseases and disorders of the stomach and intestines	Adults of all ages, children, both sexes
Geriatrics	Gerontologist	Diagnosing and treating diseases, disorders, and problems associated with aging	Older adults, both sexes
Gynecology	Gynecologist	Diagnosing and treating diseases and disorders of the female reproductive tract; strong emphasis on preventive measures	Female adolescents and adults
Hematology	Hematologist	Diagnosing and treating diseases and disorders of the blood and blood-forming tissues	Adults of all ages, infants and children, both sexes
Infertility	Infertility Specialist	Diagnosing and treating problems in conceiving and maintaining pregnancy	Married couples who desire to have children but cannot
Internal Medicine	Internist	Diagnosing and treating diseases and disorders of the internal organs	Adults of all ages, children, both sexes
Nephrology	Nephrologist	Diagnosing and treating diseases and disorders of the kidney	Adults, children, both sexes
Neurology	Neurologist	Diagnosing and treating diseases and disorders of the central nervous system	Adults, children, both sexes

(continued)

TABLE 1-1

MEDICAL SPECIALTIES (Continued)			
SPECIALTY	**TITLE OF PRACTITIONER**	**AREA OF SPECIALIZATION**	**TYPES OF PATIENTS SEEN**
Nuclear Medicine	Nuclear Medicine Specialist	Diagnosing and treating diseases with the use of radionuclides (Figure 1–14)	Adults, both sexes
Obstetrics	Obstetrician	Providing direct care to pregnant females during pregnancy, childbirth, and immediately thereafter	Pregnant females
Occupational Medicine	Occupational Medicine Specialist	Diagnosing and treating diseases or conditions arising from occupational circumstances (e.g., chemicals, dust, or gases)	Adults of all ages, both sexes
Oncology	Oncologist	Diagnosing and treating tumors and cancer	Adults of all ages, children, both sexes
Ophthalmology	Ophthalmologist	Diagnosing and treating diseases and disorders of the eye	Adults of all ages, children, both sexes
Optometry	Optometrist (Optometrists are not physicians, but are licensed in their field of practice. They hold the degree of OD, or Doctor of Optometry.)	Measuring the accuracy of vision to determine if corrective lenses are needed	Adults of all ages, children, both sexes
Orthopedics	Orthopedist	Diagnosing and treating disorders and diseases of the bones, muscles, ligaments, and tendons, and fractures of the bones	Adults of all ages, children, both sexes
Otorhinolaryngology	Otorhinolaryngologist (commonly referred to as an ENT Specialist)	Diagnosing and treatment of disorders and diseases of the ear, nose, and throat	Adults of all ages, children, both sexes
Pathology	Pathologist	Analysis of tissue samples to confirm diagnosis	Usually has no direct contact with patients
Pediatrics	Pediatrician	Diagnosing and treating diseases and disorders of children; strong emphasis on preventive measures	Infants, children, and adolescents
Physical Medicine	Physical Medicine Specialist	Diagnosing and treating diseases and disorders with physical agents (physical therapy)	Adults, children, both sexes
Podiatry	Podiatrist (Podiatrists are not physicians, but they are licensed in their field of practice. They hold the degree of DPM, or Doctor of Podiatric Medicine.)	Diagnosing and treating diseases and disorders of the feet	Adults, children, both sexes
Psychiatry	Psychiatrist	Diagnosing and treating pronounced manifestations of emotional problems or mental illness that may have an organic causative factor	Adults of all ages, children, both sexes. (Note: Child Psychiatry is a further specialized field dealing exclusively with children and adolescents.)
Psychology	Psychologist (Psychologists are not physicians, but they are licensed in their field of practice. They hold the degree of PhD, or Doctor of Philosophy.)	Evaluating and treating emotional problems. These professionals give counseling to individuals, families, and groups	Adults, children, both sexes

(continued)

TABLE 1-1

MEDICAL SPECIALTIES (Continued)			
SPECIALTY	**TITLE OF PRACTITIONER**	**AREA OF SPECIALIZATION**	**TYPES OF PATIENTS SEEN**
Pulmonary Specialties	Pulmonary/Thoracic/ Cardiovascular Specialist	Diagnosing and treating diseases and disorders of the chest, lungs, heart, and blood vessels	Adults, both sexes
Radiology	Radiologist	Diagnosing and treating diseases and disorders with roentgen rays (X rays) and other forms of radiant energy	Adults of all ages, children, both sexes
Sports Medicine	Sports Medicine Specialist	Diagnosing and treating injuries sustained in athletic events	Adults, especially young adults (athletes), both sexes
Surgery	Surgeon	Diagnosing and treating diseases, injuries, and deformities by manual or operative methods	Adults of all ages, infants, children, both sexes
Traumatic Medicine	Emergency Physician (commonly referred to as ER or trauma physician since most work in hospital emergency rooms)	Diagnosing and treating acute (traumatic) illnesses and injuries	Adults of all ages, infants, children, both sexes
Urology	Urologist	Diagnosing and treating diseases and disorders of the urinary system of females and genitourinary system of males	Adults of all ages, infants, children

SUBSPECIALTY (S)/ SPECIAL INTEREST (SI) AREAS

In the following you will be introduced to the subspecialties or special interest areas that branch off from a particular specialty practice. A brief description and definition of each area will give you a basic idea of the roles they play in the health care team. As you learn and study the duties and responsibilities of the medical assistant, you may realize a particular area of interest of your own. When the time comes for your internship and then later for you to begin the job search for gainful employment, you will have a basic understanding of the variety of practices so that you will be better prepared to make a decision of where to apply.

Adolescent Medicine

This area branches from pediatrics and specifically deals with youngsters aged eleven to twenty years, or the years of puberty to maturity. (S)

Acupuncture

This method of treatment originated in the Far East and has been gaining in popularity in western countries since the 1970s. This procedure involves the insertion of fine thin needles into specific sites of the body to alleviate pain or to treat a specific body system or area (its use is still controversial). (SI)

Aerospace Medicine

Physicians who extend their practice of medicine to this area do research in the effects of the environment in space on people. The areas of greatest concern are pathology, physiology, and psychology. (SI)

Alcoholism (Chemical Dependency)

These physicians treat patients who have addiction to alcohol and drugs. (SI)

Allergy and Immunology

An **allergy** is an acquired hypersensitivity a person exhibits to a substance that normally does not cause a reaction. Physicians interested in allergies sometimes combine these areas because they are closely related. **Immunology** is the study of how the body deals with immunity to disease (it is a subspecialty sometimes practiced alone). (S)

Cardiology (Cardiovascular Disease)

A **cardiologist** is a physician who specializes in treating diseases and disorders of the heart. Because the heart is the center of the circulatory system, a cardiovascular specialist is one who treats only patients with heart and blood vessel problems. (S)

Diabetes

As implied, these physicians have a special interest in treating only patients who have been diagnosed with diabetes. (SI)

Emergency Medicine

Physicians practicing this subspecialty are concerned with the diagnosis and treatment of patients with conditions that have resulted from injury or trauma or from sudden illness. (S)

Gynecology

The subspecialty of gynecology that deals with the diagnosis and treatment of cancer of the reproductive tract of females of all ages is called GYN Oncology. (S)

Hypertension

A physician who subspecializes in this area treats patients who have high blood pressure (hypertension). (SI)

Hypnosis

This method of treatment is becoming more popular with physicians. This procedure is used mainly in **psychotherapy** in which the patient is induced into a trancelike sleep to help change the memory or the **perception** of something in that person (such as unwanted behavior, i.e., smoking or weight control). Its use in medicine is to help patients deal with pain and stress, which affect their overall health. (SI)

Nutrition

This area of special interest includes patients with disorders or diseases related to how the body utilizes food and drink for growth and maintenance. (SI)

Pediatric Allergists

These physicians deal only with treating children who have allergies. (S)

Preventive Medicine

This branch of medicine deals with the prevention of both mental and physical illness and disease. It is sometimes referred to as General Preventive Medicine (GPM). (S)

Rheumatology

Physicians in this subspecialty treat inflammatory disorders of the connective tissues and related structures. (S)

Sleep Disorder

As the name implies, physicians who deal with these patients are interested in the various stages of sleep and the effects of sleep **deprivation**. (SI)

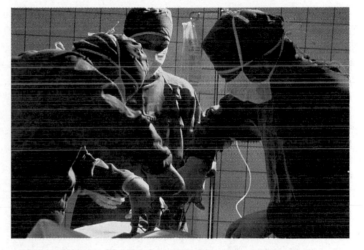

Figure 1–14   A successful operation requires the cooperation and expertise of the surgeon and the entire surgical team.

Surgery

Most of the subspecialty areas of this branch of medicine and **osteopathy** are listed below:

- Cardiovascular
- Colon (and Rectal)
- Cosmetic (Plastic and Reconstructive)
- Hand
- Head and Neck
- Neurological
- Orthopedic
- Pediatrics
- Spine
- Thoracic
- Urological
- Vascular

With the great strides that medical science achieves, the field of medicine continues to evolve with remarkable new treatments, medications, and discoveries. Being an integral part of the health care team is exciting, Figure 1–14. New areas of special interest and subspecialties are ever changing with the latest findings. Keeping abreast of these changes by attending ongoing educational programs to increase your knowledge will help you to become not only more confident in your work, but a most valuable medical assistant as well.

A NOTE REGARDING DOCTORS

As you progress in the field of medical assisting, a basic understanding of the frequently misused term *doctor* will be helpful. The term comes from Latin; it means *to teach*. Persons who hold doctoral degrees (**doctorates**) are entitled to be addressed as "Doctor" and to write the initials that stand for their doctorate after their name. The abbreviation "Dr." is the proper way to address a physician or any other type of doctor who has earned this title. In the medical field, the abbreviation "Dr." denotes that the person is qualified to practice medicine. In other fields, it means that the person has achieved the highest academic degree awarded by a college in the particular discipline. The doctors with whom you will be coming into contact include:

- Doctor of Chiropractic (DC)
- Doctor of Dental Medicine (DMD)
- Doctor of Dental Surgery (DDS)
- Doctor of Medicine (MD)
- Doctor of Optometry (OD)
- Doctor of Osteopathy (DO)
- Doctor of Philosophy (PhD)
- Doctor of Podiatric Medicine (DPM)

Doctor of Medicine and Doctor of Osteopathy

One of the areas of greatest confusion is the differentiation between MDs and DOs. Holders of either degree are licensed physicians. The degrees themselves originate from somewhat different schools of thought. (Interestingly enough, it was an MD who founded the osteopathic movement that now produces DOs.) Physicians of both schools must satisfactorily complete board examinations in the state where they wish to practice medicine. In schools of osteopathy, **manipulation therapy** is an additional skill included in their curriculum. In years past, the scope of practice of DOs was greatly limited by state medical boards. However, in most of the United States today, medical licensing boards permit DOs to perform the same duties as MDs. Should you find employment with either a DO or MD, you will be able to apply the same administrative and clinical knowledge and skills.

Although you are training primarily to assist physicians, with a little adaptation, you could also move into assisting chiropractors, psychologists, or podiatrists. To move into the dental or optometric field would require additional training.

Complete Chapter 1, Unit 3 in the workbook to help you meet the objectives at the beginning of this unit and therefore achieve competency of this subject matter.

REFERENCES

The American Medical Association Family Medical Guide. New York: Random House, 1987.

Diagnostic Tests, Nurse's Ready Reference. Springhouse, PA: Springhouse Corporation, 1991.

Encyclopedia of Medicine. Editor: Charles B. Clayman, M.D. New York: Random House, 1989.

Ebony. "Neurosurgery," September 1983, Johnson Publishing Company.

Hastings, R.P. (1974). *Medicine: An International History.* New York: Praeger Publishers, Inc.

Marks, Geoffrey, and Beatty, William K. *The Story of Medicine in America,* New York: Scribners, 1973.

Mitchell, Paula R., and Grippando, Gloria M., *Nursing Perspectives and Issues*, 5th Ed. Albany: Delmar, 1993.

Mosby's Medical, Nursing, and Allied Health, 4th ed. St. Louis: C. V. Mosby, 1994.

Raven, Susan, and Weir, Alison. *Women of Achievement.* New York: Harmony, 1981.

Reader's Digest Illustrated Encyclopedic Dictionary. Boston: Houghton Mifflin Lexical Databases, 1987.

Sicherman, Barbara, and Green, Carol Hurd. *Notable American Women: The Modern Period.* Cambridge, MA: Belknap Press, 1980.

Taber, Charles W. *Taber's Cyclopedic Medical Dictionary,* 17th ed. Philadelphia: F.A. Davis, 1993.

2

The Medical Assistant

The American Association of Medical Assistants describes the profession of medical assistant as follows: "The Medical Assistant is a professional, multi-skilled person dedicated to assisting in patient care management. This practitioner performs administrative and clinical duties and may manage emergency situations, facilities, and/or personnel. Competence in the field also requires that a Medical Assistant display professionalism, communicate effectively, and provide instruction to patients."

UNIT 1
Training, Job Responsibilities, and Employment Opportunities

UNIT 2
Personal Characteristics

UNIT 3
Professionalism

During the evolvement of the practice of medicine, physicians have come to realize the value of medical assistants. Many years ago, physicians could treat patients alone. There was no need for appointments, filing of insurance forms, or extensive record keeping. There was rarely any thought of a lawsuit.

Times have changed dramatically. It is now necessary to document every transaction between the physician or the office staff and the patient to validate appropriate and responsible care. Accurate and comprehensive records are vital. Attention to every office management detail is essential as well.

This chapter discusses the training opportunities and job responsibilities of a medical assistant. It also describes highly desirable personal characteristics that will help make you a valuable asset to the physician. In addition, it identifies those attributes of professionalism which elevate your working experience to a higher level and provide you with personal satisfaction.

UNIT 1

Training, Job Responsibilities, and Employment Opportunities

■ OBJECTIVES

Upon completion of the unit, meet the following terminal performance objectives by verifying knowledge of the facts and principles presented through oral and written communication at a level deemed competent.

1. Name the two factors that are causing increased employment opportunities in the health care field.
2. Identify three types of schools that offer programs in medical assisting.
3. Explain the purpose of the DACUM and the Role Delineation Study.
4. List the ten areas of competence identified by the Role Delineation Study.
5. Explain the term "career laddering."
6. Identify the fifteen fastest growing health occupations, according to the United States Department of Labor.
7. Spell and define, using the glossary at the back of the text, all the words to know in this unit.

■ WORDS TO KNOW

administrative
analysis
associate degree
bookkeeper
certificate of completion
clinical
competency
compliance
confidential
curriculum
DACUM
hygienist
license
methodical

nuclear medicine
   technologist
professional
proprietary
radioactive agents
receptionist
rehabilitation centers
rehabilitative therapy
Role Delineation Study
secretary
therapeutic
therapist
ultrasound technologist

You have chosen to become a medical assistant. In a brochure published by the American Association of Medical Assistants (AAMA) entitled "Plan Your Career as a Medical Assistant," a series of questions is listed to help the interested individual decide whether to pursue the career. The questions are:

- Do you like people?
- Do you want variety in your work?
- Can you "take hold" and get things done?
- Are you **methodical** and accurate in what you do?
- Can you be trusted with **confidential** information?

If you can answer yes to these questions, you may have the appropriate characteristics of a medical assistant. You will be pleased to learn that according to the United States Department of Labor this occupation is one of the fifteen health care occupational areas identified to experience significant growth in the near future. In this unit, you will learn about the training and responsibilities of a medical assistant. You will also read about opportunities for employment in medical assisting as well as how that experience, together with additional training, can qualify you for other health care jobs in the future.

Health care occupations have developed from the physician's need to enlist the help of other persons in order to provide technical and efficient care for greater numbers of patients. In addition to medical assistants who work directly with the physician, a large number of highly technical and **professional** people perform a great number of diagnostic and supporting functions. In the 1994–2005 Employment Occupational Outlook Bulletin, the United States Department of Labor data indicated that fifteen health care related occupations would be growing faster than the average overall workforce through the year 2005. Opportunities would be plentiful in these broad occupational groups, with a predicted average growth rate of 34%, which translates into approximately fourteen million new jobs. A summary of the projected health care growth rates for the fifteen fastest growing assistant, technician, and specialist occupations is listed in Table 2–1. The general overall job growth rate is anticipated to be about 22% during this period.

Seven of the twenty overall fastest growing occupations are concentrated in the health services industry: home health aides, physical and corrective therapy assistants and aides, occupational therapy assistants and aides, occupational therapists, physical therapists, medical assistants, and medical records technicians. Refer to Table 2–2 which lists data available from the United States Department of Labor. The first two columns show the 1994 and the 2005 projected employment figures of representative health care occupations. The third and fourth columns show the increase percentage of employment (except for EKG technicians) and the number of jobs anticipated within the eleven year period. Note: All data are listed in thousands, so three zeroes need to be added to each number. The last two columns show the total number of new employees needed within the eleven years and indicate the most frequent source of education for the job.

The health occupations boom is due to two factors: the extended lifetimes of Americans and the furiously evolving medical technology. Data has shown that the population over

TABLE 2–1

PROJECTED PERCENTAGES OF GROWTH IN FIFTEEN HEALTH OCCUPATIONS	
OCCUPATION	**PROJECTED GROWTH**

Service Occupations
  Dental Assistant
  Medical Assistant
  Nursing Assistant
  Psychiatric Assistant
	33% Increase

Professional Specialties
  Physician Assistant
  Recreational Therapist
  Respiratory Therapist
	37% Increase

Technicians
  Dental Hygienist
  Emergency Medical Technician (EMT)
  Electroencephalogram (EEG)
    Technologist
  Licensed Practical Nurse (LPN)
  Medical Records Technician
  Nuclear Medicine Technologist
  Radiological Technician
  Surgical Technician
	32% Increase

age eighty-five is growing at a rate of four times the total population. As people age, they develop more health problems and therefore require more services. With the development of new diagnostic tests and methods of treatment, someone must be trained to operate the equipment and provide the service. Occasionally, it means that a completely new field of employment is needed, such as has occurred with **nuclear medicine technologists**.

Another shift has resulted from the changing nature of how health care services are being delivered. A good example of this is the explosion of home health care, see Table 2–2. Employment in this area is expected to increase 102%, in other words, more than double. This reflects the fact that the growing population of the elderly and the disabled will need assistance, but the trend will be toward providing it in their homes instead of within a more expensive health care facility. Note: It may be speculative on the author's part, but it seems that the family physician may once again need to visit these persons at home if they are to be served. If a financial incentive from insurance companies were offered to physicians, home visits would probably occur.

TRAINING

Since you are reading this text, you are probably enrolled in a formal training program to acquire the knowledge and skills needed to become a medical assistant. Thirty years ago it was relatively easy to be hired and trained on the job. This may still take place in some offices, usually where there are multiple employees so work can continue while a new person learns. But today, with the fast paced, complex level of skills required to provide medical care and conduct the business affairs of the practice, the value of a trained employee is recognized as a real asset by the physician.

Training programs vary in length and design. In many states, vocational education offers medical assisting programs. It can be an educational option in public high schools, usually for junior and senior students. Vocational programs may also be offered at the adult level to meet the needs of post-high school individuals. Many technical and commu-

nity colleges may offer training as well. Programs leading to a **certificate of completion** are usually one year in length. An **associate degree** program would require two years of course work and include subject areas which complement the **curriculum**. Another major source of training is available from private **proprietary** schools. This training may also vary in length and content depending upon the school's philosophy, affiliation, and educational goals.

TABLE 2–2

CURRENT AND PROJECTED EMPLOYMENT* IN EIGHTEEN HEALTH OCCUPATIONS (FROM U.S. DEPARTMENT OF LABOR, BUREAU OF LABOR STATISTICS BULLETIN 2472)					
Occupation	**Employment**		**Employment Change, 1994–2005**		**Total Job Openings Due to Growth and Net Replacements, 1994–2005**	**Most Significant Source of Training**
	1994	**Projected 2005**	**Percent (increase)**	**Number (increase)**		
cardiology technologists	14	17	22%	3	6	associate's degree
clinical lab technologists and technicians	274	307	12%	33	86	bachelor's degree
dental assistants	190	269	42%	79	137	OJT moderate term
dental hygienists	127	180	42%	53	74	associate's degree
EKG technicians	16	11	−30%[†]	−5[†]	3	OJT moderate term
emergency medical technicians (EMT)	138	187	36%	49	72	postsecondary-vocational training
home health aides	420	848	102%	428	488	OJT short term
licensed practical nurses (LPN)	702	899	28%	197	341	postsecondary-vocational training
medical assistants	206	327	59%	121	155	OJT moderate term
medical records technicians	81	126	56%	45	59	associate's degree
medical secretaries	226	281	24%	55	103	postsecondary-vocational training
nursing aides, orderlies, attendants	1,265	1,652	31%	387	566	OJT short term
occupational therapy assistant, aides	16	29	82%	13	16	OJT moderate term
pharmacy assistants	52	64	23%	12	22	OJT short term
pharmacy technicians	81	101	24%	20	33	OJT moderate term
physician assistants	56	69	23%	13	22	bachelor's degree
registered nurses (RN)	1,906	2,379	25%	473	740	associate's degree
surgical technologists	46	65	43%	19	27	postsecondary-vocational training

Note: OJT = On-the-Job Training
*Numbers are listed in thousands
[†]Note surplus

TABLE 2–3

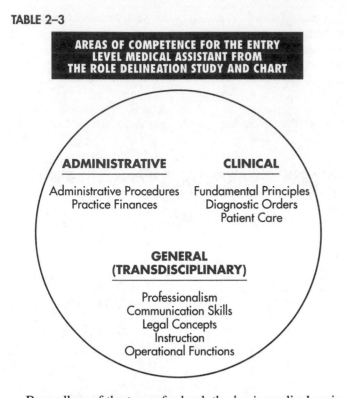

AREAS OF COMPETENCE FOR THE ENTRY LEVEL MEDICAL ASSISTANT FROM THE ROLE DELINEATION STUDY AND CHART

ADMINISTRATIVE
Administrative Procedures
Practice Finances

CLINICAL
Fundamental Principles
Diagnostic Orders
Patient Care

GENERAL (TRANSDISCIPLINARY)
Professionalism
Communication Skills
Legal Concepts
Instruction
Operational Functions

Performing clinical skills are an extension of the physician's role of assessment, examination, diagnosis, and treatment. Performing administrative skills help manage the business affairs of the practice. The performance of general skills are concerned with legal, ethical, moral, and professional conduct in the execution of your duties.

The following lists are examples of the variety of skills to be acquired in administrative, clinical, and general areas.

ADMINISTRATIVE	CLINICAL
Schedule appointments	Take medical histories
Prepare correspondence	Take vital signs
Handle telephone calls	Assist with medical procedures
Complete insurance forms	Prepare patient for examination
Obtain initial patient data	Prepare medications

GENERAL (Transdisciplinary)	
Demonstrate initiative and responsibility	Teach methods of health promotion
Treat all patients with compassion and empathy	Work as a team member
	Maintain confidentiality
Use medical terminology appropriately	Document accurately
	Follow federal, state, and local legal guidelines

Regardless of the type of school, the *basic* medical assistant curriculum should be similar. From 1979 through 1996 The American Association of Medical Assistants (AAMA) maintained a document called the DACUM (*Develop A Curriculum*). This publication identified the areas of practice and the competencies required for the occupation of medical assistant. This document was updated in 1984 and 1990. In 1997, the DACUM was revised by the Role Delineation Study. Two groups of practicing CMA's were surveyed by the National Board of Medical Examiners and AAMA. Based upon the group's practical experiences, they listed all current competencies essential for medical assistants. The lists of competencies were combined with the 1990 DACUM to form a survey instrument which was sent to a random sample of CMA's who represent many areas of practice, geographic locations, and a variety of backgrounds. The responses were evaluated and became the content for the areas of competence for entry-level medical assistants which was the outcome of the Role Delineation Study. The AAMA Curriculum Review Board will finalize the list of competencies which will be included in the *Standards and Guidelines of an Accredited Educational Program for the Medical Assistant* and will replace the previous *Essentials*.

The Role Delineation Study identified three broad areas of practice, Administrative, Clinical, and General (Transdisciplinary). These were further divided into 10 areas of competence as listed in Table 2-3. The Complete Medical Assistant Role Delineation Chart illustrating all skills (standard and advanced) within each area of competence is shown on the inside back cover of this book.

JOB RESPONSIBILITIES

The role of the medical assistant is to provide skillful execution of administrative, clinical, and general duties as an integral and supportive part of the physician's practice.

Many other tasks are performed regularly. A particularly important one is patient teaching. It is a task that requires special attention to the patient's response in order to ensure there will be compliance with the instruction. The assistant must carefully explain and/or demonstrate the procedure or activity and follow up with questioning to confirm understanding. The assistant should not assume something has been learned until the patient can explain or perform it.

It is also important for medical assistants to have a basic understanding of the anatomy and physiology of the human body. This knowledge helps in the comprehension of the need for diagnostic and treatment procedures ordered by the physician. A working knowledge of medical terminology is also essential in order to communicate with other health care professionals and to assist patients in understanding information or instructions given to them.

Another major responsibility of a medical assistant is the legal, moral, and ethical issues which are confronted on a daily basis. The medical assistant must be constantly aware of these concerns in order to respect the values of others and to eliminate the chance for personal or employer liability. This subject matter is more fully discussed in Chapter 3. To get an overview of all the tasks a medical assistant will be expected to perform, look through the "Procedures" list in the front pages of this book (page xi). Job responsibility, however, goes beyond just the execution of procedures; it includes a personal commitment to assist the physician in every way possible in order to provide total quality patient care.

EMPLOYMENT OPPORTUNITIES

The practice of medicine has changed dramatically. In earlier times, physicians could treat patients without any assistance. Today, medical assistants work in physicians' offices, clinics, hospitals, and other facilities, performing both administrative and clinical duties, under the supervision of the physician. The efficient medical practice requires much attention to detail to provide the best care possible to patients. It is essential to keep thorough records. The need for a **receptionist, secretary, bookkeeper**, and technician, in addition to a medical assistant or nurse may be required. Some small individual practices may still be able to operate with only one support person and that individual will handle all the administrative, clinical, and operational duties alone.

Some physicians like to manage their office operations themselves, but most prefer to concentrate on patient care and give office management responsibilities to a professional member of their staff. This person can discuss fees, arrange collection of accounts, order supplies, perform banking activities, schedule staff hours, pay office expenses, and many other operational duties. Medical assistants who have office experience and administrative ability are often given the responsibility of performing the duties of the office manager.

CAREER LADDERING

You may be completely satisfied as a medical assistant and find great pleasure in your work. This is very admirable—you are providing a valuable service. But perhaps, after a period of time, you decide you would like to pursue another occupation, for personal reasons, achievement needs, or financial gain. The term career laddering refers to other occupations in which you might be employed based upon your interest, training, and experience. The "ladder" can be lateral or vertical. In addition to the advancement to a medical office manager, there is hospital based employment which medical assistants can fulfill. Examples of lateral jobs are ward clerks, admissions clerks, medical records clerks, medical secretaries, phlebotomists, and EKG technicians.

Other job opportunities may be possible with some additional instruction, and you may already possess a portion of the skills. Patient care technician, a newly developing job category, is seen as an alternative position for a medical assistant. It is also hospital based and incorporates skills from medical, nursing, and medical laboratory assisting. The job tends to be defined by the employing facility who also is currently providing the training. At this time, there is no recognized criteria or standards of practice.

The following brief descriptions cover seven of the fifteen "hottest jobs" mentioned at the beginning of the unit. Each of these positions would require additional training but would also provide you with a personal challenge and reward your efforts. NOTE: The salary scales are based on 1996 figures and may vary widely according to geographic area.

Licensed Practical Nurse (LPN)

Where Employed LPNs work under the supervision of registered nurses and physicians. They work in hospitals, nursing homes, private home care, and physician's offices and clinics. The growing elderly population will increase the need for LPNs in nursing homes, group homes, and residential care facilities, Figure 2–1.

Training Usually a one year program of classroom and clinical practice. All LPNs must pass a state licensing examina-tion in order to begin practice. Training is available at approved Schools of Practical Nursing operated by voca-tional-technical schools and community colleges. A current license is required in order to work as an LPN. Renewal is subject to continuing education credits in most states.

Salary Average annual salary is approximately $23,000 for a forty hour week excluding shift differentials.

Emergency Medical Technicians (EMT)

Where Employed EMTs work for private ambulance services or municipal fire, police, or rescue squads. EMTs provide immediate, on-site care in cases such as auto accidents, heart attacks, drownings, injuries, and shootings. EMTs transport patients to a medical facility, Figure 2–2. They work in teams under the direction of a dispatcher. There are three levels of practice: basic, advanced, and paramedic. The growing population and an increase in elderly people will increase the need. There is a high turnover rate for EMTs because of the stressful nature of the job.

Training The basic training course is from 100 to 120 hours of classroom instruction plus ten internship hours in a hospital emergency room. Training is provided by vocation-technical schools and community colleges in conjunction with hospitals, police, fire, and health departments. There are certification exams for each level which must be passed to work in that capacity.

Salary Salaries vary according to the level of expertise and the employer. An average basic EMT earns approximately $23,000 to $24,000 annually. The average paramedic EMT earns $28,500 to $30,000.

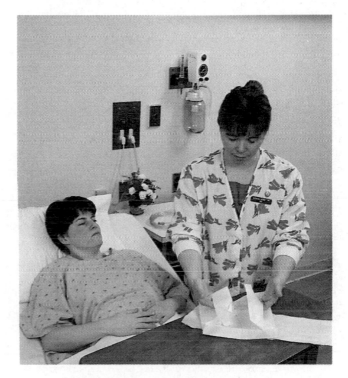

Figure 2–1 Licensed practical nurse.

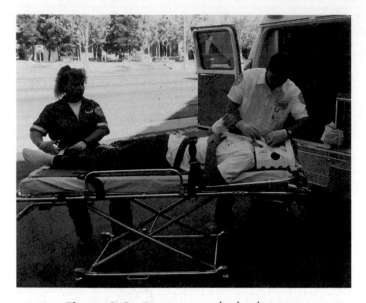

Figure 2-2   Emergency medical technicians.

$23,000 to $24,000 annually. The average paramedic EMT earns $28,500 to $30,000.

Recreational Therapists

Where Employed   Therapists work in hospitals, **rehabilitation centers**, nursing homes, senior citizen facilities and community recreational departments. They may assess an individual patient's condition by consulting medical records, the family, and the patient. A **therapeutic** program of individual or group activities is developed and may contain sports, arts, crafts, music, or outings. With advances in medical technology, more people survive illness and trauma and require **rehabilitative therapy**. Again, the increased number of elderly will require a larger amount of services.

Training   A bachelor's degree is the usual but an associate's degree program may be sufficient for some positions such as a nursing home director of activities, Figure 2–3. Cer-

tification by the National Council for Therapeutic Recreation requires a bachelor's degree.

Salary   A recreational therapist earns approximately $26,000 to $27,500 annually. Nursing home activity directors range from $16,500 to as much as $26,500 per year. Federal government employment of recreational therapists earn about $35,000 annually.

Respiratory Therapists

Where Employed   Respiratory therapists normally work forty hours per week but may work irregular night and weekend hours. Almost all work is in either respiratory care, anesthesiology, or pulmonary care departments of a hospital, Figure 2–4. Some may be employed by medical rental companies, home health care providers, and nursing homes. The increasing elderly population and the rapid rise in the number of AIDS patients will increase the need for therapists.

Training   Most programs are two years in length. There are four year and advanced two year programs which are helpful for acquiring a supervisory position. In addition, there is a one year technician program which permits employment in some settings. Most employers require all levels to obtain the Certified Respiratory Therapy Technician credential (CRRT). An advanced level certification is a Registered Respiratory Therapist (RRT).

Salary   The respiratory therapist's average annual salary is approximately $30,000.

Dental Hygienists

Where Employed   Almost all **hygienists** work in private dental offices. Some may work in public health agencies, schools, hospitals, or clinics. They regularly work forty hours per week but often part-time in more than one office. Hygienists provide preventive dental care by examining,

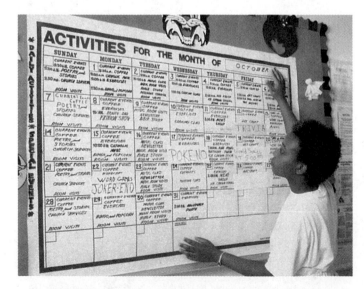

Figure 2-3   Recreational therapists/activity director.

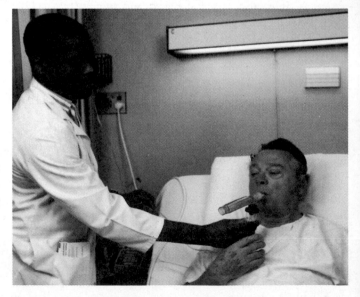

Figure 2-4   Respiratory therapist (RT) administering intermittent positive pressure breathing (IPPB) treatment.

cleaning, and taking x-rays of the teeth. They also remove sutures, teach oral hygiene, and provide restorative work. Population growth, higher incomes, and more elderly with natural teeth will increase the demand for dental services.

Training   Training is obtained at accredited dental hygiene programs of two or four year length. All hygienists must pass the American Dental Association's National Dental Examination in order to be licensed in their state.

Salary   The average annual salary is approximately $35,000, but varies greatly in relation to the number of hours worked.

Nuclear Medicine Technologist

Where Employed   About 90% of nuclear medicine technologists work in hospitals with the remaining 10% working in clinics and physician's offices. Hospital employees usually work irregular hours and "on-call" rotations. Technologists locate and track **radioactive agents** that have been introduced into a patient's body as part of a diagnostic examination. The radioactive material, absorbed by a specific organ, produces images which are recorded on the photographic film of high-tech cameras. Technological advances will increase nuclear medicine practice and the number of procedures, therefore requiring more technicians.

Training   There are different levels of training varying from one to four years in length, which permit performance of various functions. **Ultrasound** and radiologic **technologists** complete one year certificate programs, Figure 2–5. Advanced practice in nuclear medicine technology requires a two year certificate or associate's degree. Many states require licensure. Federal standards covering administration and operation of radiation detection equipment must be met.

Salary   The average technologist salary for a forty hour week, excluding shift differentials, is approximately $33,000 annually.

Physician Assistant (PA)

Where Employed   PAs are employed primarily in physicians' offices and clinics and work about forty hours per week, Figure 2–6. Some hospitals employ PAs in their emergency rooms, on two twenty-four-hour or three twelve-hour shifts per week. Approximately 30% work in smaller communities where physicians are scarce. PAs treat minor injuries, suture wounds, apply splints and casts, examine patients, order and interpret lab and x-ray procedures, and make preliminary diagnoses.

Training   The average program is two years in length and is offered by medical schools, vocational-technical schools, and four year colleges. Graduates from accredited programs may become certified by an examination and use the letters PA-C following their name. Almost all states require certification. Recertification every six years plus 100 hours of continuing education every two years is required to maintain the certificate.

Salary   The average annual salary is approximately $42,000 annually with surgeons paying a slightly higher wage.

Obviously, there is much opportunity within the health care field. Regardless of whether you remain a medical assistant or choose to practice in another field, you must be prepared to continue with life-long learning in order to maintain competency in your area of practice. At the present time, it appears your efforts will be rewarded with the security of employment opportunities in the future. You are fortunate—this is not true in many fields of work.

Complete Chapter 2, Unit 1 in the workbook to help you meet the objectives at the beginning of this unit and therefore achieve competency of this subject matter.

Figure 2–5 Registered diagnostic medical sonographer performing fetal ultrasound.

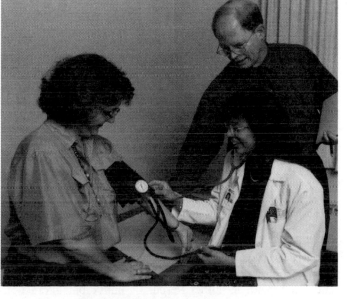

Figure 2–6 Physician assistant.

UNIT 2
Personal Characteristics

■ OBJECTIVES

Upon completion of the unit, meet the following terminal performance objectives by verifying knowledge of the facts and principles presented through oral and written communication at a level deemed competent.

1. List the seventeen highly desired character traits of health care workers.
2. Identify five personality qualities.
3. Name the four voice characteristics.
4. Give two reasons why health care providers need to be concerned about their appearances.
5. List the nine things that contribute to a professional appearance.
6. Spell and define, using the glossary at the back of the text, all the words to know in this unit.

■ WORDS TO KNOW

accurate	intelligence
adapt	monotone
appearance	patience
attitude	perceive
cooperate	perseverance
courteous	personality
dependable	posture
discreet	punctuality
empathy	reliable
enthusiasm	respectful
flexible	self control
honesty	tact
initiative	trait
innate	

HIGHLY DESIRABLE CHARACTERISTICS FOR HEALTH CARE WORKERS

There are many personal character **traits** that are highly desirable for health care workers. Some characteristics seem to be almost **innate**, while others must be learned. All traits can be enhanced by consciously making an effort to improve them. Your ability to work well with your employer, supervisors, and co-workers and your effectiveness in dealing with patients is greatly influenced by your personal characteristics.

First, let us examine some character traits as they relate to the manner in which job responsibilities are performed. As you read and consider the content, try to *honestly* examine your own character traits. Then we'll look at a few of the **personality** qualities and consider the messages they send when there is either verbal or nonverbal interaction with others.

Character Traits

For each of the following character traits, rate yourself on a scale of 1, 2, or 3: 1 = not usually, 2 = usually, and 3 = always. Can you score at least 30?

Accuracy (detailed correctness, exactness): Performing procedures in the correct manner is extremely important. Findings may be inaccurate or the process unsafe if you are careless. The **accurate** recording of patients' remarks and findings from vital signs or other assessments is extremely important, as is the preparation of medications and injections. Hopefully, you will always be conscious of accuracy, Figure 2–7.

Adaptable (the ability to adjust, to make fit): In employment, it will often be necessary to **adapt** to a change in a situation in order to benefit the operation of the office, such as changing your schedule to work for someone or perform duties not usually your responsibility. Your willingness to be **flexible** and to **cooperate** will be noticed by your employer or supervisor and, in the future, if you should need someone to adapt to your situation, they will be more willing to work it out.

Conservative (to be cautious, prudent; to handle with care; not wasteful): You will be handling equipment, materials, and supplies daily. It is important that you conserve office equipment usefulness and not carelessly waste products. Treat the things in the office as if they were your own. Waste is lost profit.

Courteous (to be polite, well-mannered): You will be a representative of your employer and expected to be **courteous** to co-workers, patients, and office visitors. This will not always be easy. It is never easy to be nice to someone who has been making it difficult for you. But, be courteous in spite of difficulties, and you will know you acted properly—it might even change the situation for the better.

Dependable (can be relied upon, responsible): Can people depend on you to carry out your responsibilities without the

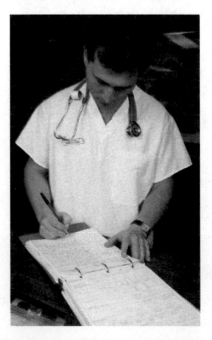

Figure 2–7 Accuracy is important when recording information.

need of constant supervision? When you agree to do something, do you always follow through? If you are **dependable,** you are at work, organized, and ready to start the day when the first patient arrives. When you are dependable, the physician and the office staff can direct their attention to other matters, knowing you are reliable.

Discreet (prudent, cautious—especially in speech): You must use good judgment in any discussion regarding a patient. You have access to confidential information that is not for discussion outside the office. The only exception is when there is a need to share information with other health professionals to whom you are making a referral for therapy or treatment, Figure 2–8. Always be **discreet**—never give out information about a patient over the phone or in writing without the patient's written permission. Even the completion of their insurance claims requires the patient's authorization.

Empathy (trying to identify one's feelings with those of another): Empathy is not the same as sympathy. Most patients do not want you to feel sorry for them, just try to understand how they feel. **Empathy** is the ability to put yourself in another person's place. Imagine you are wheelchair-bound with a condition that requires you to depend upon others for all your needs, Figure 2–9. Everyone feeling sorry for you will not be of any benefit, but, if everyone could see the situation from your viewpoint, they would realize that you just need physical assistance and their support.

Enthusiasm (zeal, intense interest): **Enthusiasm** shows in your facial expressions and the general manner in which you carry out your responsibilities. Your **posture,** voice, and mannerisms all indicate the fact that you like what you are doing. You usually will look your best and do your best when you are enthusiastic, and people will enjoy being around you. Enthusiasm must be genuine however, or it becomes an effort for you and it won't convince anyone else.

Honesty (trustworthy; the quality of being truthful): You know the saying "honesty is the best policy." In health care

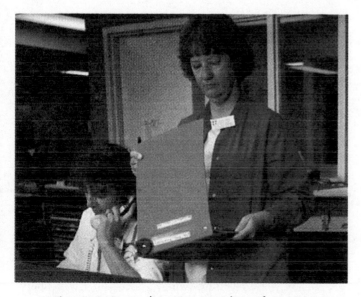

Figure 2–8 Be discreet in providing information.

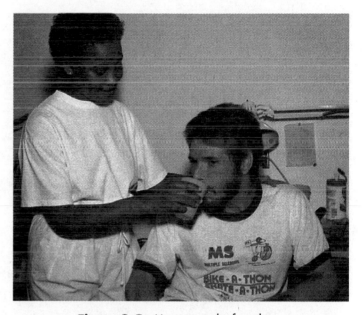

Figure 2–9 Have empathy for others.

this is extremely important. You cannot lie about something you did or did not do for a patient because you are dealing with a living human being. You cannot use "white out" to correct a mistake but you can admit to it so that it can be amended or counteracted. **Honesty** also refers to being trustworthy. You will have access to office equipment and supplies, co-workers' personal belongings, and perhaps money; you *must* be trustworthy. No business can tolerate or afford a thief or a liar.

Initiative (ambition; hustle; set something in motion): A person with **initiative** is a self-starter and a valuable member of a health care team. They recognize work to be done—even though it may not be their assigned job—and either do the work or offer their assistance. They do not have to be told or reminded of routine tasks. A person with initiative will also volunteer to take on a task or project in order to learn something new.

Patience (calmness in waiting; tolerant): It is very hard to be "patient" with a patient when you have many tasks to do. The elderly, especially, require **patience** because they are often slow to move and need assistance, Figure 2–10. If they are also lonely, they may take advantage of having someone to talk to. You are sure to have a "chronic complainer" who goes on and on about their symptoms or need for treatment until it begins to bother you. In your haste to stay on schedule and keep ahead of the physician, you will have to learn how to *politely* explain to patients that another person or duty needs your attention now and you must move on. The physician cannot afford for you to be impolite or impatient.

Perseverance (persistent effort; continue; prolong): **Perseverance** means to stick with a task until it is completed. Posting financial information, completing insurance forms, or filing can be postponed at times, until it becomes a real task to accomplish and requires self discipline to persevere until it is done. You may also need this quality when having difficulty getting a piece of equipment to function properly

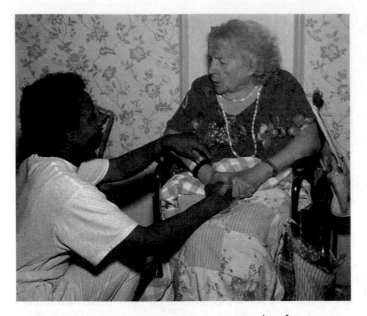

Figure 2-10 Some patients may require a lot of patience.

or performing a certain procedure. In this manner, perseverance and patience go hand in hand.

Punctual (in exact agreement with appointed time):   You are expected to be at work and on time every day, Figure 2–11. **Punctuality** is a part of being dependable. When you arrive at the established time and are ready to assume your responsibilities, the entire office will operate more smoothly. In contrast, when you are late, it often seems you never get "caught up" and your whole day goes poorly. This is a trait you definitely can acquire with self discipline.

Reliable (trustworthy, dependable, responsible): This trait is like being dependable. If you are **reliable**, the physician knows you can be expected to perform in the same consis-

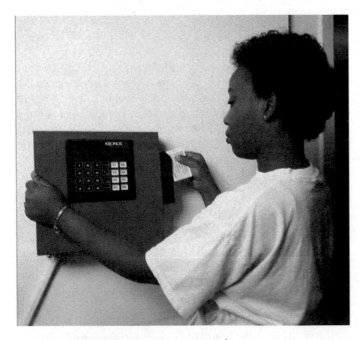

Figure 2-11 Being punctual is important.

tent manner as you have in the past. In both your personal and professional life, you know how important it is to have someone who is reliable, someone who will always be there should you have the need.

Respectful (showing regard for; considerate; courteous): Being friends with everyone with whom you work will probably not happen. You will have differences of opinion at work and at home, about how people act or what they say. You don't have to agree with them, but realize they have a right to their actions and respect that right. Even if you do not care for someone personally, it is important to be courteous and **respectful**. That is the "mark" of a mature, civil person. There will also be patients with whom you'll have difficulty, but you must always be tolerant and considerate. The trait of being respectful is necessary for good human relations.

Self control (show restraint, in check): Being in control of your actions is very important. There will be times when you may be tempted to blurt out remarks or display some negative action, but it is not appropriate in the workplace. **Self control** is also very important when there is something "trying" that has to be done. Then, you must concentrate even harder on not losing your composure. Losing self control usually makes matters worse because then you must apologize for your actions. Lack of self control could result in the termination of your employment.

Tact (delicate skill in saying or doing the right thing): **Tact** is a trait that may not be easy to acquire. Often, we respond to actions and statements *before* we think. Tact is being able to perceive a situation and knowing the right thing to say or do when dealing with people in a difficult situation. Tact is especially difficult and important when dealing with ill people. You must be very careful about what you say when responding to their questions.

This is the end of the discussion of highly desirable character traits. How do you rate?

PERSONALITY QUALITIES

In addition to the character traits discussed, there are other personality qualities that affect the way character traits are **perceived** by others. An individual could show initiative, dependability, honesty, and other traits, but if they are not "likeable," they will not get along well with their co-workers. These qualities might be more difficult to acquire since they seem to be connected to one's personality. Webster's 10th edition defines personality as "existence as a person; the assemblage of qualities, physical, mental, and moral, that set one apart from others." Let's look at some of these qualities that we like in people.

Friendly Attitude and Genuine Liking of People (real, concerned, caring viewpoint): A friendly **attitude** will be recognized by the persons with whom you deal in the office. You should know and use the names of your patients while carrying on conversations with them. Be friendly, but at the same time maintain a professional relationship. You can show a true concern for their welfare without becoming personally involved. For example, if an elderly person needs assistance but has no family support, you cannot take this on personally but you can contact community resources to arrange for the assistance. Good interpersonal relations require dealing with people so that your self-image and theirs remain positive and intact. Courtesy is never out of style. A simple "please" and "thank you" is appropriate with all ages.

Intelligence (ability to apply the mind effectively to any situation; clear thinking plus good judgment): **Intelligence** is not just a high IQ or a college degree, for neither of these are of value if the owner can't appropriately apply their knowledge to life situations. You can acquire knowledge from study and experience. There is no end to what you can learn. That information, effectively applied, is intelligence. Everything you learn affects you and, in turn, the people with whom you interact. Use every opportunity to expand your knowledge—not only of health care, but also of the world of information that is available, Figure 2–12. You will find that a willingness to learn advances your professional status. You will also find that your professional skills will improve with experience and new technology. Your knowledge can be expanded by observation, reading, and attending seminars. Physicians often sponsor attendance at workshops and educational seminars if you show an interest in learning.

Pleasant Personality (cheerful, agreeable personal qualities): A pleasant personality is tremendously important because of the continuous stream of persons with whom you will come into contact. Because of their illness, the situation will not always be the best, but if your contact with them is cheerful and pleasant, it will make their time in your office a little easier to bear. Your interaction with the physician and other team members will be much more enjoyable if you are pleasant. No one enjoys being around someone who is always complaining or is negative about everything. It has been said that success is 90% personality. Impressions about people are, at least initially, formed from the way we perceive their personality. A chance at success may not occur if the perception is negative.

Pleasant Voice (pleasing to hear): A voice has four characteristics: pitch, force, quality, and rate. The pitch of your voice refers to its highness or lowness. If you have a medium pitch, you are fortunate because it is considered the most pleasing to hear. If you are told your voice sounds high, consider exercises to lower its pitch. Record your voice and listen to it. You can also determine your pitch by using a piano. Sing "ah" to find the lowest note you can sing, then sing up the scale four whole notes. This will be your best speaking voice pitch. If you currently speak above it, practice reading aloud at the new note pitch. This will also allow you to develop variety in the range of your pitch. Without variation, your speech will be in a **monotone** which is unpleasant to hear. The force of your voice makes it possible for you to be heard. You generally need little force in office communications; in fact, you must guard against being overheard by patients. If you do find it necessary to increase the intensity of your voice, be careful it does not become irritating. The quality of your voice is reflected in the manner in which you pronounce vowels. Relaxation exercises will improve vocal quality. A good exercise for the jaw muscles is a yawn. The rate of your speech is determined by how long you hold sounds and by the pauses between words and phrases. Most of us speak too rapidly. Communication requires understanding and it is extremely hard to understand someone who runs their words together and who does not enunciate clearly. Again, you can improve your rate by listening to your recorded voice as you read aloud. With practice, you can adjust your rate and improve your communication skills. Practice is also needed to eliminate using "uh," "er," and "you know" when you speak. A simple pause, while you think of what to say, is much more pleasant for the listener.

Genuine Smile (real expression): A genuine smile is a welcome sight to anyone entering a physician's office. It conveys that you acknowledge them and are interested in being of service. You may be surprised by how many smiles you receive in return. Besides, it's hard to be unpleasant with someone who is smiling at you.

PERCEPTION AS A PROFESSIONAL

There are two other observations about you that speak very loudly, yet do not require a word to be spoken. Since you are a health care provider and consider yourself to be a professional, you are expected to "look the part."

Good Health (state of wellness): The patients and visitors coming into a physician's office gain the first impression of the practice from the medical assistant or receptionist who greets them. A neat, attractive person has a good psychological effect on everyone. To look your best, you must be in good health. This requires a routine of rest, well-balanced meals, exercise, and recreation. As a health care professional, you are perceived as an example. What message are you sending? If you need medical attention, you should see your personal physician without delay. No patient wants to receive medical attention from someone who appears unhealthy. Patients may resent, and rightly so, any exposure

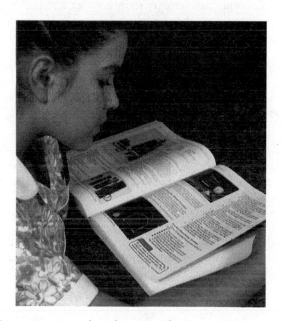

Figure 2–12 Take advantage of opportunities to learn.

to illness. Many people are in a rather fragile state of health. They come to the physician to get assistance with their own illness or injury; they do not need to "pick up" additional problems.

Personal Appearance (individual image; a look; visible): Your **appearance** says volumes about you. Neat, well-groomed professionals look self-confident, display pride in themselves, and give an impression of being capable of performing whatever duties need to be done, Figure 2–13. Not only does the patient feel the provider is competent, but the provider also feels good. We have all experienced days when we didn't feel good about the way we looked and that, in turn, affected our performance. In order to present yourself in the best possible light, you must adhere to some general guidelines for a professional appearance:

1. *Cleanliness* is the first essential for good grooming. Take a daily bath or shower. Use a deodorant or antiperspirant. Shampoo your hair at least two to three times a week, depending upon its oiliness. Brush and floss your teeth daily.
2. *Handcare* is critical. Take special care of your hands. Keep hand cream or lotion in convenient places to use after washing your hands. Since this is done frequently, hands tend to chap and crack which can allow organisms entry into your body—a risk you cannot afford. Also, keep your fingernails at a moderate length and use clear or light shades of polish if you wear a uniform.
3. *Hair* must be clean and away from your face. Long hair should be worn up or at least fastened back. It is not a good idea to have to keep pushing your hair out of the way while working with patients. You only add their organisms to your environment, and perhaps take them home with you. Patients may also be sensitive to "receiving" something from your hair when you touch them after arranging it.
4. *Uniforms* must be clean, fit well, and free from wrinkles. Uniform shoes should be kept clean with clean shoestrings. Hose are to be free of runners. It is a good idea to keep an extra clean uniform and pair of socks or hose at the office in case of accidents. Attention must also be given to undergarments worn beneath the uniform. Bright colors and patterns can usually be seen through the fabric. Underwear is best disguised if it closely matches your skin coloring because the contrast with your body is not as visible. Test different shades to see which looks the best.
5. *Jewelry,* except for a watch or wedding ring, is not appropriate with a uniform. Small earrings may be worn but still may get in the way when you use the telephone. Not only does jewelry look out of place, it is a great collector of microorganisms.
6. *Fragrances,* such as perfume, cologne, and aftershave lotions, may be offensive to some patients, especially if they are suffering from nausea. If you feel it necessary to wear something, use one with a light, clean smelling fragrance. Leave the heavy aromas for after work.
7. *Cosmetics* should be tasteful and skillfully applied. All major department stores have sales people who can help you select and learn to apply products that will enhance your appearance. Save bright eye shadows, false eyelashes, and vivid lipsticks for leisure times.
8. *Gum* chewing can be very unprofessional. A large piece interferes with speech and cracking gum is totally unacceptable. If you feel you need gum for a breath concern, use a breath mint or mouthwash instead.
9. *Posture* affects not only your appearance but also the amount of fatigue you experience. The ease at which you move around reflects your poise and confidence. To check your posture, back up to a wall, place your feet apart, straight down from your hips, and try to insert your hand through the space between your lower back and the wall. If you can, you need to improve your posture. Pull your stomach in, tuck under your buttocks, and try to place your spine against the wall. Your shoulders should be relaxed with your head held erect. This will probably feel very unnatural, but practice keeping your body straight and head erect when you walk and you will see how much better you look and feel.

A lot of different elements make up our personal characteristics and have a definite effect upon how we feel about ourselves and how others perceive us. This discussion should help you evaluate yourself and help you identify things you can do to improve your effectiveness when interacting with people.

Complete Chapter 2, Unit 2, in the workbook to help you meet the objectives at the beginning of this unit and therefore achieve competency of this subject matter.

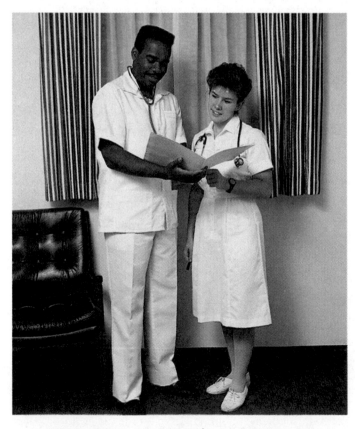

Figure 2–13 Present a professional appearance.

UNIT 3
Professionalism

■ OBJECTIVES

Upon completion of the unit, meet the following terminal performance objectives by verifying knowledge of the facts and principles presented through oral and written communication at a level deemed competent.

1. Discuss the origin of the medical assistant profession.
2. Describe the history and purpose of the American Association of Medical Assistants (AAMA) and the American Registry of Medical Assistants (ARMA).
3. Discuss the definition of medical assisting according to the AAMA and the ARMA.
4. Describe and discuss the AAMA logos: original and current.
5. Discuss the three levels of membership of AAMA and the value of same.
6. Define and discuss the meaning of professionalism.
7. Discuss the *Standards of Practice* set by the American Medical Technologists.
8. Discuss the purpose of continuing education and how to acquire it.
9. Identify the qualifications for and methods of acquiring medical assistant certification from AAMA, AAMT, and ARMA.
10. Describe methods for revalidation of medical assistant certification from AAMA, AAMT, and ARMA.
11. Discuss advantages of membership in one or more of the professional organizations contained in this unit.
12. List additional purposes of the AAMA and the ARMA besides membership.
13. Spell and define, using the glossary in the back of this text, all the words to know in this unit.

■ WORDS TO KNOW

accreditation	professionalism
autonomous	pro tem
certification	registry
competent	revalidation

HOW MEDICAL ASSISTING BEGAN

In *A Brief History of Medicine* in Chapter 1, you learned about the many pioneers in this field. These leaders in the practice of medicine obviously had the best interest of their patients in mind as they treated them as efficiently as they could with what little was available. The sick went to be treated without an appointment and they waited as long as necessary to be seen by the physician. Payment for medical care was a barter-type, often with food or whatever the patient or the family had of value. If one had no means of payment, the doctor treated the person anyway. No medical records were kept as they were not even thought to be necessary in those days. Since the physician was considered to be a valuable close family friend and was well respected by the entire community for his/her knowledge and life-saving skills, it was very rare for a lawsuit to be filed against the physician.

Since those days, times have changed dramatically in the practice of medicine. Accurate and comprehensive records are vital in managed care of patients. Documentation of every transaction between physician and patient is a must. The efficiently run medical practice requires absolute attention to every detail to protect the reputation of the physician and to make it possible to render the best care possible to the patient. Since medical school offers little or no background for physicians in the realm of managing the "business of medicine," s/he must entrust this responsibility to a competent individual. Even today, a common term "my office nurse" is often used by physicians in reference to a member of their office personnel. This can often be misleading as there may in actuality be no nurses employed in the facility. Using this term casually is not a wise practice because it is deceiving to the public. The art and skill of nursing is for the most part aimed toward the critically ill and those patients requiring bedside care. Obviously, in an ambulatory setting such as an office or clinic, and in some departments in medical centers and hospitals, medical assistants can be and are employed in a wide variety of positions. This person, who works under the supervision of the physician, performs a wide variety of administrative and clinical duties and has given rise to the title of medical assistant. During this evolvement in the practice of medicine, physicians have realized the value of both administrative and clinical medical assistants to run their offices and assist in many other roles with appropriate instruction and evaluation. Unit 1 of this chapter discusses the many roles and responsibilities that await the medical assistant in the wealth of opportunity in the medical field.

HISTORY OF PROFESSIONAL ORGANIZATIONS
The American Association of Medical Assistants

In 1955, medical assistants from fifteen states met in Kansas City, Kansas, and adopted the name American Association of Medical Assistants (AAMA). The representatives elected **pro tem** officers and made plans for an organizational meeting to be held the following year. In October of 1956, physicians and advisors of the American Medical Association (AMA) met with 250 members of medical assistant societies from sixteen states. At this meeting, the AAMA was officially founded with advice, assistance, and moral support from the AMA. The founder and first national president of the American Association of Medical Assistants was Maxine Williams, Figure 2–14. The primary purpose of the AAMA was to raise the standards of the medical assistant to a professional level. Physicians realized then, as they do now, that health care professionals were needed to assist them in the multitude of office duties for which nurses had not been

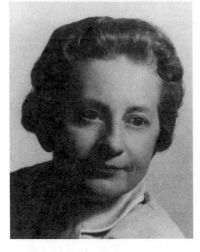

Figure 2–14 Maxine Williams, founder and first national president of the AAMA.

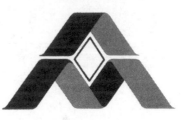

Figure 2–16 Current logo of the AAMA.

trained. They also needed help in the physician/patient relationship. Another concern was that of instilling in young people a desire to carry the profession of medical assisting into the future. The *Maxine Williams Scholarship Fund* was established to award several $500 scholarships annually to students who were seriously interested in pursuing a career as a medical assistant. NOTE: The scholarships are awarded on the basis of interest, need, and aptitude. Applications are available from the AAMA executive office. Applicants must have the completed form postmarked no later than May 1 of the year in which the scholarship will be used.

In 1958, a national emblem was selected for use on AAMA stationery and official publications, Figure 2–15. The current logo for AAMA, introduced in 1978, is shown in Figure 2–16. The American Association of Medical Assistants received word from the United States Department of Health, Education, and Welfare that medical assisting had been formally recognized as an allied health profession and that its educational programs were eligible for federal funding by the Bureau of Health Manpower.

The AAMA Board of Trustees approved the current definition of medical assisting in February of 1991: "Medical Assisting is a multi-skilled allied health profession whose practitioners work primarily in ambulatory settings, such as medical offices or clinics. Medical assistants function as members of the healthcare delivery team and perform administrative and clinical procedures."

The American Registry of Medical Assistants (ARMA)

The American Registry of Medical Assistants was established in 1972. This organization was also instituted to provide a means of continuing education to its members and to promote the professional recognition of medical assistants. The ARMA is operated under the direction of the American Medical Technologists. A national board of directors is elected to conduct the business of the organization such as educational programs, legal concerns, certification, and other national issues. The ARMA maintains a placement service conducted without fee for qualified members. Members are appointed by the national board to state and local council positions. These members of leadership status work directly with the needs of the membership. Members receive a professional publication, *AMT Events,* which provides timely information regarding educational seminars, the annual meeting held in late June, test sites for certification, and home education programs for continuing education units. The certification examination for registry is given twice each year. Applicants must be a graduate of an Accrediting Bureau of Health Education School (ABHES) program and generally sit for the exam at their school with a monitor present who has been approved by the ARMA. Successfully passing this exam awards the applicant with the title "Registered Medical Assistant" and the abbreviation of RMA after their signature. This title signifies that the person is a qualified medical assistant.

Registered Medical Assistants (RMA)

The purpose of the RMA organization is to advance the standards and profession of medical assisting and to promote educational and social advantages for its members. Continuing education is necessary for the medical assistant of today, as this is one of the fastest growing and changing career fields. Through American Medical Technologists Institute for Education (AMTIE) a five year revalidation process has been developed with the first five year cycle having been completed in 1987.

Currently, the definition of a medical assistant, as approved by the Board of Directors of the ARMA, is "A medical assistant is an integral member of the health care delivery team, qualified by education and experience to work

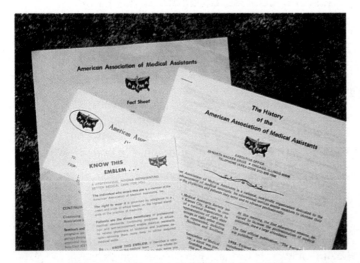

Figure 2–15 Original logo of the AAMA.

in the administrative office, the examining room and the physician's office laboratory. The medical assistant, also a liaison between doctor and patient, is of vital importance to the success of the medical practice."

American Association for Medical Transcription (AAMT)

One who interprets and transcribes patient information from oral to printed form by typing or with the use of a word processor is known as a medical transcriptionist. These professionals are medical language specialists who must possess excellent skills in the areas of listening, English grammar and punctuation, spelling, and transcription technology. Additionally, the medical transcriptionist must have a solid foundation in anatomy and physiology, disease processes, medicolegal and ethical areas, and professionalism.

The AAMT is the professional organization for the advancement of medical transcription and for the education and development of medical transcriptionists as medical language specialists. This organization was incorporated in 1978 in Modesto, California. The AAMT publishes a bimonthly journal to inform association leaders of important relevant information. State or regional component associations offer members delegate representation at the national convention, and local chapters offer educational opportunities. Voluntary certification by examination is offered by the AAMT. This certification is valid for three years. The certified medical transcriptionist must achieve 30 continuing education credits (CEU) in each three year cycle for recertification or successful reexamination. The AAMT offers a national convention, continuing education programs, workshops, and seminars for members. This organization also publishes materials specifically for those in the medical transcription profession.

Professional Secretaries International® (PSI)®

This organization offers the administrative medical assistant many benefits. PSI® promotes competence and recognition of the professional and represents the interests and welfare of persons working in and preparing for secretarial and related positions. Certified Professional Secretary® (CPS)® is the registered service mark for the rating that has become the recognized standard of measurement of secretarial proficiency. To attain the CPS® rating, a secretary must meet certain education and work experience requirements, and pass the two-day examination. The six-part examination is administered in May and November by the Institute for Certifying Secretaries, a department of PSI®. The CPS® examination has six parts: behavioral science in business, business law, economics and management, accounting, office administration and communication, and office technology.

PROFESSIONALISM

On your journey of study to become a medical assistant you must also become aware of just what a professional is and

what that means to you. One who is trained and skilled in the methods of the profession is the coined definition which can apply to *any* profession regarding technical and ethical standards of the particular skill area. In an article in the January/February 1987 issue of AAMA's *The Professional Medical Assistant* magazine, Barbara Smith defined **professionalism** as "a state of mind. It is a particular blend of self-esteem, self-confidence, enjoyment of life, respect for the feelings of others, as well as specific knowledge and skills."

The American Medical Technologists outline the requirements of professionalism in their *Standards of Practice*, Figure 2–17. All members and RMAs, as well as every member of the health care delivery team, are urged to follow these standards.

True professionalism goes well beyond a mere definition. Standards of conduct are certainly a noble consideration, especially in this revered field of medicine. The physician and the field of medicine in general have always been highly respected and admired by society. And, rightfully so, those who seek the services of professionals in the health care field have expectations of being treated with respect and dignity. It takes a certain type of person to work with the sick and injured day in and day out. You have been introduced to the personal characteristics that health care professionals should possess. Those necessary attributes are used perpetually in patient care. It is all part of being a professional. In the AAMA Role Delineation Study, there are nine areas of competency under Professionalism which are identified as follows:

- Project a professional manner and image
- Adhere to ethical principles
- Demonstrate initiative and responsibility
- Work as a team member
- Manage time effectively
- Prioritize and perform multiple tasks
- Adapt to change
- Promote the CMA credential
- Enhance skills through continuing education

Professionalism is a complex issue. It is your personal standard of conduct, morality, and ethics. It is having the will to excel in your vocational aspirations and to go above and beyond what is expected of you. Professionalism is seen in those who aspire to become certified and **revalidate** when the time comes. The professional is one who seeks out the ways and means to grow personally as well as professionally and encourages others to do the same. The leaders of these organizations, the pacesetters of the AAMA and the ARMA, have paved the way of the professional medical assistant. You are learning a fine tradition of the example they set for the future of the profession of medical assisting and in the establishment of the AAMA and ARMA continuing education programs. You have a great opportunity because of the efforts of a few medical assistants who saw the vision of the profession and had the desire to do something about it. That is what professionalism is all about. They did something above and beyond their 9 to 5 job.

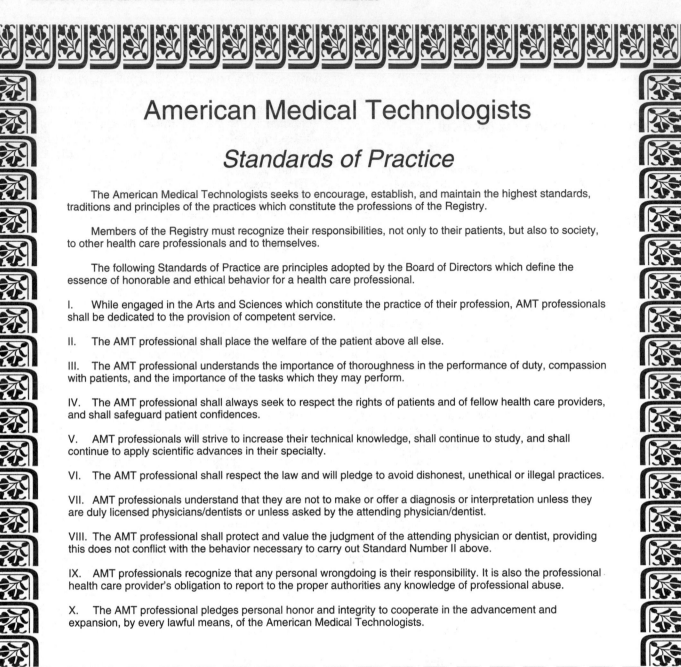

American Medical Technologists

Standards of Practice

The American Medical Technologists seeks to encourage, establish, and maintain the highest standards, traditions and principles of the practices which constitute the professions of the Registry.

Members of the Registry must recognize their responsibilities, not only to their patients, but also to society, to other health care professionals and to themselves.

The following Standards of Practice are principles adopted by the Board of Directors which define the essence of honorable and ethical behavior for a health care professional.

I.   While engaged in the Arts and Sciences which constitute the practice of their profession, AMT professionals shall be dedicated to the provision of competent service.

II.   The AMT professional shall place the welfare of the patient above all else.

III.   The AMT professional understands the importance of thoroughness in the performance of duty, compassion with patients, and the importance of the tasks which they may perform.

IV.   The AMT professional shall always seek to respect the rights of patients and of fellow health care providers, and shall safeguard patient confidences.

V.   AMT professionals will strive to increase their technical knowledge, shall continue to study, and shall continue to apply scientific advances in their specialty.

VI.   The AMT professional shall respect the law and will pledge to avoid dishonest, unethical or illegal practices.

VII.   AMT professionals understand that they are not to make or offer a diagnosis or interpretation unless they are duly licensed physicians/dentists or unless asked by the attending physician/dentist.

VIII. The AMT professional shall protect and value the judgment of the attending physician or dentist, providing this does not conflict with the behavior necessary to carry out Standard Number II above.

IX.   AMT professionals recognize that any personal wrongdoing is their responsibility. It is also the professional health care provider's obligation to report to the proper authorities any knowledge of professional abuse.

X.   The AMT professional pledges personal honor and integrity to cooperate in the advancement and expansion, by every lawful means, of the American Medical Technologists.

Figure 2–17 AMT *Standards of Practice.*

The seeds they planted have taken root and bloomed into a formally recognized profession.

The AAMA and ARMA Examinations

Furthermore, both the AAMA and the ARMA certification/recertification examinations also cover content on professionalism. Areas from which questions may be derived are:

- professional organization
- accepting responsibility for own actions
- performing within ethical boundaries
- AMA, AAMA and ARMA code of ethics
- patients' rights
- current issues in bioethics
- maintaining confidentiality
- releasing patient information
- intentional tort
- invasion of privacy
- slander and libel
- promote competent patient care
- working as a team member to achieve goals
- team member responsibility

Keeping all these points in mind as you learn and practice your skills will help you toward your goal of becoming a concerned and **competent** medical assistant.

COMPETENCY OF PROGRAMS

The AAMA has established an **accreditation** process for programs that prepare individuals to become medical assistants. Over 221 medical assisting programs at the postsecondary level in various schools and colleges nationwide have been accredited by the Committee on Allied Health Education and Accreditation (CAHEA), an **autonomous** committee of the AMA and an accrediting body sanctioned by the United States Department of Education.

All schools and colleges that offer accredited medical assisting programs must follow the AAMA's Occupational Analysis/Role Delineation Study outcomes in designing their curriculum. These statements of competence are an integral part of the document called *The Standards and Guidelines of an Accredited Educational Program for the Medical Assistant.* It is this document that specifies the requirements an educational facility must meet in order to be accredited by the AMA/AAMA review boards. *The Standards and Guidelines* are the minimum standards for accrediting educational programs that prepare individuals to enter into an allied health profession recognized by the American Medical Association. It is this level of quality that qualifies medical assisting as a profession.

BECOMING CERTIFIED

At the 1995 AAMA Convention in San Antonio, Texas, the certification board voted that as of February 1, 1998, only those individuals who have successfully completed an accredited medical assistant program may sit for the national certification examination. The AAMA certification exam is designed to evaluate entry-level competency in medical assisting. Administrative and clinical skills, anatomy and physiology, human relations, medical terminology, professionalism, communication, and medicolegal are included in this exam. It is offered twice each year at over 100 test centers nationwide. The National Board of Medical Examiners serves as an educational test consultant and works with the AAMA in preparing the examination. To be eligible for the certification exam you must be a graduate of a CAHEA accredited medical assistant program.

Beginning in 1998, certified medical assistants (CMA) must recertify every five years to demonstrate current knowledge of administrative, clinical, and general medical information. A CMA remains current through December 31 of the fifth year following certification or recertification. Recertification reinforces the validity of the CMA credentials and helps maintain continued acceptance by physicians, patients, and other health care professionals. This requirement may be met in one of two ways:

1. By earning sixty recertification points through continuing education courses or academic or other formal credit that has relevancy to medical assisting, with the points dis-

tributed equally among the three areas covered in the examination.
2. By taking the certification examination.

Those who sit for the exam and are successful in achieving a passing score are entitled to the CMA designation following their names. Figure 2–18 shows a photo of the official certified medical assistant pin from AAMA. NOTE: There are also attractive pins sold in uniform shops around the country that say "medical assistant" or "certified medical assistant" as accessory items. Even though they inform the onlooker that one is a medical assistant, they are not authorized by AAMA and do not reflect the wearer's credibility regarding AAMA certification.

In addition to sitting for the national certification exam after completing studies in medical assisting, you should carefully consider the many benefits of joining AAMA. An active member must be a certified medical assistant or an individual who was an active member on December 31, 1987 and who maintains continuous active membership. An associate member is one who is not eligible for another category of membership but who is interested in the profession of medical assisting. Those enrolled in a medical assistant program may become student members at a reasonable cost. Student membership may be retained for dues one year after graduation if active or associate membership is not chosen.

One of the best and most appropriate ways for you to continue your education is through AAMA tri-level membership (local, state, and national levels). Hundreds of educational programs offering continuing education units (CEU) are conducted throughout the year. Physician advisors are among the professionals who speak at the monthly meetings and other educational activities. Many physician employers and/or office managers offer financial assistance to employees to encourage attendance and participation in seminars, workshops, and conventions where important current topics are shared. Members are entitled to special rates for all educational pursuits offered by the organization as well as many other financial advantages (such as group rates). Soon after joining, members automatically begin receiving AAMA's bimonthly journal, *The Professional Medical Assistant,* which is devoted to educational articles

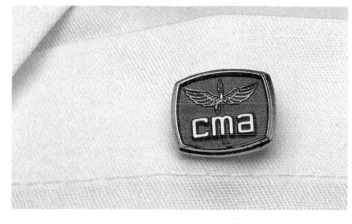

Figure 2–18 CMA pin.

that are written by experts in allied health and related fields. This magazine contains current medical research reports, the latest state and federal health legislative news, education program announcements, and articles offering CEU credit. Most organizations at the state level keep members informed with a news publication containing educational articles as well as dates for programs, meetings, and other activities relevant to the medical assistant. Many local chapters send notices to their members about meeting times and other important information.

Both the AAMA and the ARMA additionally provide guided study programs at a reasonable cost in a wide range of areas such as Human Relations, Medical Law, and Communication Skills, among others. These professionally designed courses allow medical assistants to learn and study at home at their own rate of speed. CEUs are awarded for the successful completion of the examinations accompanying each home study course.

Employers are impressed with applicants who take the initiative in belonging to one or more of such organizations. This shows your interest not only in self-improvement, but also shows your initiative in improving your skills for the welfare of the patients you serve. Most employers encourage their employees to attend seminars, workshops, and courses that offer education that relates to the medical office practice, both clinical and administrative. Some employers even pay for the costs of membership and for educational program fees. Well informed personnel provide competent care to patients and assist in quality management of administrative tasks.

Additional information may be obtained by writing to or calling the professional organizations listed at the end of this unit.

Complete Chapter 1, Unit 2 in the workbook to help you meet the objectives at the beginning of this unit and therefore achieve competency of this subject matter.

REFERENCES

American Association of Medical Assistants. *AAMA Role Delineation Study: Occupational Analysis of the Medical Assisting Profession.*

American Association of Medical Assistants. *Educational Components of the DACUM Occupational Analysis.* 1990.

American Association of Medical Assistants. *Medical Assisting Programs. Pride, Partnership, Professionalism.* 1989.

American Association of Medical Assistants. *Certified Medical Assistants. Healthcare's Most Versatile Professionals.* 1989.

American Medical Association.

American Vocational Association, Vocational Education Journal. *The Health Occupations Boom.* September 1995.

Encyclopedia of Medicine. Editor: Charles B. Clayman, M.D. New York: Random House, 1989.

Peterson, Arlin V., and Allen, Roy C. *The Humanistic Medical Assistant: A Book on Human Relations.* AAMA, 1978.

U.S. Department of Labor. Occupational Employment Statistics, Washington, DC.

Webster's Collegiate Dictionary (10th ed.) Springfield: Merriam-Webster.

PROFESSIONAL ORGANIZATIONS

American Association of Medical Assistants, 20 North Wacker Drive, Suite 1575, Chicago, IL 60606
(312) 899-1500

American Association for Medical Transcription, 3460 Oakdale Road, Suite M, P.O. Box 576187, Modesto, CA 95357-6187
(209) 551-0883

Professional Secretaries International®, P.O. Box 20404, Kansas City, MO 64195-0404
(816) 891-6600

Registered Medical Assistant of AMT, 710 Higgins Road, Park Ridge, IL 60068-5765
(847) 823-5169

3

Medical Ethics and Liability

During the past twenty years the numbers of patients bringing lawsuits against physicians have increased dramatically. Medical liability insurance rates have increased so much that physicians in some areas are practicing without liability insurance, although not all states permit this. Laws may vary in different states, but ethical standards are the same in every state. **Ethics** deals with moral choices and rules of conduct. Both the American Medical Association and the American Association of Medical Assistants have a code of ethics.

UNIT 1
Ethical and Legal Responsibilities
UNIT 2
Professional Liability

UNIT 1

Ethical and Legal Responsibilities

OBJECTIVES

Upon completion of the unit, meet the following terminal performance objectives by verifying knowledge of the facts and principles presented through oral and written communication at a level deemed competent.

1. List licensure requirements for physicians.
2. Describe methods of licensure.
3. List exceptions to the need for licensure.
4. Define the components of public and private law.
5. Recognize the differences between ethics and law.
6. Identify areas of medical ethics of particular concern to medical assistants.
7. List the five primary elements of the American Association of Medical Assistants Code of Ethics.
8. Describe the reason diagnostic related groups are causing an ethical issue for physicians.
9. Name one societal group being denied health insurance.
10. List ethical considerations surrounding the life of a fetus.
11. List and define the three categories of medical transplants.
12. Name the most common transplant.
13. Describe a living will.

14. Name four examples of tort law.
15. Define the term *emancipated minor* and give examples.
16. Describe the three parts of the physician-patient contract.
17. Define the terms *implied consent* and *express consent*.
18. Prepare common consent forms used in medical offices.
19. Define the term *privileged communication*.
20. List instances of legally required disclosure.
21. Explain the terms *defamation of character, libel,* and *slander.*
22. Describe the conditions for revocation or suspension of a medical license.
23. Spell and define, using the glossary at the back of the text, all the words to know in this unit.

WORDS TO KNOW

agent	ethics
artificial insemination	explicit
assault	fraudulent
battery	genetic
biennially	intimidation
civil law	*non compos mentis*
coercion	peer review
confidentiality	reciprocity
criminal law	revoke
defamation	senility
emancipated minor	statutes
enact	surrogate
endorsement	tort

Our founding fathers saw a need for regulation of the practice of medicine and in colonial days medical practice acts were in effect for the protection of citizens. These acts were gradually repealed because it was believed the Constitution gave everyone the right to practice medicine. This resulted in a period of time in the nineteenth century when quackery was common. After a Supreme Court decision in 1899 upheld a state's right to establish qualifications for people wishing to practice medicine, all states soon had once again established medical practice acts. Most state statutes define two basic elements that constitute the practice of medicine. One is diagnosis and the other is the prescribing of treatment. Only a licensed physician can engage in the diagnosis and prescribing of treatment for the physical condition of human beings. In general terms, medical practice acts define the practice of medicine and establish requirements for licensure and grounds for suspending or revoking a license.

LICENSURE REQUIREMENTS

Licensure requirements are established by each state. A doctor is usually required to:

- be of legal age
- be of good moral character
- have graduated from an approved medical school
- have completed an approved residency program or its equivalent
- be a resident of the state
- have passed the oral and written examinations administered by the National Board of Medical Examiners of the state

Physicians who have all the necessary requirements for licensure may also be licensed by reciprocity or endorsement. A physician who has been licensed in one state and wishes to move to another state may be granted a license by reciprocity if it is determined that the original licensure requirements are equal to the requirements in the new state. Many physicians take the test administered by the National Board of Medical Examiners at the same time they take the first state test. The high standards of the national board make it possible to obtain a state license by endorsement when the national board examinations have been successfully passed.

Physicians are required to renew their license annually or biennially. You should be sure the physician has a record of all continuing education units (CEUs) earned since the previous renewal as this is a requirement in many states. Physicians earn CEUs by attending seminars and scientific meetings as well as university courses. The renewal notice will notify the physician of the number of CEUs necessary to renew the license.

There are some exceptions to the rule requiring a current state license to practice medicine. Any physician is free to administer first aid outside the state of residence.

Physicians in military service must be licensed to practice medicine in their home states. They do not need to be licensed in the state where they are stationed as long as they practice only on the military base.

The State Board of Medical Examiners provides procedures for revocation or suspension of licensure. In some states the board has the power to revoke a license and in other states a special review committee has this authority.

A physician may lose the license to practice medicine if convicted of a crime such as murder, rape, violation of narcotic laws, or income tax evasion. A medical license may be revoked for unprofessional conduct. The most usual offenses in this category are betrayal of patient-physician confidence, excessive use of drugs and alcohol, and inappropriate sexual conduct.

A license may be revoked because of proven fraud in the application for a license. In some cases fraudulent diplomas are used. Fraud in the filing of claims for services that were not rendered and fraud in the use of unproven treatments are also grounds for revocation of a license.

Physicians who are found to be incompetent to practice because of senility or mental incapacity may have their license revoked.

ETHICAL CONSIDERATIONS

Whereas laws concern matters enforced through the court system, ethics deals with what is morally right and wrong. The ethical standards established by a profession are administered by peer review, and violation of the standards may result in suspension of membership. The American Medical Association Principles Code of Medical Ethics was revised in 1980 and is reprinted here so that you can see what is expected of a physician.

Physician's Code

Preamble: The medical profession has long subscribed to a body of ethical statements developed primarily for the benefit of the patient. As a member of this profession, a physician must recognize responsibility not only to patients, but also to society, to other health professionals, and to self. The following Principles adopted by the American Medical Association are not laws, but standards of conduct which define the essentials of honorable behavior for the physician.

  I. A physician shall be dedicated to providing competent medical service with compassion and respect for human dignity.
  II. A physician shall deal honestly with patients and colleagues, and strive to expose those physicians deficient in character or competence, or who engage in fraud or deception.
 III. A physician shall respect the law and also recognize a responsibility to seek changes in those requirements which are contrary to the best interests of the patient.
 IV. A physician shall respect the rights of patients, of colleagues, and of other health professionals, and shall safeguard patient confidence within the constraints of the law.
  V. A physician shall continue to study, apply, and advance scientific knowledge, make relevant information available to patients, colleagues, and the public, obtain consultation, and use the talents of other health professionals when indicated.
 VI. A physician shall, in the provision of appropriate patient care, except in emergencies, be free to choose

whom to serve, with whom to associate, and the environment in which to provide medical services.

VII. A physician shall recognize a responsibility to participate in activities contributing to an improved community.

(Used with permission of the American Medical Association. From the *American Medical Association Principles of Medical Ethics.* Adopted by the AMA House of Delegates, July 1980.)

Medical Assistant's Code

As an agent of the physician, you too are governed by ethical standards. It must be remembered that the primary objective of the practice of medicine is the welfare of the patient, not the making of a profit. Some offices now notify patients of interest charges on overdue accounts in a brochure introducing the patient to the office practice. The notice of possible interest charge is also included on all billing statements. Some physicians charge for missed appointments and preparing more than one insurance form.

The physician must release patient information when the patient authorizes the release or if the release is required by law. State laws vary regarding release of information. Information that must be reported includes:

- Births and deaths
- Cases of violence such as gunshot wounds, knifings, and poisonings
- Sexually transmitted diseases
- Suspected cases of child abuse
- Cases of contagious, infectious, or communicable diseases

Medical assistants should check with local authorities for the procedures to be followed in making these reports. They need to be aware also of other required local reports. When a physician moves or retires it is important that the original records be kept until the period for filing of liability suits has expired. A copy of the records is provided to a new physician.

The American Association of Medical Assistants Code of Ethics is in many respects similar to that of the American Medical Association.

You will often find it necessary to make decisions based on the professional nature of your employment. Patients can be extremely insistent at times, but you must be firm in carrying out the expectations of your employer and your profession. A patient may, for instance, demand that you call in a prescription for medication when the physician is not immediately available. You have to stand your ground and say that only the physician can give you the orders to do this. You then carefully record on the chart the request of the patient and how it was taken care of. *Never put yourself in the position of practicing medicine.*

The Federal Drug Administration has established five categories, or "schedules," which classify chemical substances with specific regulations as to their use. The states also have laws that further define the use of drugs. It is important for the medical assistant to understand that only the physician can legally prescribe medications. The medical assistant must understand that certain medications cannot be refilled and that restrictions limit the number of times some medications can be refilled. Some drugs require written prescription only to be filled, while others can be called in by telephone.

The United States Department of Justice Drug Enforcement Administration publishes a physician's manual that gives all the information necessary for office personnel to understand the provisions of the Controlled Substances Act. This booklet is free and is furnished on request.

The Drug Enforcement Administration also publishes a *Pharmacist's Manual,* which lists seven recommendations for physicians about the care and security of prescription pads. These will help reduce the number of forged prescription orders:

1. Treat prescription pads like a personal checkbook.
2. Maintain adequate security for prescription pads.
3. Stock only a minimum number of prescription pads.

**CODE OF ETHICS
of the American Association of Medical Assistants**

The Code of Ethics of AAMA shall set forth principles of ethical and moral conduct as they relate to the medical profession and the particular practice of medical assisting.

Members of AAMA dedicated to the conscientious pursuit of their profession, and thus desiring to merit the high regard of the entire medical profession and the respect of the general public which they do serve, do pledge themselves to strive always to:

A. render service with full respect for the dignity of humanity;
B. respect confidential information obtained through employment unless legally authorized or required by responsible performance of duty to divulge such information;
C. uphold the honor and high principles of the profession and accept its disciplines;
D. seek to continually improve the knowledge and skills of medical assistants for the benefit of patients and professional colleagues;
E. participate in additional service activities aimed toward improving the health and well-being of the community.

MEDICAL ASSISTANT'S CREED

The creed of the American Association of Medical Assistants reads as follows:

I believe in the principles and purposes of the profession.
I endeavor to be more effective.
I aspire to render greater service.
I protect the confidence entrusted to me.
I am dedicated to the care and well-being of all patients.
I am loyal to my physician-employer.
I am true to the ethics of my profession.
I am strengthened by compassion, courage, and faith.

(Copyright by the American Association of Medical Assistants, Inc. Used with permission.)

4. Keep prescription pads in your possession when you are actively using them.
5. Do not leave prescription pads unattended. When not in use, place them in a locked desk or cabinet.
6. Store surplus prescription pads in a locked drawer or in a safe, appropriate place.
7. Report any prescription pad theft to local police and pharmacies as well as to the State Board of Pharmacy.

In the practice of medicine it can be difficult to distinguish between legal and ethical issues. The trend in the United States is to demand good health care as a right for everyone. However, not all citizens are willing to finance such a program. The present use of diagnostic related groups (DRGs) in determining the payment hospitals will receive for Medicare patients raises both ethical and legal questions. The problem with the system arises when patients may be discharged too early simply because the hospital will not be paid for more than the DRG-allowed number of days. The physician knows the legal responsibility is to the well-being of the patient, but the hospital must have money to stay in business. The physician wants to stay in good standing with the hospital. In a recent decision in California (Wickline versus State of California), a physician was held liable for releasing a patient too early. In fact, the physician had failed to protest the third party's decision to shorten the patient's recommended hospital stay. In this case, the third party payer was a California Medicare agency called Medi Cal.

Insurance companies are presenting more ethical questions to medical care providers when they refuse insurance to individuals who have acquired immune deficiency syndrome (AIDS), human immunodeficiency virus (HIV), and the AIDS-related complex (ARC).

Many ethical considerations surround the life of a fetus, an infant's birth, and the newborn. New technologies allow us to have more control over birth by detecting *in utero* abnormalities. The improved techniques of **artificial insemination** bring before the court system the problems associated with **surrogate** motherhood and paternal responsibility. Many advances have been made in the use of fetal tissue in transplants. Our society must study the ethical and emotional considerations of ending a pregnancy if a serious **genetic** deficiency is found before birth or allowing the infant to be born handicapped. We seem to have more questions than answers at the present time.

The use of transplants has added another series of ethical problems. Medical transplants are divided into three categories:

- Autograft transplantation of a person's own tissue (can also be used to describe transplant between identical twins)
- Homograft transplantation of tissue from one person to another
- Heterograft transplantation of animal tissue to humans

The blood transfusion is the most common transplant. Nearly all the major organs of the body may be transplanted, and research continues to improve these possibilities.

THE UNIFORM ANATOMICAL GIFT ACT

The Uniform Anatomical Gift Act was passed in 1968. By 1978 it was reported that all fifty states had established some system of organ and tissue donor identification once an individual died. Any person of sound mind and legal age may give any part of the body after death for research or transplant. The family may make this decision for the donor if the donor has not done so while living. The time of death must be determined by a physician who will not be involved in the transplant in any way. No money can be exchanged for making an anatomical donation. Many states allow residents to mark and sign a donor card on the back of the driver's license.

Different ethical problems affect the use of organs from living donors. As the technology of transplantation becomes more readily available, the demand for organs will grow. Human organs should never be sold for profit, but our western ethics are not always followed worldwide. In a book titled *Law, Liability, and Ethics for Medical Office Personnel,* Myrtle Flight discusses the medical community's concern over the sale of human organs for transplant. One source has estimated that by the year 2000, most of the poor in India will learn to survive with only one kidney as the result of the common practice of selling kidneys to wealthy foreigners.

LIVING WILL

The health care team will provide a larger percentage of care to geriatric patients as the quality of care extends our life expectancy. It is important that everyone in the office listen to elderly patients and allow them to make decisions regarding a living will, Figure 3–1, page 45. A majority of the states now have laws that define policies on withholding life-sustaining procedures from hopelessly ill patients. The will is signed when the patient is competent and must be witnessed by two individuals. The effect of this will is to protect the wishes of the patient who may become incompetent and thus unable to make rational decisions. The patient and all family members should discuss these issues while the patient is still rational and can fully comprehend the implications. A chosen family member should then be made aware of the responsibility of carrying out the patient's wishes as it becomes necessary. Copies of the document should be filed with the family, the primary physician, and the family's attorney. The family of the patient and the physician should receive a copy of the document.

Choice in Dying, Inc. now stresses the importance of also completing a Durable Power of Attorney for Health Care, authorized by either your state's statute or some other legal authority. This allows you to appoint another person (known as your **agent**) to make health care decisions for you if at any time you become unable to make them yourself. It is strongly advised that an individual appoint an agent, assuming there is someone who can be trusted to make the decisions you would make if you could, and who is willing to act for you in this way. The appointed proxy (agent) must be aware of your wishes and understand the complete document before giving consent to carry out the agreement. It may be helpful

THE FOLLOWING IS AN EXAMPLE OF A LIVING WILL FOR THE STATE OF FLORIDA. PLEASE CONTACT CHOICE IN DYING AT (212) 366-5540 TO RECEIVE A COPY OF APPROPRIATE ADVANCE DIRECTIVES FOR YOUR STATE.

FLORIDA LIVING WILL

INSTRUCTIONS

PRINT THE DATE

Declaration made this _____ day of _____, 19_____.

PRINT YOUR NAME

I, _____, willfully and voluntarily make known my desire that my dying not be artificially prolonged under the circumstances set forth below, and I do hereby declare:

If at any time I have a terminal condition and if my attending or treating physician and another consulting physician have determined that there is no medical probability of my recovery from such condition, I direct that life-prolonging procedures be withheld or withdrawn when the application of such procedures would serve only to prolong artificially the process of dying, and that I be permitted to die naturally with only the administration of medication or the performance of any medical procedure deemed necessary to provide me with comfort care or to alleviate pain.

It is my intention that this declaration be honored by my family and physician as the final expression of my legal right to refuse medical or surgical treatment and to accept the consequences for such refusal.

In the event that I have been determined to be unable to provide express and informed consent regarding the withholding, withdrawal, or continuation of life-prolonging procedures, I wish to designate, as my surrogate to carry out the provisions of this declaration:

PRINT THE NAME, HOME ADDRESS AND TELEPHONE NUMBER OF YOUR SURROGATE

Name: _____

Address: _____

_____ Zip Code: _____

Phone: _____

© 1995
CHOICE IN DYING, INC.

FLORIDA LIVING WILL — PAGE 2 OF 2

PRINT NAME, HOME ADDRESS AND TELEPHONE NUMBER OF YOUR ALTERNATE SURROGATE

I wish to designate the following person as my alternate surrogate, to carry out the provisions of this declaration should my surrogate be unwilling or unable to act on my behalf:

Name: _____

Address: _____

_____ Zip Code: _____

Phone: _____

ADD PERSONAL INSTRUCTIONS (IF ANY)

Additional instructions (optional):

I understand the full import of this declaration, and I am emotionally and mentally competent to make this declaration.

SIGN THE DOCUMENT

Signed: _____

WITNESSING PROCEDURE

Witness 1:

Signed: _____

Address: _____

TWO WITNESSES MUST SIGN AND PRINT THEIR ADDRESSES

Witness 2:

Signed: _____

Address: _____

© 1995
CHOICE IN DYING, INC.

Courtesy of Choice In Dying
200 Varick Street, New York, NY 10014 1-800-989-WILL
9/95

Figure 3–1 Sample living will form (Reprinted by permission of Choice In Dying, 200 Varick Street, New York, NY 10014, Phone 212-366-5540).

---

to record the wishes of a living will and power of attorney on a video tape so there could be no doubt the patient made the statements regarding care.

A medical "Miranda warning" law approved by Congress and signed by President Bush gives patients legal options for refusing or accepting treatment if they are incapacitated. The law, which took effect in November 1991, applies to hospitals, hospices, nursing homes, health maintenance organizations (HMOs) and other health care facilities that receive money from Medicare and Medicaid programs. Under the law, patients must receive written information explaining their right-to-die options according to their state laws. The law stipulates that hospitals and other providers must note on medical records whether patients have legal directives on treatment. Providers also must have procedures to ensure they comply with a patient's wishes.

Every member of the medical care team should be current in Cardiopulmonary Resuscitation (CPR) certification. An ethical question arises when the elderly or terminally ill patient does not wish to receive CPR in the event of a cardiopulmonary arrest. The courts have held that individuals have the right to make decisions that affect their own deaths.

LEGAL CONSIDERATIONS

In the United States the laws are divided into the categories of public law and private law. The various branches of public law include **criminal law**, constitutional law, administrative law, and international law. Criminal law deals with offenses against all citizens. The practice of medicine without a license is an offense under the criminal law. Constitutional law defines the powers of the government and the rights of its citizens. Each state has a constitution which defines its powers over matters not covered by the federal government, which are spelled out in the United States Constitution. Administrative law is concerned with the powers of government agencies. International law is concerned with agreements and treaties between countries.

The practice of medicine is primarily affected by private law or **civil law**, specifically by contract law and torts law. The patient-physician relationship is considered a contractual one. A **tort** is defined as any of a number of actions done by one person or group of persons that cause injury to another. Violations of tort law may be intentional or negligent. Negligence is an act or failure to act as a reasonably prudent physician under the same or similar circumstances that directly or proximately causes injury to a patient. The negligent causing of an injury, when committed by a physician in the course of professional duties, is commonly referred to as *malpractice*. Intentional torts also result in professional liability suits. Libel and slander are two forms of **defamation**. Libel refers to written statements, slander to oral remarks. **Assault** is defined as a deliberate attempt or threat to touch without consent. Another intentional wrong is **battery**, which is the unauthorized touching of another person. A patient has a right to refuse treatment. Other civil laws govern property ownership, corporations, and inheritance.

The contract between a patient and a physician has three parts, Figure 3–2. They are the offer, the acceptance, and the consideration. The offer takes place when a competent individual indicates a desire to become a patient. The acceptance takes place when an appointment is given and the physician examines the patient. The consideration is the payment given in exchange for services. When a child is a patient, the parent is expected to pay. A young person is considered to be a minor until reaching full legal age, known as the age of majority. The statutes defining the age of majority vary from state to state. The medical assistant needs to be aware that the rights of minors in medical treatment are changing. More than half of the states allow minors the right to consent to treatment or consultation for pregnancy, contraception, venereal disease, drug abuse, or alcoholism.

An **emancipated minor** is an individual who is no longer under the care, custody, or supervision of parents. The emancipated minor may be married, in the armed forces, or self-supporting and living apart from parents. An emancipated minor can legally consent to medical care.

An individual who has been judged by the courts to be mentally incompetent must have an appointed guardian. The general legal term for all varieties of mental illness is *non compos mentis*. The guardian is responsible for both the payment of bills and the care of the patient. In this case the parents are not responsible for payment. When a patient-physician contract is entered into, the physician is responsible for the care of that patient until the physician officially withdraws from the case or the patient discharges the physician.

The contract between the patient and the physician may be either implied or expressed. An express, or written, contract must be entered into if a third party is to be responsible for payment. If this agreement is not in writing, it is not possible to press for payment. There are also implied consent and express consent agreements between patients and physicians. The fact that the patient has come to see the physician implies consent for treatment. The instances when express consent is required are:

- proposed surgery or other invasive treatments such as cerebrospinal taps, sigmoidoscopies, biopsies, etc.
- use of experimental drugs
- use of unusual procedures that may involve high risk

3 Parts Of Patient-Physician Contract

1. The offer—desire to become patient

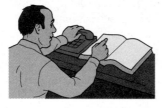

2. Acceptance

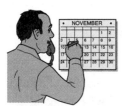

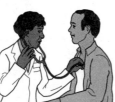

a. Appointment is given   b. Physician examines patient

3. Consideration—payment made for services

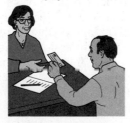

Figure 3–2 This cartoon illustrates the three parts of the patient-physician contract.

FORM P-2

CONSENT TO OPERATION, ANESTHETICS, AND OTHER MEDICAL SERVICES (ALTERNATE FORM)

Date_____ Time_____ A.M. P.M.

1. I authorize the performace upon_____ (myself or name of patient)

of the following operation _____ (state name of operation)

to be performed under the direction of Dr._____

A. The nature of the operation_____ (describe the operation)

_____

_____

B. The purpose of the operation _____ (describe the purpose)

_____

C. The possible alternative methods of treatment _____

(describe alternative methods)

D. The possible consequences of the operation _____

(describe the possible consequences)

E. The risks involved_____

(describe the risks involved)

F. The possible complications _____

(describe the possible complications)

3. I have been advised of the serious nature of the operation and have been advised that if I desire a further and more detailed explanation of any of the foregoing or further information about the possible risks or complications of the above listed operation it will be given to me.

4. I do not request a further and more detailed listing and explanation of any of the items listed in paragraph 2.

Signed _____ (patient or person authorized to consent for patient)

Witness _____

Figure 3–3 Consent to operation, anesthetics, and other invasive services (Courtesy American Medical Association).

Form P-22
CONSENT TO TREATMENT

Date ________ Time ________ A.M. P.M.

I have been informed by Dr. ________________ of the nature, risks, possible alternative methods of treatment, possible consequences, and possible complications involved in the treatment by means of ________________

____

____

for the relief of ________________

____

Nevertheless, I authorize Dr. ________________ to administer such treatment to me.

Signed ________________
(Patient or person authorized to consent for patient)

Witness ________________

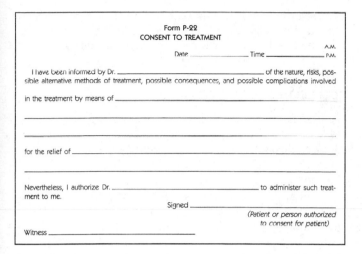

Figure 3–4 Consent for treatment (Courtesy American Medical Association).

Form P-17
REQUEST FOR STERILIZATION

Date ________ Time ________ A.M. P.M.

We, the undersigned husband and wife, each being more than twenty-one years of age and of sound mind, request Dr. ________________, and assistants of his choice, to perform upon ________________, the following operation: ________
(name of patient)

____
(state nature and extent of operation)

It has been explained to us that this operation is intended to result in sterility although this result has not been guaranteed. We understand that a sterile person is NOT capable of becoming a parent.

We voluntarily request the operation and understand that if it proves successful the results will be permanent and it will thereafter be physically impossible for the patient to inseminate, or to conceive or bear children.

Signed ________________
(Husband)

Signed ________________
(Wife)

Witness

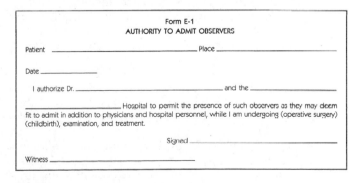

Figure 3–5 Request for sterilization (Courtesy American Medical Association).

There are exceptions to the rule for surgery. Minor procedures generally involve explanation by the physician and oral consent of the patient. The notes regarding this conversation need to be entered by the physician in the patient record.

The American Medical Association has developed recommended standardized forms to be used by physicians, Figure 3–3. It will be your responsibility to know what consent forms your employer uses. The physician may wish to develop forms individualized for the practice. It is important that these be **explicit** as to what is to be done. Experiments have been conducted using a tape recorder to keep a record of the information given the patient before a consent form is signed. These were discussions with patients who had to be told they had cancer. Most of these patients had little or no memory of what had been discussed because they were extremely upset by the diagnosis. In some of these cases the patients were certain they were not fully informed, but the replay of the tape proved they had been. The medical assistant should understand that the physician must be legally responsible for obtaining informed consent from a patient. You should not be given that responsibility. Informed consent is necessary to avoid a claim of assault and battery. The law describes this as a threat to make a physical attack on someone and carrying out the attack. You will be expected to prepare consent forms and ideally be present to listen so that you may help determine whether the patient understood before signing the consent form.

If an all-purpose form is used, it is important to cross out the paragraphs that do not apply. You may be asked to sign as a witness. What you say when you ask a patient to sign after the physician has explained the risks is important. A suggested statement is: "If you have no further questions for the doctor and you understand the consent form, will you please sign it?"

If a physician is to treat a patient with unusual or experimental medication, it is best to use a Consent to Treatment form, Figure 3–4. When a physician is to perform a sterilization procedure, it is preferable to have both husband and wife sign a Request for Sterilization form, Figure 3–5.

Patients have the right to privacy when they are being examined and treated. Many physicians have arrangements with medical facilities to offer training opportunities for medical students or residents, but the patient has the right to refuse to have observers present. Patients must first be asked if it is okay with them for observers to be present during the examination. If the patient refuses, no **intimidation** or **coercion** should be expressed to make the patient change the decision. Therefore, physicians may protect themselves by having an Authority to Admit Observers form signed, Figure 3–6.

Information contained in a patient medical record and information exchanged between a physician and a patient are considered to be privileged communications. Every patient has a legal right to privacy and **confidentiality**. Information disclosed to the health care team must be kept in the strictest confidence, and you must be ever mindful of the legal implications of handling patients' records. Information concerning patients may be given to another member of the health care team, such as a laboratory technician or referring physician, only when it pertains directly to the course of treatment. Another medical office may telephone to inquire about a patient's medical history for diagnostic purposes, to confirm symptoms, or to verify birthdate. In complying with referral appointments or scheduled tests, patients will have given implied consent for necessary information to be transmitted concerning their condition.

Form E-1
AUTHORITY TO ADMIT OBSERVERS

Patient ________________ Place ________________

Date ________

I authorize Dr. ________________ and the ________________

________________ Hospital to permit the presence of such observers as they may deem fit to admit in addition to physicians and hospital personnel, while I am undergoing (operative surgery) (childbirth), examination, and treatment.

Signed ________________

Witness ________________

Figure 3–6 Authority to admit observers (Courtesy American Medical Association).

Medical information may be given to parties not concerned in the patient's treatment only when the patient has signed a release of information form.

A large number of states have privileged communication statutes that have been **enacted** to offer additional protection to the patient. You will find that curious and well-meaning friends and relatives ask about patients and you must remember to give only information that has been authorized by the patient. Each time a patient authorizes release of information the form must state specifically who is to receive what information covering what time period. This authorization must be kept in the medical record.

All health care providers must be aware of any state regulations governing the reporting of HIV positive tests. At issue is the right of the AIDS patient to confidentiality and the rights of citizens to be protected from accidental exposure to the HIV virus. Such exposure might occur when police, fire, emergency medical personnel, or any medical personnel come into direct contact with the blood or body fluids of a patient whose diagnosis of AIDS is not known to the personnel.

In all fifty states, confirmed cases of AIDS/HIV constitute a reportable condition either by statute or administrative regulation.

Complete Chapter 3, Unit 1 in the workbook to help you meet the objectives at the beginning of this unit and therefore achieve competency of this subject matter.

UNIT 2

Professional Liability

▪ OBJECTIVES

Upon completion of the unit, meet the following terminal performance objectives by verifying knowledge of the facts and principles presented through oral and written communication at a level deemed competent.

1. List rights of the physician in providing medical care.
2. List rights of the patient in receiving medical care.
3. Describe the correct procedure for terminating the physician-patient contract.
4. Define and give examples of abandonment.
5. Define and give examples of professional negligence.
6. Give an example of an implied agreement.
7. Describe the precaution that should be observed in giving written instructions to a patient.
8. List the reasons for keeping medical records.
9. Describe who owns medical office records and who has a right to the information in them.
10. List the record keeping necessary to provide legally adequate records.
11. Discuss the kinds of notes that are not appropriate in a patient chart.
12. Name the six basic principles for preventing unauthorized disclosure of patient information.
13. List six office procedures that can cause problems when the physician is involved in a lawsuit.
14. Describe the acceptable method for making changes in medical records.
15. Spell and define, using the glossary at the back of the text, all the words to know in this unit.

▪ WORDS TO KNOW

abandonment	enumerate
breach	harmonious
chronological	liability
competent	mores
confrontation	obligate
criterion	procrastination
defamation	rapport
deposition	*res ipsa loquitur*
doctrine	*respondeat superior*
encompass	*subpoena duces tecum*

PHYSICIAN AND PATIENT RIGHTS

Physicians have the right to determine whom they will accept as patients. Physicians who have been in practice for a long period of time may build up a patient load that is as large as one person can adequately care for. Since a physician must care for all patients accepted, it is not unusual to have to decide to see no new patients. A physician may not, on the other hand, refuse to provide emergency service if assigned to an emergency service, and most physicians will provide emergency service whenever the need exists, since they do not have to continue the patient's treatment. Physicians have the right to decide what types of medicine they wish to practice and where. They have the right to establish their own working hours, to charge for their services, and to take a vacation if they provide names of qualified substitutes to care for their patients while they are unavailable. Physicians have the right to change the location of their office but must notify patients in advance to give them adequate time to make alternate plans for medical care.

Patients have the right to receive care equal to the standards of care in the community as a whole. Patients have the right to choose the physician from whom they wish to receive treatment, from the listing of physicians who are enrolled in their particular insurance plan. Of course, a patient may always see any physician desired as long as they take full responsibility for payment of services rendered, meaning that the patient pays cash at the time of service if the patient's insurance plan will not cover the services of that particular physician. However, if a patient becomes a member of an HMO, the right to choose a physician may be restricted to physicians who are members of the chosen HMO. A patient has the right to accept or reject treatment, and to know when treatment is prescribed whether it has side effects, what the prognosis is, what effect the treatment will have on the body, and any alternatives to treatment.

A physician may choose to withdraw from the care of a patient who does not follow instructions for treatment or follow-up appointments or who leaves a hospital against advice. Withdrawal must be by means of a letter sent by certified mail with return receipt requested as proof the letter was received. The return receipt should be filed in the patient record. The letter may state the reason for the withdrawal and needs to state the date the withdrawal will become effective, Figure 3–7. If the patient needs follow-up, the letter should

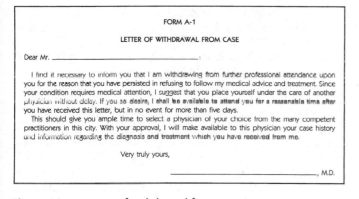

FORM A-1

LETTER OF WITHDRAWAL FROM CASE

Dear Mr. _____ :

I find it necessary to inform you that I am withdrawing from further professional attendance upon you for the reason that you have persisted in refusing to follow my medical advice and treatment. Since your condition requires medical attention, I suggest that you place yourself under the care of another physician without delay. If you so desire, I shall be available to attend you for a reasonable time after you have received this letter, but in no event for more than five days.

This should give you ample time to select a physician of your choice from the many competent practitioners in this city. With your approval, I will make available to this physician your case history and information regarding the diagnosis and treatment which you have received from me.

Very truly yours,

_____ , M.D.

Figure 3–7   Letter of withdrawal from case (Courtesy American Medical Association).

recommend that the patient make an appointment with another physician. It is appropriate to indicate that a copy of the medical records will be sent to the new physician if the patient sends written authorization to do so. The letter should be signed by the physician.

A patient has a choice and a right to change physicians. The patient should notify the physician but if this does not take place in a written form the physician may send a letter confirming the dismissal. This letter should also be sent by certified mail, return receipt requested, and a copy of the letter and the receipt should be filed in the patient chart.

A physician who has begun care of a patient must carry through until the patient no longer needs treatment or decides to see a different physician, or the physician has withdrawn from care. A physician who has undertaken care of a patient and is then not available to continue that care may be sued for **abandonment** unless coverage for the patient by some equally qualified physician is provided. If a patient is admitted to the hospital and the physician does not see the patient right away to check on condition and order treatment, the physician may risk being accused of abandonment by the patient or by a family member of the patient. If a physician is ill, the office staff must refer patients who need care to other qualified physicians who will care for them.

Physicians are not **obligated** to provide follow-up care when they see a patient for preemployment or insurance examinations or on other occasions when the request comes from someone other than the patient, as when a school athletic department requests assessment of a potential athlete.

Medical Assistant Rights

The medical assistant has the right to be free from sexual discrimination. This may involve a man or woman being refused employment because the job is usually filled by someone of the opposite sex. It can involve promotions, paying less for the same work, or being treated as inferior in any way.

Title VII of the Civil Rights Act of 1964 defines sexual harassment as "Unwelcome sexual advances, requests for sexual favors, and other verbal or physical conduct of a sexual nature when submission or rejection of this conduct explicitly or implicitly affects an individual's employment, unreasonably interferes with an individual's work performance or creates an intimidating, hostile or offensive work environment." Sexual harassment can occur in a variety of circumstances. It may include but is not limited to:

- The victim as well as the harasser may be a woman or a man. The victim does not have to be of the opposite sex.
- The harasser can be the victim's supervisor, an agent of the employer, a supervisor in another area, a co-worker, or a nonemployee.
- The victim does not have to be the person harassed but could be anyone affected by the offensive conduct.
- Unlawful sexual harassment may occur without economic injury to or discharge of the victim.
- The victim has a responsibility to establish that the harasser's conduct is unwelcome.

It is in the victim's best interest to directly inform the harasser that the conduct is unwelcome and must stop. Each instance reported to authorities is handled on a case-by-case basis and involves a thorough investigation.

Negligence

Torts is the branch of private law that deals with **breach** of legal duty. Torts **encompass** such wrongs as invasion of privacy, personal injury, malpractice, and slander or libel. The tort of negligence is a primary cause of malpractice suits.

Physicians are expected to be as well trained and to exercise the same degree of skill with the same degree of judgment as other physicians in similar circumstances. These criteria are used in determining the standard of care. In lawsuits involving specialists, the standard of care is that practiced nationally rather than that in a given community.

In a case of negligence the patient must establish that he or she was examined by the physician, that the physician did or did not do something another physician under similar circumstances would or would not have done, whichever the case may be, and that the negligence injured the patient. Testimony of a physician as an expert medical witness is almost always necessary in a case of negligence. In some cases the testimony of an expert witness is not required. In these instances the **doctrine** is *res ipsa loquitur*, or *the thing speaks for itself*. These cases involve such situations as a sponge or instrument left in the patient during surgery, an injury done to the bladder while performing a hysterectomy, and an infection caused by the use of unsterilized instruments. This doctrine has different interpretations in different states.

Physicians are responsible for the actions of their employees. This **liability** is expressed in the doctrine of *respondeat superior (let the master answer)*. This is the law of agency, and you are an agent for the physician. Any individual entering the profession of medical assisting is considered to be accepting a position as a health care professional. If you violate the standard of care, you create the basis for a medical malpractice lawsuit. The physician is responsible for the acts of the medical assistant in the care of patients, and it is reasonable to expect the care to be as professional as the care given by the physician. A medical assistant is not licensed to practice medicine and cannot decide for a patient what care should be given.

After a Roche Laboratories medicolegal seminar, the Los Angeles County Medical Society sent the following directive to its doctors:

When you ask your office assistant to instruct or refill a prescription, you are placing both the assistant and yourself in jeopardy. The physician's aide who directs a pharmacist to fill or refill a prescription becomes guilty of practice of medicine without a license. A physician who directs his assistant to do this places his license in jeopardy by assisting an unlicensed person to practice medicine. The conclusion of this directive is that when you want a pharmacist to fill or refill a prescription, let him or her hear the doctor's own telephone voice, or better, have written orders on a regular prescription blank.

Negligence is doing or not doing something that a reasonable person would do or not do in a given situation. Malpractice is a professional's negligence. Under ordinary circumstances, a medical assistant performing the administrative duties of a receptionist or secretary would be considered a person who could be charged with negligence. A medical assistant performing clinical procedures such as drawing blood or administering injections would be considered a professional and charged with malpractice.

Medical assistants who have had special training are expected to perform at a higher standard of care than those with no special knowledge or training.

The medical assistant is not always covered by the physician's insurance, but insurance is available for the protection of medical assistants.

Good Samaritan Act

The Good Samaritan Act originated in California in 1959 to protect the physician who gives emergency care from liability for any civil damages. The physician could help in an emergency without fear of being charged with neglect or abandonment for follow-up care. Now all states have Good Samaritan statutes. The statute requires that the emergency care be given to the best ability of the person providing the care. In some states, the statute includes coverage for any health professional or citizen with first aid skills. The Good Samaritan law does not cover physicians if they receive compensation for the emergency care.

An implied agreement is considered to be a legal contract in a medical office. The medical assistant should never make a promise of a cure. You should be certain the patient understands the instructions you give come directly from the physician or from written instruction sheets. When you hand a patient a written instruction sheet you need to be certain the patient can read the instructions. Illiterate people are often reluctant to let anyone know that they cannot follow the directions for use of medications or preparation for a diagnostic test. Informative videos that present detailed instructions regarding procedures, tests, and examinations for patient education are available from many pharmaceutical companies (or you can make them yourself) for patients to view while they are waiting to see the physician. Their questions and any further explanation can then follow at the end of their office visit. One indicator of illiteracy might be the patient who becomes a "pest" by asking over and over for office staff to explain the instructions given by the physician. This patient might also ask you to explain a printed instruction sheet as a means of getting you to read it aloud.

The importance of doing everything possible to avoid a medical malpractice suit cannot be overemphasized. Simply being accused can have severe effects and repercussions on the physician and his/her practice and family. Those physicians who are wrongly accused of serious charges of neglect or malpractice can have ongoing problems with public mistrust and other issues depending on the extent of publicity. This misfortune can affect the livelihood of the physician, therefore ruining his/her medical practice. A physician can be ethical, honest, and **competent**, and still be sued for medical malpractice by a single patient who for some reason did not realize the expected result of treatment. Thus, another reason why the medical assistant is vital in providing patient education to supplement the physician's orders. The great increase in malpractice cases has caused physicians to order more tests and X rays than are really necessary because they need to protect themselves from the possibility of missing a diagnosis and therefore being sued by the patient. The medical assistant is an extremely important person in the practice of preventive medicine in the medical office. When a friendly, **harmonious** interpersonal relationship is found in the office (known as **rapport**), the patient is much less likely to feel angry about anything associated with the care received. The well-trained medical assistant will understand the basic skills in good human relations and will then avoid **confrontations** that could lead to lawsuits against the office.

The following is the beginning of a chapter regarding medical office staff written by Melvin Belli, an internationally known attorney:

> A woman once came to me with a complaint that she'd been incorrectly treated by a "dumb doctor."
>
> "How do you know he's dumb?" I asked her.
>
> "Because everybody who works for him is dumb."
>
> It's common for patients to relate a doctor to his or her staff. Therefore, quite often, patient dissatisfaction with an office assistant will put the doctor on a malpractice spot.

(Reproduced with permission from Melvin M. Belli, Sr., and John Carlova. *For Your Malpractice Defense,* Oradell, New Jersey: Medical Economics Company, Inc., 1986.)

The patient who suffers nerve damage as the result of a medical assistant giving an improperly administered injection may sue both medical assistant and physician under this doctrine. You should always inform the physician immediately of any mistakes you have made in the care of a patient so that corrective measures may be taken. You should never attempt to perform a procedure for which you have not been trained. Finally, you should be sure you understand your job responsibilities as outlined in a written procedures manual, which should be periodically updated.

You must be especially careful what you say about a patient within hearing of anyone but the physician or other office personnel. Statements regarding patients may be considered **defamation** of character and a breach of confidentiality. If you should make public the fact that a patient has a venereal disease, for example, this could be damaging to the patient.

You play an important role in preventing negligence by scheduling appointments for careful follow-up, knowing how and where to reach the physician at all times during the day, and making sure that the telephone is adequately covered at all times. The patient who feels well cared for will not be anxious to sue the physician. The patient who can never reach the physician for advice or who has difficulty obtaining an appointment will be much more apt to sue on the grounds of negligence.

The medical assistant should investigate use of an arbitration agreement procedure by contacting your local or state medical society. Not all states have an arbitration statute at the present time but it is well worth investigating as a possible way to settle legal problems without going to court.

Because the incidence of malpractice suits has increased, the medical assistant may need to be involved in preparing materials for court. This may include the professional training and experience of the physician as well as the patient medical record.

The attorneys may agree to taking the testimony of the physician by **deposition**. A deposition is oral testimony and may be taken in the attorney's office, or the physician's office in the presence of a court reporter.

A medical assistant may also receive a *subpoena duces tecum* to appear in court with patient records. This occurs when the physician is not available at the time needed in court.

Statutes of Limitations

A statute of limitations is a law that designates a specific limit of time during which a claim may be filed in malpractice suits or in the collection of bills. Each state is obligated to protect individuals by establishing the statutes that regulate the time period. It is important to research the current law by contacting your state medical association.

MEDICAL RECORDS

The medical office staff must understand the importance of maintaining accurate, up-to-date records on all patients. You must have complete records to give adequate care to patients. Your records may be used in research into certain illnesses or forms of treatment, and your records must be complete for protection in case of a lawsuit. A patient record that would meet this criterion would include (1) personal information such as full name, address, occupation, marital status, and insurance carrier; (2) patient's personal family sociocultural and medical history; (3) all details of physical examinations, laboratory and X-ray findings, diagnoses, and treatments; and (4) consent forms for procedures done and authorization forms for release of medical information. **Procrastination** cannot be tolerated in handling medical records. As legal documents, they are subject to critical inspection at any time, Figure 3–8.

You should always take a medical history in a private room or ask the patient to complete the information. Make entries on the patient medical record only as requested by the physician. All entries should be factual. All results of findings on a patient should be recorded even if they are normal or negative. Errors on a medical record must be corrected by drawing a single line through incorrect material and adding your initials, the date, and the reason for the change. All prescription refills should be noted along with missed appointments, the reason for the missed appointment, and follow-up. Requests for medical information should be noted along with the information given. Any failure to follow the treatment or advice of the physician should be noted. All notations should be in blue or black ink, as pencil is too easily erased. Blue ink, as well as other colors, and pencil do not copy well. This is a concern for duplicating reports and records for referrals.

Standard abbreviations should be used. Upon the death of a patient, a copy of the death certificate should be filed in case of subsequent requests for information. A quality medical record indicates quality medical care.

Medical records are considered the property of the physician who treats the patient. No record should be shown to a patient without the knowledge of the physician, as there may be some reason the patient should not see all of the record.

Each office should have a written policy regarding releasing information from a medical record. This policy must take into consideration local or state statutes. In some states, the legislature has given the patient, his or her physician, or authorized agent the right to examine or copy the medical record. The requirement of confidentiality regarding the medical record is no longer recognized when the patient initiates a malpractice claim against a physician.

Physicians cannot agree on whether patients should be allowed to review their own records. The physician must be careful of personal opinion notes placed in the chart if there is a possibility the patient will be reading it. The following are two examples of patients reading medical records that were not recorded for their viewing:

A female patient was being professionally treated by a young physician when the doctor was suddenly called away from his office and left her medical record open on his desk. The patient read the first sentence: "This woman is a crock." Needless to say, she became very distraught and angry. (From "Personal Comments in Medical Records May Cause Trouble," *Medical World News,* Jan. 12, 1976, 128.)

While waiting to see a physician, a patient had been given her own record. Curious, she took out the notes and read them only to find that the doctor had written on the heading of the page, "Beware, hysterical and manipulative, determined to be unwell." She left immediately. (From "Case Conference: Fain Would I Change That Note," *Journal of Medical Ethics,* 4 [1978] 207–209.)

Any review of the chart by the patient should be done when the physician is present to interpret medical terms or abbreviations. Some physicians give patients a copy of their

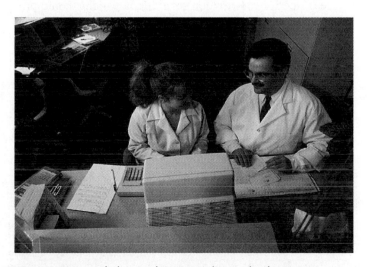

Figure 3–8 To help avoid an error, this medical assistant checks with her supervisor to clarify information regarding a patient's condition before recording it on the permanent record.

medical records and believe this reduces any anxiety regarding their health.

The following are six basic principles for preventing unauthorized disclosure of information:

1. When in doubt, err by not disclosing rather than by disclosing. There are exceptions to this principle but a mistaken refusal to disclose confidential data is, at least, reversible.
2. Remember that the owner of the privilege to keep information confidential is the patient, not the doctor. If the patient is willing to release the data, the physician may not ethically decide to withhold it even 'for the patient's own good.'
3. Apply the concept of confidentiality equally to all patients despite the physician's assessment of their goals, **mores**, and lifestyles. A physician cannot ethically inform an insurer of suspicions that a patient is trying to defraud an insurer.
4. Be familiar with the federal, state and local law plus ordinances, rules, regulations and administrative decrees of various agencies such as public health departments.
5. When required to divulge a confidence, discuss the situation with the patient. When obligations to society conflict with those of the patient, the physician should discuss the conflict with the patient. When legal guidelines are absent or vague, the criteria for decision are the immediacy and degree of danger to either the patient or society.
6. Get written authorization from the patient before divulging information. To meet standard situations such as requests from third parties, have the patient sign a blanket authorization in advance to release pertinent data to specific third parties.

(Reprinted with permission from Leif C. Beck, "Patient Information: When—and When Not—to Divulge," *Patient Care,* April 15, 1972.)

The AMA has several forms for authorization for disclosure. It is a good policy to refuse to answer a telephone question as to whether an individual is a patient. A person coming to the office for information regarding a patient should produce an authorization to disclose information before any is given. It is important to check the specific details authorized to be released and to ask for photo identification of the individual or organization requesting the information. The signed authorization should be placed in the patient chart with a copy of the information released. According to Myrtle Flight, "when the information requested is disclosed, it must be accompanied by a note forbidding redisclosure" (*Law, Liability, and Ethics for Medical Office Personnel,* 134).

The complete, unaltered medical record is a legal document and is the best defense for a physician who is charged with malpractice. The first step a lawyer will take in a malpractice case against a physician is to obtain a copy of the patient's records and have them examined by an independent physician. The following office procedures have caused problems in malpractice suits:

1. Procrastination or delay in filing lab test results.
2. Incomplete medical records.
3. Illegible records.
4. Unexplained altered medical records.
5. Faking or forging a document or signature.
6. Loss of records.

There are acceptable methods of making changes in medical records. A single line should be drawn through an incorrect entry. An initial of the person making the correction should be written in the margin along with the date the error was discovered. The corrections should appear in the record in **chronological** order.

The contents of a medical record have been **enumerated**. In addition to having complete, up-to-date records you must be aware of the need for keeping these records even after care has ceased or the patient has expired. Records should be kept as long as the statute of limitations is in effect on a case history. A few states designate the length of time records must be kept. You have a responsibility to see that necessary records are kept for any narcotics used in the office. You also may be responsible for keeping accurate financial records. Within the following pages of this book, whenever appropriate, points will further remind you of the medicolegal importance of the subject matter.

Complete Chapter 3, Unit 2 in the workbook to help you meet the objectives at the beginning of this unit and therefore achieve competency of this subject matter.

REFERENCES

American Association of Medical Assistants. "Law for the Medical Office—1984."

Flight, Myrtle. *Law, Liability, and Ethics for Medical Office Personnel.* Albany: Delmar, 1988.

Hasty, Frederick E., III. "Your Most Dangerous Malpractice Gamble." *Medical Economics for Surgeons.* August 20, 1984.

Horsley, Jack E. "Who Can Sue You For Not Rendering Care?" *Medical Economics.* August 20, 1984.

Isele, William. "Legal and Ethical Concerns of the Medical Assistant." *The Professional Medical Assistant.* July–August 1977.

Kinn, Mary E., and Derge, Eleanor. *The Medical Assistant: Administrative and Clinical,* 7th ed. Philadelphia: W. B. Saunders, 1993.

Lewis, Marti, and Warden, Carol. *Law and Ethics in the Medical Office,* 3rd ed. Philadelphia: F. A. Davis, 1993.

Monahan, James S. "How Your Office Staff Can Get You Sued." *Medical Economics.* August 22, 1983.

Physician's Guide to Ohio Law. Ohio State Medical Association, Columbus, 1987.

The Professional Medical Assistant. "Ethics, a Roundtable Discussion." September–October, 1979.

Thomas, J.R., Esq., Attorney-at-Law, Columbus, Ohio (personal communication, August, 1996).

The Office Environment

A physician's office should be a safe, secure, and environmentally friendly workplace. The office staff must utilize constant vigilance to maintain that status. This chapter discusses the many aspects of the office environment as they relate to both patients and staff. Safety involves not only the use or condition of the physical equipment and furnishings in the office, but also the human activities of office personnel, visitors, and patients. The protection of staff, office equipment, and materials is very important. The working environment must allow for a focus on the provision of care rather than concern about personal safety.

The efficient design of the office is also a great asset to its ability to function effectively. **Provisions** for the physically challenged make the office environment a friendlier place for these people. Having the appropriate office management equipment available allows the office to operate more efficiently and applying the principles of ergonomics assures employees will be able to function more effectively and safely. This chapter discusses the preparation of the office to receive patients and considers how important the perception of the office is to patients and visitors.

UNIT 1

Safety, Security, and Emergency Provisions in the Medical Office

OBJECTIVES

Upon completion of the unit, meet the following terminal performance objectives by verifying knowledge of the facts and principles presented through oral and written communication at a level deemed competent.

1. Name four things to check to assure safety in a reception room.
2. List four hazards in a reception/business office area.
3. Name three things in an examination room that might be unsafe.
4. List nine items that are covered by OSHA or CDC regulations.
5. Name the three elements necessary for fire.
6. List four ways a fire might start.
7. Name six items that are considered to be protective barriers to prevent skin and mucous membrane exposure to pathogens.
8. Spell and define, using the glossary at the back of the text, all the words to know in this unit.

WORDS TO KNOW

assault	precautions
barrier	prevention
biohazardous	provisions
emergency	reception
environment	safety
evacuated	security
extinguisher	universal precautions
hazard	ventilation
irrational	volatile

A SAFE, HEALTHY ENVIRONMENT THROUGHOUT THE MEDICAL OFFICE

The medical office, like the home, is a place where you should feel safe and secure. But just like a home, it takes conscious effort to assure that the office has a protective, healthy **environment**. The medical assistant is part of the team responsible for recognizing any **safety**, security, or operational **hazard**, helping to eliminate it, and warning co-workers and patients of any dangers.

Safety in the Reception Room

A safe environment begins at the front door. The **reception** room requires a safety check every morning to assure it presents no hazards for patients and visitors. Observe the condition of the furniture carefully. Pay attention to chair and table legs—they must be stable and able to support appropriate weight. Lamps and electrical cords should be examined. Bulbs should not dim or flicker and cords should be in good condition with no evidence of fraying. Be sure lighting is adequate so that even people with impaired vision can see well. Check the floor to be certain there is neither carpet wrinkles nor anything lying on the floor that might cause someone to fall. Avoid the use of decorative or throw rugs.

Safety in the Receptionist/Business Office

In the receptionist/business office area, pay special attention to file drawers and cupboard doors. NEVER open more than one file drawer in a vertical file at a time because the unbalanced weight could cause the cabinet to tip forward. Many people have sustained back and extremity injuries from the automatic reaction to "catch" a cabinet. Also, be careful with opened bottom drawers. They can easily fall over. Wall cupboards pose another safety hazard. If the door is left open, you could strike your head quite forcefully when you stand up or raise up from underneath. All electrical cords must be kept behind desks and other office furnishings so that they will not be tripped over. All equipment should operate properly and show no evidence of electrical shorts or damage.

Safety in the Examination Room

The examination table must be cleaned after each patient. The table must operate properly and the medical assistant must be thoroughly competent in its use. Assist patients as necessary to sit or lie on the table. If the use of a stool is necessary, be exceptionally cautious to guard against the patient stepping on the edges, which could cause it to tip. Very ill patients, the elderly, and children should not be left alone on an examination table where they could fall. Small children accompanying a parent are best left with another office staff member while the parent is in the examination room.

There is also a natural curiosity about "things" on the examination room cabinet or counter. Anything which might be hazardous or could become contaminated should be kept out of sight. Prescription pads should not be left lying around where they could be stolen and possibly used to obtain controlled substances. In an examination room, there is a lot of equipment with electrical cords that must be positioned where they will not interfere with movement or walking within the room.

Safety in the Laboratory Area

Chemicals kept in the office for laboratory work must be properly labeled and stored. Chemicals that could become **volatile** when kept beyond their expiration date must be monitored carefully. The testing of patients' urine, blood, and other specimens requires special procedures. Containers for the disposal of used equipment and **biohazardous** waste must be readily accessible. A strict adherence to **universal precautions** is essential to the maintenance of a safe and healthy office environment. NOTE: The United States Occupational Safety and Health Administration (OSHA) and The Centers for Disease Control (CDC) in Atlanta, Georgia, have established rules for health care workers which cover blood products, body fluids, tissue cultures, vaccines, sharps, gloves, speculums, cotton swabs, and other items. These are discussed in Section IV—The Clinical Medical Assistant.

GENERAL OFFICE SAFETY

Fire

Fire **prevention** is very important to everyone's safety. Only three elements need to be present for a fire to start: heat, fuel, and oxygen, Figure 4–1. Today, there are rare exceptions to the "no smoking" regulations in medical and public facilities. Yet, there is still a possibility of a carelessly discarded match or cigarette ash dropping into furniture or being discarded into a trash container. Some facilities provide floor model ashtrays just outside their entrance for disposal of smoking materials. If they contain sand in which materials can be placed, they are relatively safe. However, types with opening metal tops can be an ideal place for a fire since people tend to use the ashtray as a receptacle for their trash. Any regular ashtray may contain smoldering smoking materials and is best emptied into a toilet and flushed rather than into a waste basket which could later burst into flame.

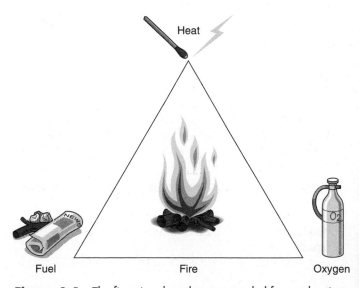

Figure 4–1 The fire triangle—elements needed for combustion (burning).

Fires can also be started by other causes. A defective outlet or frayed wires on any electrical appliance or office equipment could short out and start a fire. Coffee pots and water sterilizers can also boil dry and cause a fire. It is a good policy to unplug all electrical appliances whenever the office is closed.

The office should have an established policy regarding the procedure to follow in case of fire. There should be a planned route of escape prominently posted, Figure 4–2. All patients as well as office staff must be **evacuated** from the building and the fire department notified. Exit signs should be clearly posted. All stairways and hallways should be free from clutter to allow quick, safe passage. When appropriate, knowing the location of the fire **extinguisher** and using it properly could prevent a fire from spreading. This knowledge should be everyone's responsibility, Figure 4–3 (A-C).

Natural Disasters

A severe weather warning is another event that requires an established policy. Natural disasters such as strong electrical storms and tornados are unpredictable and can claim lives if necessary steps are not taken. In these instances, people must remain inside and take shelter in the predetermined safest area. In areas where there is danger from earthquakes, it is wise to stand in doorframes or beneath

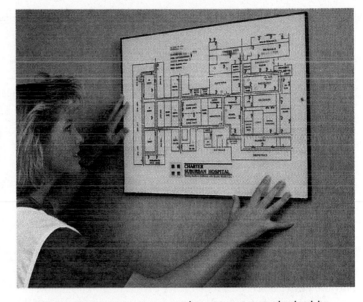

Figure 4–2 Know your quickest route to exit the building.

a sturdy structure. It may be dangerous to go outside where you could be struck by falling trees and buildings or come into contact with downed power lines. Yet, remaining in a multistory building may not be the safest policy, either.

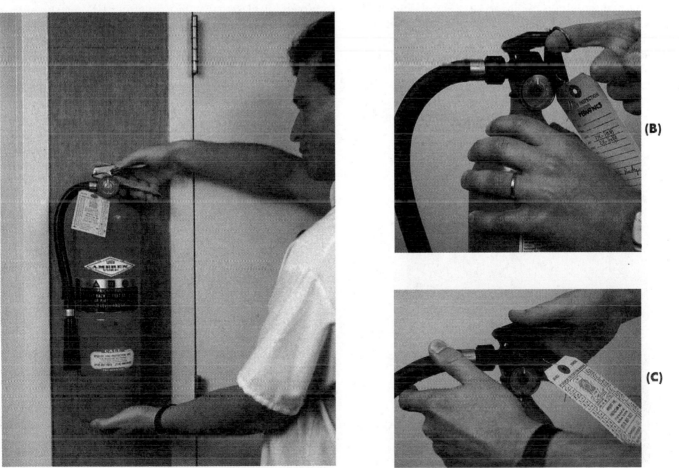

(A)

(B)

(C)

Figure 4–3 A, B, C Know the location of the fire extinguisher and how to use it.

People living in high risk areas generally know the appropriate action to take.

Electrical power is sometimes disrupted during such an **emergency**. Never use an elevator during a threatening situation because the power could go off, trapping everyone inside until power is restored or they are rescued. Large medical facilities may have electrical generators to provide emergency lighting during emergency situations. Battery-powered lights should always be available and accessible.

Routine fire and weather drills prepare people psychologically to act in a safe and responsible manner. A practical time to review drill procedures is at a staff meeting or during new employee orientation. Those who are prepared have a greater chance of surviving a crisis than those who do not know what to do or how to act. Keeping calm and confident in times of emergency helps to reduce panic and **irrational** behavior in oneself and others. It is not practical to decide at the time of such an emergency what to do with the patients and the staff. Each member of the office team should be assigned specific duties and know how to carry them out safely and efficiently.

Spills and Dropped Objects

It is very important to clean up spilled liquids immediately. When the spill involves bodily fluids such as blood or urine, universal precautions must be observed by using gloves and placing materials in a **biohazardous** bag, Figure 4–4. Objects dropped on the floor must also be picked up immediately in order to prevent falls. Glass fragments are best picked up using a brush or broom and dust pan. Glass must be discarded in such a way that it will not puncture the plastic bag liner of the waste receptacle—this could accidentally cut someone's hands when it is removed. Fragments could be carefully wrapped in layers of news-

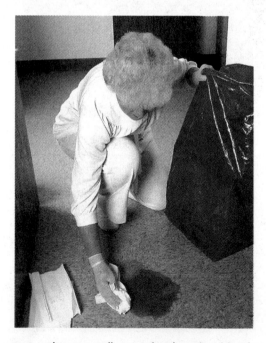

Figure 4–4 Clean up spills immediately. When blood or other body fluids are involved, universal precautions must be observed.

paper or placed inside empty cardboard or plastic containers before being deposited into the receptacle.

Emergency Phone Numbers

A list of emergency phone numbers should be posted by the phone for quick access. Such numbers may include but are not limited to: police, fire department, emergency service, poison control center, building security, utility companies, hospital emergency room, and a hospital admissions office. When an urgent situation arises, you don't want to have to search for phone numbers.

Safety Items

The installation of hand rails in hallways and bathrooms within the office assists elderly and weak or motor impaired people in moving throughout the office with greater stability and less chance of falling. Be certain the floors are clear from any materials and that carpets are smooth and secured—loose rugs are very dangerous, especially over tile or vinyl flooring. The medical assistant must always be on guard to be certain no one falls.

Personal Safety

All health care workers must practice universal precautions to protect themselves against acquiring HIV or hepatitis B infection. **CAUTION:** All patients should be considered infected because medical history and examination cannot reliably identify all patients infected with HIV or other blood-borne pathogens. Protection involves the use of appropriate **barrier** precautions to prevent skin and mucous membrane exposure when there is contact with blood or other body fluids of any patient. This means the appropriate use of gloves, face shields, masks, protective eyewear, and aprons and gowns as needed. Persons likely to be in an emergency situation also need to make use of mouthpieces, **ventilation** bags, and other ventilating devices in order to avoid direct contact with saliva or possible blood due to an injury. **Precautions** are identified later in this text as they become necessary within procedures. Look for the glove icon at the top of a procedure instruction.

SECURITY IN THE MEDICAL OFFICE

The increased incidences of crime makes security a prime concern. A criminal may think a physician's office has cash from daily receipts or from people in the office, such as employees or patients, and decide to commit a robbery. There is also the concept that large amounts of drugs are kept on site and could be easily attained. Unfortunately, sexual **assault** can also occur when the interior office is accessible from the reception area. In order to provide a degree of **security**, police recommend that doors between these areas be equipped with snap locks to prevent unwanted entry. Also, any opening between the two areas, such as a window, should be covered with a grill if it is possible to climb through it. (This author knows of an incident when an intruder crawled through the reception room window and as-

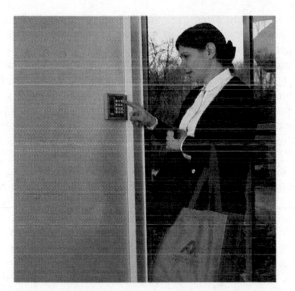

Figure 4–5 Enter the security code before opening the door.

saulted a nurse who was working alone in an office.) If there are private entry doors, be certain they are kept locked at all times. If you must enter or leave the office after dark, be especially alert. The outside area should be well lit. If building security people are available, ask for an escort.

Many offices today are equipped with electronic security systems. If you are the first staff member to arrive at work, it will be necessary to enter the code before opening the door or enter the code on an internal key pad before the entrance delay expires, Figure 4–5. Both these systems lend a feeling of safety and security, but be aware, it only takes a few seconds for someone to grab your purse or force you to hand over office money or drugs. Never enter the office if there is evidence of forced entry or if it appears that someone might either be inside or has been inside. Leave and call building security or the police at once.

Complete Chapter 4, Unit 1 in the workbook to help you meet the objectives at the beginning of this unit and therefore achieve competency of this subject matter.

UNIT 2
Efficient Office Design

▇ OBJECTIVES

Upon completion of the unit, meet the following terminal performance objectives by verifying knowledge of the facts and principles presented through oral and written communication at a level deemed competent.

1. Explain what an efficient office design is and why it is important.
2. Discuss the American Disabilities Act of 1990 in regard to a public facility.
3. Design an office setting that includes provisions for those with physical disabilities.

4. In a facility that was not originally designed to provide for persons with a disability, describe the steps that should be taken to remedy this situation.
5. List ways for dealing with disabled persons effectively and considerately.
6. Explain where to obtain information for persons who have a disability.
7. Spell and define, using the glossary in the back of this text, all the words to know in this unit.

▇ WORDS TO KNOW

anticipation	handicap
Braille system	implementation
communicable diseases	insomnia
contamination	mandate
cultivate	pantomime
design	signer
disability	triage area
feasible	

In a medical facility where patients are treated for sickness, disorders, injuries, and a variety of illnesses, safety and well-being should always be the primary concern. In providing care for those who come in and out of the office daily, many things must be considered, including the design of the facility. Quality care begins long before patients come in for appointments to see the physician. Each medical facility is the result of long hours of planning and **anticipating** the needs of all who frequent the premises.

DESIGNING THE MEDICAL FACILITY TO ACCOMMODATE THE DISABLED

The original blueprint of the facility contains the basic floor plan. Several considerations are necessary for the plan to become **feasible**.

The American Disabilities Act

According to the American Disabilities Act (ADA) of 1990, all public facilities must be accessible to all persons with physical **disabilities/handicaps**.

All offices, clinics, medical centers, and the like constructed before 1990, that were not already **designed** to accommodate persons with physical disabilities, had to be updated to comply with this federal **mandate**. The mandate stated that these public facilities must be adapted that persons with disabilities and those in wheelchairs could easily and safely . . .

. . . enter and exit buildings

. . . reach door handles to open and close doors

. . . travel from floor to floor (so elevators are a must for buildings that have more than one floor)

. . . proceed through hallways and doorways

. . . use phones, drinking fountains, and restrooms,

and all else that the general population is free to do in public places.

So that the disabled could enter any public facility, every facility must be altered, if not already designed to accommodate all persons. Ramps must be permanent so that those in wheelchairs can have access to buildings without assistance.

Provisions must be included for disabled persons regarding reception area, examination and treatment rooms, and all other areas including work stations and restrooms. Those architectural barriers which prevent the disabled from entering public facilities must be eliminated according to many state and federal laws. It is wise to check the regulations governing this matter in your area.

Accommodating the Needs of Hearing and Vision Impaired Patients

For persons with hearing and vision impairment, accommodations must also be made. The **Braille system** must be provided for the blind to give them instructions and information for directions and identification of their whereabouts. If this is not possible, office staff must escort the person to and from the facility and give appropriate instructions verbally to assist them in getting around safely.

Those who are hearing impaired need to have a **signer** (sign language interpreter) available to communicate their needs, or else they must face the person speaking so that they can read their lips. When speaking to a hearing impaired patient, stand in the light so the person reading your lips can see well enough without straining. There should not be anything in your mouth, such as gum or food, when speaking. Taking it slower than a normal conversation may also be helpful for the person. Using gestures and **pantomime** can be of great assistance, too. Body language and appearance are additionally important. It should be noted that one should talk directly to the deaf person rather than to the interpreter, just as one should speak directly to *anyone* with a disability and not just to the person(s) accompanying them. It is appropriate to ask questions necessary for adequate health care, but personal questions are inappropriate. Employees with disabilities must also be considered with the same respect and attention.

NOTE: When talking to patients, regardless of the disability, it is important to be aware of your physical presence in relation to theirs. When talking to someone who is confined to a wheelchair for any length of time, it is considerate to sit so that your eye level is the same as theirs so the person does not have to keep looking up to hold a conversation with you. This position, as you can imagine, would be quite uncomfortable for a prolonged period of time.

PLANNING THE LAYOUT OF A GENERAL PRACTICE

The reception area should have comfortable but supportive seating that is comfortably spaced for both individuals and groups. For a general practice, the area where patients are received should accommodate all ages and help them to feel at ease. Most offices supply children with safe plastic toys that can be washed after use. Soft colors which are warm and simplistic are the most appealing. Proper ventilation and moderate temperature are necessary for comfort. Lighting should be varied for those who wish to sit quietly as well as for those who would like to read while they wait for their appointments. Background music that is instrumental is most appropriate. Music soothes the soul and helps one to relax. Reading material for all ages should be available in the reception area for patients waiting to see the physician.

Figure 4–6 is an example of a layout for a general practice clinic. Notice the traffic flow from entrance to exit as a patient travels through the entire facility. Specific assistance should be provided for patients with particular needs, Figure 4–7.

Using this design as a reference, follow the traffic flow of office staff, patients, and others who visit the facility. Efficient office design allows for the traffic pattern to flow without retracing steps to eliminate unnecessary walking for the employees and others alike. It also yields to the patient a feeling of expediently advancing through the facility. A well-planned layout allows people to enter the facility and proceed with whatever may be necessary, therefore, time seems to pass more quickly. Often, patients feel as though they are in a medical facility for a lot longer than they really are—waiting to see the physician or for results of a test can seem like forever. When patients are detained in the facility either before or after their examination with the physician because of a temporary back-up in the schedule, they especially appreciate having their needs met in an orderly fashion: being called into the **triage area**, progressing to an exam room, having lab tests performed, having preliminary exam/health history information taken, receiving treatment/medication, receiving patient education provided, etc. If attention is given to the patient to make the time go faster, then the patient is more likely to be satisfied.

Facility layout has a lot to do with how work patterns flow. If a medical facility has no available waiting area for very ill patients and everyone—sick and healthy—must stay together in the reception area, it makes for an uncomfortable situation. All patients waiting for appointments are placed at risk for possible **contamination** of **communicable diseases**. However, if the facility has an interior reception area for those who are very ill, the sick patient can be removed from the general reception area as soon as they arrive. The ideal design would have a central reception area with access through two doors: one for well and ambulatory patients, and another (wheelchair width) that opens automatically for those who are very ill. With this design, the contagious and more acutely ill patients would not come in contact with those who are not really ill (those for check ups, re-checks, etc.); the healthy patients could then avoid coming into contact with an additional illness during their well visit.

Of course, a medical facility does not have to be huge with many rooms in order to be efficient. Efficiency has to do with many points. The management of the schedule is a vital part of a practice. Scheduling will be discussed in length in Chapter 6. What is important to keep in mind is the relationship between office design layout and schedule and how they affect each other. Understanding the flow process is essential in efficient use of time and space. Once the staff realizes this fact and makes the proper adjustments, **implementation** of efficiency practices is possible.

A General Practice Scenario

Follow Figures 4–8, 4–9, 4–10, and 4–11 as you read the following scenario to see how these factors can work together for optimum efficiency. This example shows small numbers, representing patients and office staff, from the point of entry throughout their completed office visit.

The physician and three full-time staff members are beginning their day of providing health care to patients in a general practice facility.

Patient #1, who is scheduled for a complete physical examination, enters the general reception area, places belongings on the coat rack, reports to the receptionist's window, and takes a seat in the reception area, Figure 4-8.

Patient #2 enters shortly thereafter and does the same as patient #1. Patient #1 is called in to the clinical area and escorted by a clinical medical assistant (A-1) to the triage area where a health history is taken. While this is taking place, patient #2 waits a few more minutes, uses the restroom, and returns to the reception area. Patient #1 is then shown to the CPE room and prepared to see the physician.

Patient #3 is a sick child with a high fever and rash who is brought into the reception area and placed on a chair near the door while the parent reports their arrival to the receptionist. The clinical medical assistant A-1 is alerted by the receptionist and calls patient #3 into the inner reception area. Triage and assessment are done for the child and the physician is informed that the child is ready to be examined in the ill patient exam room.

Patient #4 enters the general reception area. Patient #4 needs a dressing change for a burn by the clinical medical assistant. Patient #2 is taken to the clinical area for triage and assessment by clinical medical assistant A-2, where it is determined that he needs an ECG for follow-up care of a hospitalization for a heart attack that occurred a few weeks earlier. The physician reads the ECG and discusses the results with the patient. He makes an appointment for a recheck in four weeks and leaves the office.

The part-time medical assistant arrives at the rear entrance, clocks in, and puts her belongings in the staff room. She then proceeds to the appointment desk to assess the patient flow and begins her duties of preparing patients. She calls patient #4 into the second exam room on the left. The doctor checks the progress of the burn, the MA dresses it, and the patient leaves the office after making another appointment and a payment on the account.

Patient #5 enters the general reception area, reports to the receptionist that she is here for a re-check of her medications for diabetes and hypertension, and sits down in the reception area.

Patient #6 enters the general reception area coughing, sneezing, and feverish. The physician is called to see this sick patient. He is treated and leaves the office.

Patient #4 is escorted back to the treatment room for a dressing change. (See Figure 4–9.) The physician examined and treated the sick child first, then examined patient #1 and ordered an ECG, chest x-ray and lab tests. Following these procedures, patient #1 stopped at the receptionist's desk and made a return visit appointment before leaving. The parent of the sick child took care of the charges incurred by the child's visit, made a re-check appointment for the following week, and exited through the same door they had entered. (The child was only in the far end of the general reception room and the inner reception room for a very brief period. The parent was able to leave the child in the exam room for a short time while the business was handled and then the child was taken home.)

Then enters adolescent patient #7 with a knee injury. The receptionist sees her across the room and reports her arrival to clinical medical assistant A-2, who calls her in through the door near the drinking fountain. She helps patient #7 to the inner reception area to await the physician's exam for a possible x-ray of the knee. The doctor examines the patient, orders an x-ray and the patient is treated and leaves the office, following a stop at the desk for a return appointment in two weeks.

Patient #5 has a glucose test and is checked by the doctor after weight and blood pressure are measured. She stops at the desk to pay her bill, makes another appointment, and leaves the office.

Patient #8, who has had problems with stress and **insomnia**, enters and speaks to the receptionist. The MA takes her to the physician's office for a consultation appointment. Another appointment is made at the reception desk before patient #8 leaves.

Patient #9 arrives, sits and is silent. The receptionist greets the patient, calls him to the desk and asks quietly what he is to see the doctor for today. She is told that he has been having headaches and made the appointment with the physician over the phone the night before. (See Figure 4–10.) This patient is escorted to the last room on the left for an examination. The doctor refers him to a neurologist and he stops at the desk for the appointment to be made by the receptionist.

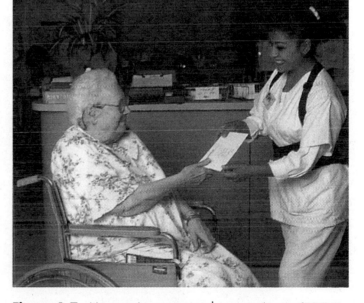

Figure 4-7 Many patients may need some assistance in getting around the facility carefully.

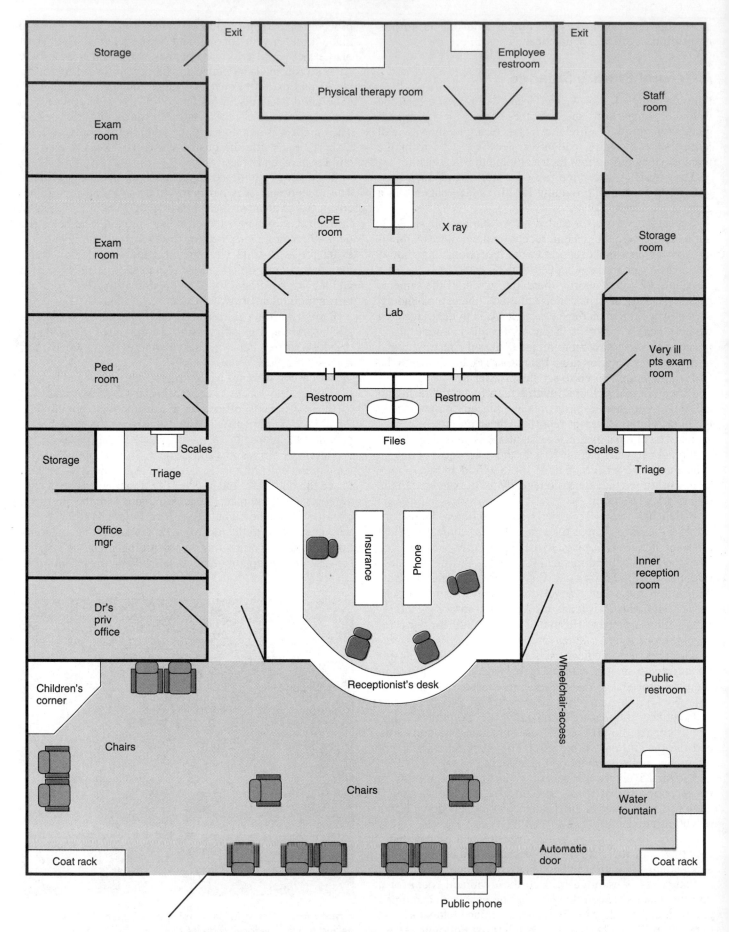

Figure 4–6 Trace the steps through this general practice facility to follow the efficient design in caring for patients.

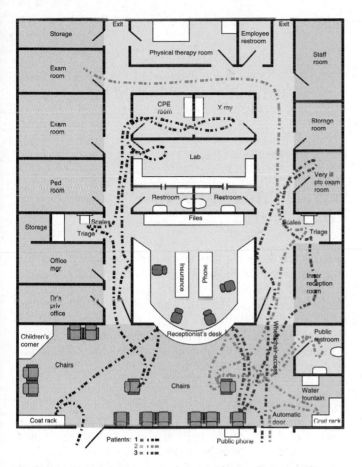

Figure 4–8 Patients 1, 2, and 3 are taken to the rooms for assessment and treatment as quickly as possible.

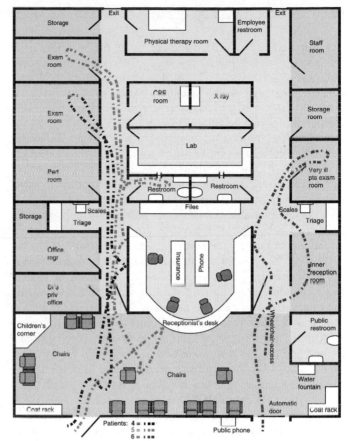

Figure 4–9 Patients 4, 5, and 6 are taken to be treated for their needs.

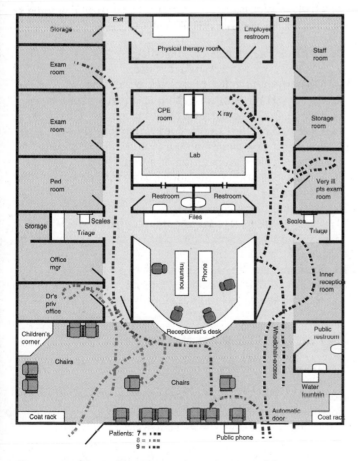

Figure 4–10 Patients 7, 8, and 9 are prepared for examination by the physician.

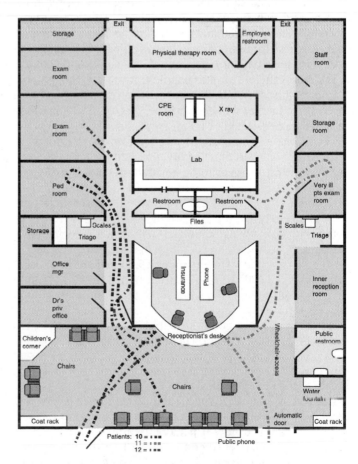

Figure 4–11 Patients 10, 11, and 12 are given necessary care.

Child patient #10 enters and reports at the reception desk that she is here for her allergy shot. The clinical medical assistant A-1 is notified. The child is brought in for the injection and requested to wait twenty minutes for observation. At the end of the time period, there are no problems noted and the patient leaves the office.

Patient #11 enters the waiting room and reports directly to the receptionist, complaining of nausea. Clinical medical assistant A-2 is notified immediately and calls the patient into the inner reception area through the door near the water fountain. The restroom is directly across from the reception area for the patients' convenience and comfort. The doctor sees this patient and he leaves.

Patient #12 enters the reception area and reports to the receptionist. The patient has a badly burned hand sustained at work the previous evening. The receptionist calls the patient to the window and begins obtaining information regarding the injury. Clinical medical assistant A-1 takes the patient to the exam/treatment room. (See Figure 4–11.)

And so on daily, until all patients are examined and treated and the business is settled.

As you follow the number patterns on the floor of the layout of the facility, you can see that most of the steps taken by both the patients and the staff are minimal. This is, of course, the goal of the designer for maximum efficiency. Infection control is more easily attained by keeping those who may be contagious in basically one area of the office. Necessary equipment and supplies should be within a few steps of where they will be used. Anticipation of needed supplies is an art and skill that needs to be **cultivated** by those who prepare patients to see the physician. This is most beneficial to the physician and the patient, as it saves time and reduces stress for both parties. Knowing what is or might be necessary for a patient *before* the physician sees the patient is the most efficient way to handle traffic flow. Sometimes, of course, this is not possible. Also, the office policy and protocol of the facility will certainly be a factor in whether procedures are performed or not.

Additionally, financial coverage of medical care must also be a consideration. Many procedures must be pre-authorized for payment to be ensured. Seeing as many patients as possible in a day will bring in the greatest amount of revenue. If the day's patient flow of the schedule gets backed up too often, it can result in a decline in the return of patients to the medical facility. Even though it is not the most pleasant thought, the consideration that medical practice is a business is a reality. Time is money, and patients in volume bring financial success to the office. When the flow of traffic goes well, so does the work force that contributes to this success. The old saying "in one door and out another brings more company" is a good thing in this arena. Having a person received in the reception area, entering an exam room for treatment, and then stopping at the appointment desk, settling payment, and exiting is a very efficient way to design traffic of the patient/staff flow.

As you continue to learn about medical assisting, you will be able to understand the effects of design layout in relation to patient care and how it personally affects your work. In Unit 4 of this chapter, ergonomics will be discussed. This topic is important because it will help you to realize the importance of the work environment in relation to yourself.

Complete Chapter 4, Unit 2 in the workbook to help you meet the objectives at the beginning of this unit and therefore achieve competency of this subject matter.

UNIT 3
Office Management Equipment

The medical assistant may be responsible for the operation of many pieces of business equipment in the process of performing administrative duties. A variety of office machines contribute to the efficiency of an office. Some are rather simple while others can be quite complicated, requiring specialized training and practice to master. This unit identifies a variety of equipment that would be found in a medical practice.

■ OBJECTIVES

Upon completion of the unit, meet the following terminal performance objectives by verifying knowledge of the facts and principles presented through oral and written communication at a level deemed competent, and demonstrate the specific behaviors as identified in the terminal performance objectives of the procedures, observing safety precautions in accordance with health care standards.

1. Demonstrate the use of a calculator.
2. Explain why a check writer is used.
3. Demonstrate the use of a check writer.
4. List seven types of material that often is photocopied.
5. Demonstrate the use of a copy machine.
6. Give two reasons why records are microfilmed.
7. Explain when dictation on a tape should be saved.
8. Demonstrate the operation of a transcriber.
9. Discuss the primary advantage of a word processor over a typewriter.
10. Define all the computer terms listed in the unit.
11. List four items known as computer hardware.
12. Explain why the backing up of computer data is necessary.
13. Demonstrate the basic operation of a computer.
14. Spell and define, using the glossary at the back of the text, all the words to know in this unit.

■ WORDS TO KNOW

acronym	microfilming
calculator	payee
computer	processor
dictation	programmed
electronic	software
hardware	technology
maintenance contract	transcription
microfiche	

A variety of machines and equipment is required to manage the business operation of a medical office. Large multi-physician offices and clinics have more employees and therefore require a greater number and larger capacity of equipment. Smaller offices and single physician practices will likely have less specialized equipment, concentrating on the essentials primarily due to costs and limited operating personnel. The following material discusses the types of common office management equipment found in a medical practice.

CALCULATOR OR ADDING MACHINE

There are many occasions when an accurate calculation of figures is necessary. Some examples are the totalling of charges when preparing a patient's statement, submitting an insurance claim for services rendered, preparation of banking deposits, and the reconciliation of a banking statement. The summation of the daily log of receipts and charges is easier and more accurate when calculating equipment is used. Of course, care must be taken to enter the figures accurately or the results will be incorrect. NOTE: when multiples of the same item are listed, it is often listed as a "single" cost, which must be mathematically converted to the total price. This is especially important when checking the accuracy of invoices for ordered items. If the **calculator** produces a hard copy, the entries can be easily reviewed. If it displays the amount digitally in the LED window, each entry can be viewed for accurate keying when entered, but it would be wise to also repeat the calculation to see if you get the same answer twice. A simple ten key calculator with a few additional function keys is adequate for general office management, Figure 4–12. Calculators are powered by various size batteries, electricity, or even light from the sun or a lightbulb. Some models can use either electricity or battery. The term "adding machine" was used before the era of electronics and refers to equipment that performs many of the same functions but is probably older, larger, and may operate manually without the aid of any power. Adding machines and printing

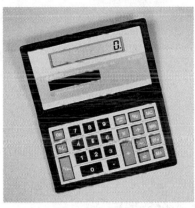

Figure 4–12
Calculator

calculators (Procedure 4–1) use a roll of narrow paper upon which the numbers are printed, similar to what you receive from the grocery store.

COPY MACHINE

The copy machine is extremely important to the efficiency of the office, Figure 4–13. A **photocopy** of a correspondence, an insurance form, a patient's record, laboratory reports, or account information is often needed (Procedure 4–2). Most machines can be set to use either letter or legal size paper. Frequently, prepared literature, information sheets, initial information forms, and so on will require copying. Newer models can produce color copies which greatly enhances information materials. Some offices may use the copier for monthly billing. The accounting record is copied, folded, and inserted into an envelope and mailed, thereby eliminating preparation of a separate statement. Remember, the copier is not for your personal use. Generally, if the equipment is owned, you will be permitted to make a few copies if necessary. Some machines are leased and have attached counters which record the number of times the camera flashes making copies. Offices are charged a rate reflective of their usage. With this arrangement, use of the

P R O C E D U R E

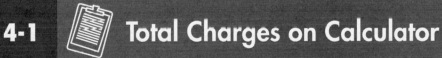

4-1 Total Charges on Calculator

PURPOSE: To accurately total and record a list of numbers using a calculator.

EQUIPMENT: Calculator, a list of 20 charges to be calculated, an invoice or ledger card, pen or pencil.

TERMINAL PERFORMANCE OBJECTIVE: Provided with necessary equipment and materials, calculate a list of 20 charges, performing any necessary mathematical functions, and correctly determine the total amount. The same correct answer must be obtained twice within a maximum of three attempts.

1. Turn on calculator.

2. Clear machine.
   Key Point: The digital display window or printed tape gives visual evidence that the machine is cleared.

3. Enter figures to be calculated and perform mathematical functions.

4. Total fees.

5. Double-check tape or refigure on digital display to be sure you get the same answer twice.

6. Record total.

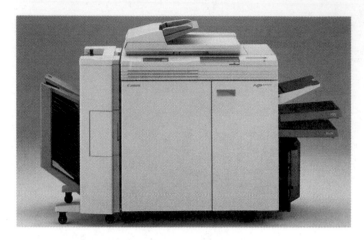

Figure 4–13 Copy machine.

copier is restricted. NOTE: Care should be taken to avoid copying material that carries a copyright protection, as this is considered illegal unless the permission to copy is obtained from the writer or publisher.

Routine maintenance will improve the quality of copies made. Offices should have service arrangements with suppliers of equipment and copy materials. Service representatives can demonstrate cleaning of the glass, feed rollers, and surfaces, and show you how to maintain the toner. Large copiers can be programmed to perform several functions such as enlarging or reducing copy size, stapling, sorting, off-set stacking, one- or two-sided copying, and insertion of cover sheets. A properly operating copier can produce a great variety of materials and is a valuable asset to the physician's office.

MICROFICHE

The medical assistant may need to be familiar with the microfilming process, Figure 4–14. Microfilming is a method of preserving material by reducing it to minute film images. **Microfilming** of office records can provide the necessary record security while using a minimum of storage space. The machine is easy to operate. The microfilmed documents may be read at any time with the use of a microfilm reader. In seconds, the reader–printer can provide a hard copy of **microfiche** material printed on plain bond paper.

You may find that some patients will present an insurance card that needs to be read with the help of a microfilm reader-printer, Figure 4–15.

P R O C E D U R E

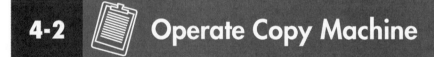

4-2 Operate Copy Machine

PURPOSE: To accurately prepare settings on a copy machine in order to produce a duplicate of the original in the size, number, and order desired.

EQUIPMENT: Copy machine, paper, and material to be copied.

TERMINAL PERFORMANCE OBJECTIVE: Given access to necessary equipment and supplies, demonstrate adjustment of settings in order to produce the specified copy or copies, while operating the copy machine accurately following the steps in the procedure.

1. Assemble material to be copied.

2. Determine number of copies needed.
   Rationale:
   a. **You usually make one file copy of every letter you send. If copies are to be sent with the letter, you need additional copies.**
   b. **Two copies of most medical legal reports are needed.**
   c. **If you are making copies of instruction sheets for patients, copy enough for a month's use at one time.**

3. Turn on copy machine.
   NOTE: Some offices leave the machine on all the time because it requires a warm-up period before it can be used. If this is not your office policy, turn the machine off when finished.

4. Adjust settings for what you want to copy.
   Note:
   a. **Legal or letter size paper.**
   b. **Regular copy/lighter/darker may be adjusted on some machines.**
   c. **Regular, reduced, or enlarged copy.**
   d. **Number of copies.**

5. Check paper supply.
   Rationale: Assure adequate supply. Some machines will jam when supply becomes too low. Also, check paper type. The last person using the copier may have used colored paper, a different size, or letterhead paper.

6. Raise lid and place material to be copied, one sheet at a time, face down on glass.
   NOTE: On self feeding models, place material on feeder tray. If more than one page, arrange in proper order.

7. Close lid.

8. Press button or key pad to activate copier.

9. Remove original(s) and copy/copies. Remove special paper, if used, from supply.

10. Return machine to "standard" settings if changed.

11. Turn off machine (if policy).

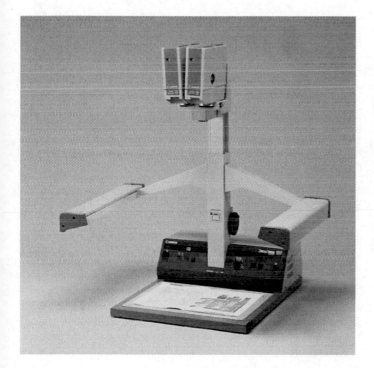

Figure 4–14   Microfilm machine (Courtesy of Canon, Inc.).

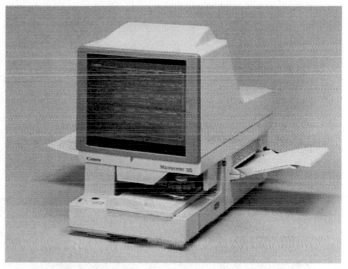

Figure 4–15   Microfilm reader-printer machine (Courtesy of Canon, Inc.).

DICTATION-TRANSCRIPTION MACHINE

The most common units to be used in the physician's office are the desktop machines, Figure 4–16. Several kinds of units are available: a unit for **dictation** only, a unit for **transcription** only, or a combination unit that can be used for both purposes. Many physicians use a portable dictating machine, which can be operated by battery or electricity. The physician may use this machine in the office, in the car, at home, or while attending meetings. The medical assistant can help the physician use the equipment more efficiently by tactfully discussing any problems encountered while transcribing. Tell the physician when the dictation is good. If you are experiencing difficulties due to dictation or mechanical reasons, explain precisely the problem and offer specific solutions. Sometimes a list of helpful hints to improve dictation and reduce the chance of error can be used to help both the physician and the transcriptionist. The list might include the following:

1. Check machine to be sure it is recording.
2. Indicate date and what is being dictated (chart note, letter, research paper, report, and so on).
3. Recognize that you are talking to a person through the machine.
4. Dictate the name of the patient and the name of the person or firm who will be the recipient of the message.
5. Dictate the street address, city, state, and zip code to which correspondence is to be sent and the number of copies needed.
6. Dictate punctuation such as "period," "comma," or "paragraph."
7. Encourage the physician to refrain from eating, drinking, or listening to loud music or television while the dictation is being done.

8. Speak in a normal clear voice.
9. End with an appropriate message to indicate the dictation is completed.

The machine which is carried out of the office must be kept in operating order at all times—you never know when the physician will put it to use. When it is in the office, check to be certain it is ready for use. Replace the batteries as needed and maintain a supply of erased tapes for reuse.

The transcription machine (Procedure 4–3) has a foot control that starts the machine. When the pedal is released the machine stops. It also has a backup pedal that allows you to relisten to the transcription if you need to hear it again before you transcribe. You will learn to press the pedal, listen, then begin typing the sentences with a minimum of time. With practice and speed, you may be able to type and listen almost simultaneously. The machine has controls for automatic rewind and fast forward. The speed control can be adjusted to either slow or speed up the voice message. The speed control should generally be adjusted for the normal voice quality for the physician making the dictation.

If you are using a standard typewriter, transcription presents an additional challenge since the typed copy cannot be viewed prior to printing as with word processing equipment. Because you cannot judge the length of the message when you begin, it may be advisable to run the tape to determine its content before typing. You may also need to make an initial rough draft copy, setting your margins, headings, and tabs later according to content involved.

WORD PROCESSORS

The word **processor** can be an electronic typewriter with the added features of fast daisy wheel printing, spelling checks, and spelling corrections similar to computer capabilities. These are equipped with insertable disk drive units for either line or add on screen display. This allows you to store text on a microfloppy disk for later use. They may also allow an auto-cut sheet feeder and tractor feeder to be added.

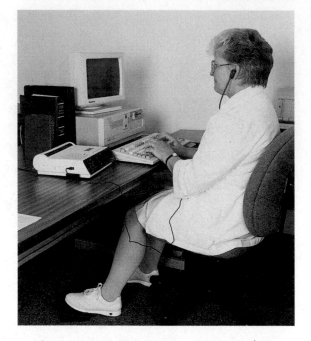

Figure 4–16 Dictation-transcription machine.

Word processing software is available on almost all desktop computers, Figure 4–17. These have functions such as automatic correction, adding or deleting words, centering, margin alignment, decimal tabs, column layout, automatic indent, and table features. Word processors offer special features such as word or single letter underline, boldface type, subscripts, and superscripts. Because you can visualize the copy on the screen and move words, lines, or paragraphs with special key functions, it is possible to proof the copy and to see a "print view" version on the screen BEFORE actually printing the document.

THE COMPUTER

In a text titled *Computer Fundamentals for an Information Age,* authors Shelly and Cashman define a computer as follows:

> A **computer** is an **electronic** device, operating under the control of instructions stored in its own memory unit, which can accept and store data, perform arithmetic and logical operations on that data without human intervention, and produce output from the processing.

PROCEDURE

4-3 Operate Transcriber

PURPOSE: To operate transcriber equipment in order to produce a printed copy from recorded material.

EQUIPMENT: Transcriber, dictation tape, headset, foot control, a typewriter, wordprocessor, or computer, and paper.

TERMINAL PERFORMANCE OBJECTIVES: Given access to equipment and supplies, operate the transcriber, correctly following all steps in the procedure. Complete an accurate transcription within a specified time period.

1. Turn on the transcriber.

2. Verify that headset with earphones and the foot control are attached to the unit.

3. Select tape.
   Rationale: Type rush reports or oldest dictation first.

4. Adjust headset with earphones. **NOTE: Earphones should not be shared. Rationale: Prevents the spread of organisms.**

5. Insert tape. Press play tab or the pedal to listen for the beginning of the dictation.

6. Listen for physician's instructions. **NOTE: The material to be typed will guide you in selecting the appropriate paper. It may be a chart note, a report, or a letter requiring letterhead paper.**

7. Adjust volume, tone, and speed controls for clearest communication reception.

8. Set typewriter or computer margins and tabulator stops.

9. Insert paper in typewriter or bring up blank screen on computer and type recorded information.

10. Alternately press and release foot pedal to listen and transcribe the recorded message. **NOTE: Consult a dictionary, if a word is unfamiliar. If you are unable to understand a word or words, leave a blank, note the place on the tape and ask someone else to listen. If necessary, ask the dictating physician for assistance so you can complete the work.**

11. Turn off the machine and place accessory items in proper storage space.

12. Save the dictation on the tape. **Rationale: In case questions should arise before the physician will approve the report or sign the letter.**

13. Erase tape following the report approval or signature of physician on letter, so it can be used again.

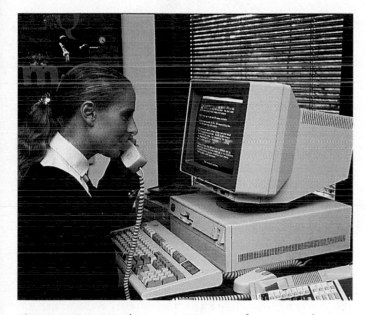

Figure 4-17 Word processor (Courtesy of International Business Machines Corporation).

Computers come in a variety of makes, styles, sizes, capacities, and price ranges. However, they all perform about the same way. Some can be carried like a small notebook, others are large, designated primary network machines. Many have the capacity to convey sound and some are capable of responding to voice commands. Computer **technology** advances so rapidly that those last two statements will seem outdated by the time this book is published. This device has changed the way information is processed and stored. An individual with computer skills can be a valuable employee. But, with technology constantly changing, it is necessary to update and learn new applications almost continuously. It would be wise to take every opportunity possible to acquire additional skills.

Physicians are aware of the advantages of using computers in the office. Large clinics often have direct-line insurance reporting by computer: the necessary information is **programmed** into the clinic computer and travels directly to the insurance company computers. This eliminates paper work, and the speed of processing claims is enhanced considerably.

Computer Terms

With the development of the computer came a whole new vocabulary of technical terms as well as new meanings for old words. In order to communicate with other users, it is important to understand and use the language. The following are some of the most commonly used terms relating to the computer and its components. Become familiar with them quickly.

- **backup**—duplicate of data files made to protect information. Records should be backed up daily. Some experts recommend twice daily.
- **batch**—an accumulation of data to be processed.

- **boot**—to start up a computer.
- **bug**—an error in a program.
- **catalog**—a list of files on the storage media.
- **CD-ROM**—Compact disk read only memory. The term which indicates the computer is capable of playing compact disks.
- **characters per second**—term used to measure printer output.
- **CPU**—central processing unit, or the brain of the system. The memory is made up of **bits.** A bit is a single **BI**nary digi**T.** *Binary* refers to a situation in which there are only two choices: for example, yes/no, on/off, pass/fail. Digit refers to a single number. A bit is either 0 or 1. A **byte** is the fundamental group of bits that a computer will treat as a word. A byte consists of 8 bits. A 16-bit processor is twice as fast as an 8-bit processor. One **K** is equal to 1,024 bytes. A 64-K computer can handle 65,536 bytes. The greater the number of bytes, the greater the memory.
- **cursor**—a marker on the screen that shows where the next letter, number, or symbol will be placed (may be an underline dash or a blinking rectangle or square).
- **data**—information that can be processed or produced by a computer.
- **debugging**—finding errors and correcting them in computer programs.
- **disk**—a magnetic storage device made of rigid material or flexible plastic (floppy disk).
- **disk drive**—the device used to get information on and off a disk.
- **DOS**—(Disk Operating System) a program that tells the computer how to use the disk drive.
- **dot matrix printer**—printer that uses dots to form letters and numbers.
- **downtime**—a period of lost work time during which a computer is not operating or is malfunctioning because of machine failure.
- **electronic mail**—the transmission of letters, messages, or memos from one computer to another over telephone lines.
- **external memory**—recording on floppy disks.
- **file**—a single, stored unit of information that is given a file name so it can be accessed.
- **font**—a family or assortment of characters of a given size or style.
- **GB**—gigabyte, approximately one billion (1,000,000,000) bytes. (1,073,741,824 bytes to be more exact.)
- **hard copy**—the readable paper copy or printout of information.
- **hardware**—the electronic, magnetic, and electromechanical equipment of a computer system (keyboard, disk drive, monitor, and printer).
- **initialize**—to prepare a diskette to receive data. This is usually referred to as *formatting* the disk.
- **input**—data processed from peripheral equipment into the machine via the keyboard or the floppy disk for internal storage.
- **interface**—the hardware and software that enable individual computers and components to interact.

- **K**—computer shorthand for 1,024 bytes; a term used to measure computer memory capacity.
- **keyboard**—an input device resembling a typewriter keyboard that converts keystrokes into electrical signals which are displayed on the screen as words or symbols.
- **kilobyte**—one thousand bytes.
- **main memory**—the internal memory of the computer.
- **MegaByte**—approximately one million (1,000,000) bytes. (1,048,576 bytes to be more exact.)
- **memory**—data held in storage.
- **menu**—a display of available machine functions for selection by the operator.
- **microcomputer**—a self-contained computer system that uses a microprocessor as the central processing unit. Often called a desktop or personal computer (also known as PC). Has limited capacity for internal memory.
- **microprocessor**—a single chip where the computer computes.
- **minicomputer**—a computer significantly smaller in size, capacity, and software capability than its larger mainframe counterparts.
- **modem**—**MO**dulator/**DEM**odulator. A peripheral device that enables a computer to communicate with other computers or terminals over normal telephone lines.
- **monitor**—visual display unit with a screen called a cathode-ray tube (CRT).
- **mouse**—a hand-held computer input device, separate from a keyboard, used to control cursor position on a VDT (video display terminal).
- **output**—what the computer produces after recorded information is processed, revised, and printed out.
- **peripheral**—anything you plug into a computer; for example, a printer, a disk drive, CRT terminal, or printer.
- **printer**—a device that produces hard copy. It may be dot matrix, letter quality, or laser.
- **program**—a set of instructions written in computer language.
- **prompting**—messages issued to a user requesting information necessary to continue processing.
- **RAM**—**acronym** for **R**andom **A**ccess **M**emory. This is temporary, or programmable memory. You can put new information into RAM. When you turn off the computer, this memory is gone.
- **ROM**—acronym for **R**ead **O**nly **M**emory. This is permanent memory. You cannot put new information into ROM. It has been determined by the computer manufacturer.
- **scrolling**—moving cursor up, down, right, or left through information on a computer display to view information otherwise not visible.
- **security code**—a code the operator must enter in before procedure may be completed. Used to prevent unauthorized access to data in system.
- **software**—computer programs necessary to direct the hardware of a computer system to perform specific tasks.
- **terminal**—a device used to communicate with a computer, usually a keyboard and monitor. Terminals depend on the main (host) computer for their abilities. An office may have several terminals and a host computer physically removed from any of them.
- **write-protect**—process or code that prevents overwriting of data or programs on a disk.

Input into a computer is by means of a keyboard very much like that on a typewriter. There are added keys to give you expanded capability. You do not need to be an expert on computer technology or programming to make good use of a computer.

Any computer, like a typewriter, will occasionally require service. When this becomes necessary, contact is made with the supplier's service department and arrangements are made. Usually, a faulty system component must be taken in for service. Large business central systems will be serviced on site.

When discussing computers, reference is made to hardware and software. The **hardware** refers to the hard disk drive, the CPU, the monitor, and the keyboard. **Software** is the programs containing instructions to the computer that enable it to perform tasks. You interact with the software to produce correspondence, maintain records, calculate financial statements, and many other tasks. Software is available on disks to be transferred to the computer's hard drive. A great deal of software is now available on CD-ROM. When you input data with a software program, you can enter it into the memory and store it on the hard drive or on a floppy disk inserted into the disk drive. Floppy disks are usually covered with hard plastic and are 3½". This hard type is preferred and more durable. Figure 4–18 provides guidelines for handling floppy disks. Disks come in different capacities and densities to match different hardware.

The information stored on a disk is called a *file*. It is necessary to assign a code to information to be saved on a file so that it may be *called up* from the storage disk by using the code. Computer manufacturers usually provide basic software programs that are compatible with the hardware. Many companies design special programs of software for use with specific computers. A computer is useless without the software instructions for accessing and inputting data.

The main storage component for a computer is its hard drive, an oxide-coated metal platter that is sealed inside a housing to ensure dust-free operation. The hard drive can store enormous amounts of information which can be retrieved almost immediately. PCs store their software programs as well as input data on their hard drive. In offices with several work stations, the individual computer or terminals can be networked with a service or mainframe computer. This central unit will contain the software programs and the data banks of information to be shared in the office. Each terminal can access information from the central computer, thereby freeing up hard drive space at each work station. A properly networked system permits input and updating of records from all stations and allows the information to be accessed from all stations.

Electrical surges and power outages can destroy information currently being used by the computer if it has not yet been saved by the operator or automatically by the program. This is most likely to occur during a severe storm. Loss of data due to electrical surges and power outages can be pre-

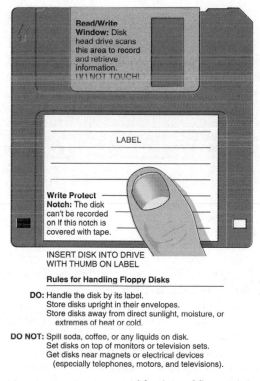

Figure 4–18 Care and feeding of floppy disk.

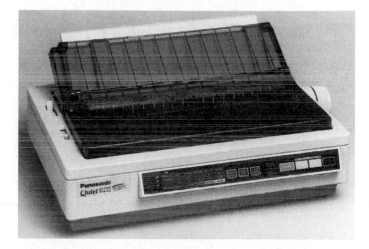

Figure 4–19 Dot matrix printer (Courtesy of Panasonic Communications & Systems Co.).

vented by the installation of a protective device known as an Uninterrupted Power Supply (UPS), which contains a battery backup system. UPS is capable of sensing a surge or outage, and automatically switches to a backup battery to preserve the data. The size of the battery determines the length of time the equipment can be sustained. The prime purpose is to allow you time to save your document, exit the program, and shut down your system until the power is again stable.

It is very important to establish a "backup policy" to make copies of office programs and data. Often this is performed each night. Data on the hard drives of individual PCs can be copied onto floppy disks if the data is not too extensive. Computer hard drives can "crash," causing the loss of all programs and stored data. Programs and extensive data can be copied by a tape backup device which is a peripheral to the computer, thereby providing a durable copy of information. All central computer data should be backed up on tape daily. Some offices may even contract to have materials backed up in an off-site facility in order to protect against loss of files from fire or natural disaster.

COMPUTER PRINTERS

To produce hard copy, you must have a printer. Printers may be equipped with a single-sheet feeder or a tractor feeder that automatically advances the paper. Three types of printers are appropriate for a medical office: dot matrix, ink-jet, or laser. The dot matrix, Figure 4–19 produces print made up of pin-head dots and can produce "near letter quality" printing. Depending on the type of printer you have, you may set "draft mode," and the printer will print more than twice as fast as it will on letter quality. For example, one popular

model prints 180 characters per second in draft mode and sixty characters per second in letter quality. The print wheel in most cases will be bidirectional (prints from left to right and right to left) as this offers more speed. The letter-quality printers may have many print styles built in, and more can be loaded into the printer. Ink-jet printers produce letter quality copy by "spraying" letters onto the paper. A variety of type fonts allow great variation of print styles and many interesting features can be added to your office's print communications.

Laser printers are more expensive but the print quality is comparable to typeset material. A toner cartridge inside the printer contains the printer's powered "ink" material which produces the type or graphic images. The cartridge will last for approximately 4000 pages of text. The laser can also have postscript capability which allows infusion of many graphic applications to customize office correspondence, patient information sheets, reports, and professional papers, Figure 4–20.

USE OF COMPUTER SOFTWARE

Computer software capabilities are virtually limitless. Software companies are continually designing programs that make it possible to direct a computer to produce different prescribed outcomes. It takes anywhere from twelve to twenty-four months to research, write, and test a comprehensive software program. When the project is begun, the newest technology is used. By the time the project is completed and fully tested, the newest technology is now two years or more outdated. It is important to keep this in mind if you are in a position to recommend use of specific software.

Medical management software is available from many different companies. An example is the MEDWARE program available from Computer Solutions. The software programs make it possible to keep patient information with no limit to the number of patients except the capacity of the computer memory. It provides information needed for billing such as primary and secondary insurance. It is easy to look

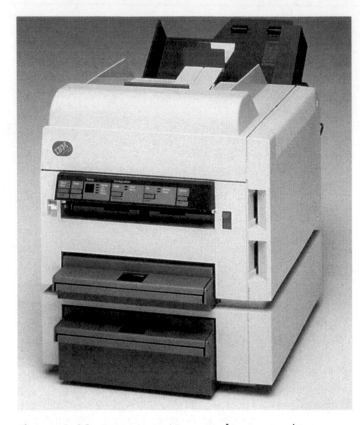

Figure 4–20   Laser printer (Courtesy of International Business Machines Corporation).

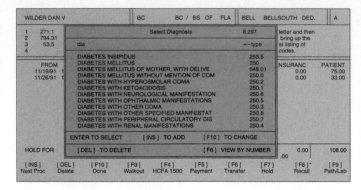

Figure 4–21   Diagnosis and procedure codes may be quickly called up alphabetically or numerically (Courtesy of Computer Solutions, New Smyma, FL).

up patient treatment or payment history, print patient mailing labels, phone listings, or set up a recall/reminder system.

The number of procedure and diagnosis codes that may be entered is limitless, Figure 4–21. The codes may be searched by number or by description.

The computer program allows all posting charges and payments to be completed. The input screen is modeled from the standard insurance form (HCFA-1500), Figure 4–22. The program allows the medical assistant to input the necessary information and then push one key to print a completed insurance form. The information in the computer may be retrieved at any time.

Reports can be prepared with a minimum of effort when data is regularly put into the computer. Accounts receivable

may be printed by date or aging, or alphabetically. Accounts receivable may be broken down between insurance company and patient. A detailed summary of income between two given dates may be easily prepared. The report of charges between any two dates may be accessed in detail or summary. A day sheet can be easily prepared. Physicians may find a need for a statistical report of diagnosis and procedure code usage, which can be retrieved from the stored data. Reports can also be sorted and output by individual patient, physician or insurance company.

Figure 4–23 shows a new patient entry screen. This screen provides for the entry of account information for each patient or family group. All the data needed to properly bill the account are included. Note the ability to enter aged balance information for each account. This means that you can begin your computerized system with all accounts properly aged.

Figure 4–24 illustrates the daily transactions entry screen. This is where all charge entries are done, as well as the entries for payments made at the time of service. Up to five entries may be made on each screen. During charge entry, a running total of the account is displayed at all times. When you have finished making entries for the patient, the account updates

Figure 4–22   Screen modeled on the HCFA-1500 layout (Courtesy of Computer Solutions, New Smyma, FL).

Figure 4–23   New patient entry screen (Courtesy of Artificial Intelligence, Inc., Renton, WA).

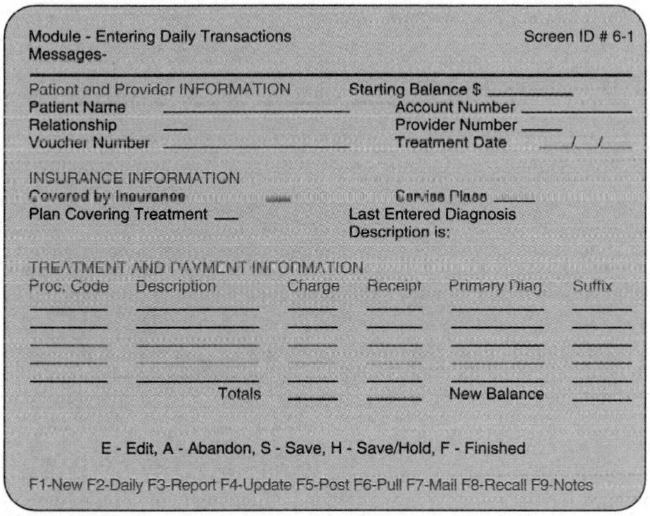

```
Module - Entering Daily Transactions                    Screen ID # 6-1
Messages-

Patient and Provider INFORMATION        Starting Balance $ _____
Patient Name      _____            Account Number _____
Relationship      ___                   Provider Number _____
Voucher Number    _____            Treatment Date    __/__/

INSURANCE INFORMATION
Covered by Insurance     ___            Service Place _____
Plan Covering Treatment ___             Last Entered Diagnosis
                                        Description is:

TREATMENT AND PAYMENT INFORMATION
Proc. Code  Description   Charge   Receipt   Primary Diag   Suffix
  ___        ___           ___      ___        ___           ___
  ___        ___           ___      ___        ___           ___
  ___        ___           ___      ___        ___           ___

              Totals       ___      ___      New Balance     ___

        E - Edit, A - Abandon, S - Save, H - Save/Hold, F - Finished

F1-New F2-Daily F3-Report F4-Update F5-Post F6-Pull F7-Mail F8-Recall F9-Notes
```

Figure 4–24 Daily transactions entry screen (Courtesy of Artificial Intelligence, Inc., Renton, WA).

immediately. When you have finished your entries for each patient, you will be given the option of printing an insurance claim form, a patient statement, or both. Prompt billing of patients means faster payment, and efficient, accurate submission of claims means a higher payment ratio.

Figure 4–25 is an example of a medical office daily transactions report which shows charges and receipts for daily records.

Figure 4–26 is an example of a utility menu screen. This screen gives you access to all the functions that let you set up and maintain the custom files to be used by the system,

establish the format for your custom forms, and do the maintenance work to keep your system running efficiently. Among the files set up in utility code are the procedure codes, diagnosis codes, provider, insurance company, hospital, and referring doctor. Once these files are established, the data in them is a keystroke away when the system is in use. For additional information on computer billing see Chapter 8, Unit 4.

These illustrations of computer screens are only a sampling of the many office procedures possible with computers. It is important to note that many of the software manufacturers make programs which are compatible with more than one brand of computer. Many of the software systems run on IBM® computers. MAI Systems Corporation has developed its own computer and the software for medical offices. Healthcare Communications™ makes software exclusively for Macintosh™ SE.

Some believe that in the future it will be common practice to use a hand-held scanner (like those used in department stores) to scan the bar code on the patient charge slip and thus automatically enter the code number of the procedure or illness and the charge for service. This would eliminate the possibility of error in typing the figures into the computer.

The computer should be useful for inventory control of office supplies, to personalize form letter mailings for collections, to reschedule annual checkups, and to gather research data.

Some physicians find the computer essential if they are engaged in research and need to quickly identify all patients with a specific diagnosis. It is also valuable in the quick identification of patients taking a particular drug if the manufacturer should issue a warning about side effects.

DAILY CHARGES AND RECEIPTS REPORT - Thur March 8, 1990

Mode of operation - Daily data only

Page 1

DATE	ACCNT #	ACCOUNT NAME	PAT NAME/ PMT. SOURCE	DOCTOR	PROC	DIAG	VOUCHER	CHARGES	RECEIPTS	TODAYS BALANCE	BILLED P	I	INS
03/08/90	2	Brown	Rachael	1	82996	V22.2	2	$18.00	$0.00	$134.00	N	N	Y
03/08/90	4	Gonzales	Joseph	1	93000	785.1	1	$36.00	$0.00	$36.00	N	N	Y
03/08/90	6	O'Brien	Janet	1	85022	285.9	3	$23.00	$23.00	$75.00	N	N	N
03/08/90	9	Williams	Ryan	1	90071	780.7	7	$44.00	$0.00	$144.00	N	N	Y
03/08/90	1	Takamoto	Credit Adj.	1	MO2		5	–$18.00	$0.00	$78.00	N	N	Y
03/08/90	10	Young	David	2	73090	848.9	6	$54.00	$54.00	$0.00	N	N	N
03/08/90	15	Anderson	Nancy	1	86300	075	4	$18.00	$0.00	$62.00	N	N	Y
03/08/90	12	Lightfoot	James	2	92551	389.9	8	$36.00	$0.00	$36.00	N	N	Y
03/08/90	11	Roberts	Debit Adj.	1	MO1		9	$0.00	–$25.00	$75.00	N	N	N
03/08/90	13	Paulson	Jon	2	95000	477.9	10	$44.00	$0.00	$144.00	N	N	Y
03/08/90	14	Bond	PAYMENT	1	M91		11	$0.00	$75.00	$200.00	N	N	Y

| | | | | | | | | $255.00 | $127.00 | | | | |

TOTALS
Total interest included in Charges $0.00
Total Debit Adjustments   - $25.00
Total credit Adjustments   - $18.00
Mode of operation - Daily data only

Figure 4–25 Daily transactions report (Courtesy of Artificial Intelligence, Inc., Renton, WA).

Module - PAS-3 PLUS Utility Module   Screen ID # 11-1
Message -

THE FOLLOWING REPORTS ARE AVAILABLE

1 - Procedure Codes
2 - Diagnosis Codes
3 - Copy of Files to Backup Disk
4 - Delete Patient Record
5 - Reconstruct Hash/Key Tables
6 - Selective Activity Purge
7 - Move Record to Inactive Disk
8 - Change Billing Forms Format
9 - Set Up Practice Data Files
10 - File Checker
11 - Reclaim Backup Files
12 - Sort Procedure/Diag/Key Code File
13 - Split the Disk

14 - Enable Rebill Insurance/Patient
15 - Create and Add Records to Files
16 - Provider Files
17 - Unlock All Files
18 - Insurance Company File
19 - Hospital/Facility Files
20 - Referring Doctors File
21 - Encounter Form Setup
22 - Dunning Messages Establish
23 - Change Insurance Forms Format
24 - Relationship Cross Reference
25 - Format User Defined Data Screen
26 - Format Third Party Billing Forms

Warning Do not Run Utility options while another terminal is using files.

Enter number of option wanted ____

F1-New F2-Daily F3-Report F4-Update F5-Post F6-Pull F7-Mail F8-Recall F9-Notes

Figure 4–26 Utility menu (Courtesy of Artificial Intelligence, Inc., Renton, WA).

You may be involved in the use of a computer for patient education. This is similar to the television programs used by some offices. The medical assistant may load the programs into the computer, discuss with patients what they will see, and ascertain whether patients have further concerns after they complete the viewing. Information programs have been developed for diabetes, cancer, pregnancy, health hazards of smoking, and many other conditions.

Most word processing software has a standard built-in dictionary that helps with spelling. Misspelled words are highlighted when the spell-check is activated. You still must read carefully to be sure you typed the correct words for the message you wish to convey. You must be accurate in your proofreading. Medical dictionaries are also available as enhancements to the standard dictionary.

Continuous letterheads and new continuous envelopes make your work much faster. There is no need for a typewriter to address envelopes.

You have learned in this unit that using computers in medical offices can be extremely important in helping to complete your work. You should use any opportunity you have to practice with the computer. You should learn the vocabulary and how to read and understand an instruction manual. You need to practice on a typewriter if a computer is not available so that you will have accurate keyboarding skills.

All computer systems and word processors have instructions to help you utilize the equipment. Some are in

P R O C E D U R E

4-4   Operate Office Computer

PURPOSE: To operate a computer system in order to enter, revise, delete, save data, and print a hard copy of document.

EQUIPMENT: Computer, peripherals, printer paper, prepared material to be entered.
(Suggest a list of 12 "patient" names to be scheduled from 1:00-3:00 PM on an electronic appointment sheet)

TERMINAL PERFORMANCE OBJECTIVE: Given access to equipment and material to be entered, operate system following steps in the procedure to produce an accurate print copy of a schedule.
NOTE: This exercise is generic, loosely based on Word Perfect . . . specific steps must be performed as required by available software and computer system.

1. Turn on power to computer
2. Position cursor on appropriate program on main menu, key ENTER or click mouse
3. Position cursor on scheduling software program, key ENTER or click mouse
4. Locate cursor or click on first cell to be completed
5. Enter 1:00 PM appointment for first patient on list
6. Enter remaining names at 15 minute intervals

7. SAVE data
   NOTE: If input is not saved, it will be lost when computer is turned off. Some programs save automatically at intervals. Others will save data as part of the EXIT process.
8. Exit scheduling program to main menu
9. Exit from main menu
10. Re-enter main menu
11. Bring up scheduling software
12. Locate cursor at 2:30, enter patient as work-in who is currently scheduled for 1:30
13. Locate cursor at 1:30, cancel appointment
14. Scroll through schedule to view and proofread
15. Turn on printer, allow time for test sheet, if appropriate
16. Check paper supply
17. Key or click on PRINT
18. Select from available options
19. PRINT document
20. Exit program
21. Exit Main Menu and system
22. Turn off power to printer and computer

the form of books, known as documentation, which are helpful references for both beginners and experienced operators. With large programs requiring much information, it will probably be available on-line or on a CD which can be easily accessed from your screen. Most computer dealers offer basic training with the purchase of new equipment and provide "pay for instruction" classes on the use of specific software applications for the general public. Many public schools and community colleges provide adult education classes which are very beneficial. Procedure 4–4 discusses operation of the office computer.

IMPORTANT STEPS IN SELECTING A COMPUTER SYSTEM

The medical assistant employed in the office planning to consider automation with computers will be able to look forward to the experience if there is an opportunity to take part in the planning.

It is important to research the kinds of software available, the kinds of computers the software can be used with, the costs, how long the supplier has been in business, and the kinds of support offered after installation.

A good source for this information is *The Computer Talk Directory of Medical Computer Systems,* which is published semiannually by:

Computer Talk Associates, Inc.
482 Norristown Road, Suite 112
Blue Bell, PA 19422
(610) 825-7686

There are hidden costs to consider. It will be necessary to provide electrical outlets at the areas where the computer terminals and printers will be located. The office will need desk space for both computers and printers. A **maintenance contract** should be available. Investigate the costs and availability of insurance to cover theft, natural disasters such as a tornado, and internal disasters such as fire or flood damage. Determine the availability and cost of a consultant to supervise the training of the office staff.

It is always important to obtain cost estimates from at least three companies. The companies should also refer you to current users to help you determine the reliability of the software and hardware. Find out if the software company can furnish new formats when needed.

When the physicians decide what they want to accomplish with the system and the costs have been obtained, a decision must be made as to whether the return will justify the cost.

If the determination is made, the first task is to select software that will meet the needs of the office. It should meet the needs of the office in word processing, accounting and office management, and should permit a database for research. The software can then be matched with a compatible computer system.

Complete Chapter 4, Unit 3 in the workbook to help you meet the objectives at the beginning of this unit and therefore achieve competency of the subject matter.

UNIT 4
Ergonomics in the Office

▮ OBJECTIVES

Upon completion of the unit, meet the following terminal performance objectives by verifying knowledge of the facts and principles presented through oral and written communication at a level deemed competent.

1. Discuss ergonomics as it relates to the medical office.
2. Explain the reasons for and the importance of including ergonomics in planning for any facility.
3. List the main concerns for employment sites regarding ergonomics.
4. Discuss the use of light and color in regard to the medical office.
5. List ways to prevent problems related to repeated use of computers and VDTs.
6. Explain the importance of adjustable components at a work station.
7. Describe the relation between proper back support and posture.
8. Discuss the importance of noise control.
9. Spell and define, using the glossary in the back of the text, all the words to know in this unit.

▮ WORDS TO KNOW

aesthetic	ergonomics
amenity	evoke
carpal tunnel syndrome	glare screen
(CTS)	ocular accommodation
controversial	precise
cumulative trauma disorder	renovate
(CTD)	video display terminal
discipline	(VTD)

THE SCIENCE OF ERGONOMICS

Ergonomics has finally come to the forefront of the workplace in the '90s even though this science has been around for over fifty years. Its origin was during World War II when attention to the success of pilots was vital to the outcome of the war. In order to make the duties of the pilots as effective as possible, a team of designers and planners were called upon to determine the detailed changes that had to be made to make the pilot's job easier and more **precise** and therefore improve performance.

This scientific **discipline** continues to advance and is becoming very highly technical regarding the well-being, safety, and productivity of employees. A 1994 poster from the Division of Safety & Hygiene in cooperation with the Society of Ohio Safety Engineers states, **"Make Sure that Your Job Fits You . . . Ergonomics is the answer."** The picture that goes along with this statement shows a male blue collar worker in uniform being measured for the job with a tape measure by a seamstress. There is another male worker in the background wearing safety glasses at a work station sitting on a chair that is of comfortable height for his job. The picture **evokes** thought regarding the purpose of ergonomics. Ergonomics is the applied science of being concerned with the nature and characteristics of people as they relate to design and activities with the intention of producing more effective results and greater safety. In industry in general this science applies to both the workers and the products that are produced.

Research has shown that in order for humans to be productive and efficient in the workplace, the health and safety of employees is a primary concern. In another definition the science of ergonomics also includes study and analysis of human work as it is affected by individual anatomy, psychology, and other human factors. Attention is also geared to convenience and comfort. This science also includes the skills and abilities of workers as well as their shortcomings. In the field of medicine, for the most part, employees are by nature interested in the well-being of others. So it is fitting that those who care for others should first have their own health and safety assured as they provide services to others.

All of us require the same basic physical needs: oxygen, food, water, and protection. As you will study, these basic needs must be met before other needs and desires can be realized. These basics satisfy our human needs and make it possible for us to share feelings and care for ourselves and others.

In a service based business such as the medical profession, the number of persons necessary for an efficient patient flow that brings in steady income varies from facility to facility. There are those offices or clinics where it seems that there are so many employees that they are tripping over each other, yet they are always behind schedule, while other offices are understaffed yet have the same problem. The fault may be more complex than one may realize at first glance.

THE ERGONOMIC DESIGN OF A MEDICAL FACILITY

Often, the inefficiency of the staff lies in the design of the facility. If the planners were not aware of the nature of the business that was to take place there, the problem may never be completely solved. Some medical practices are moved into an office space where another type of business totally unrelated to medicine previously resided. Valiant attempts are made to **renovate** the facility to accommodate a productive practice. However, many spaces are just not easily adapted and do not accommodate the practice of medicine efficiently. Sometimes the answer may be to bring in an efficiency consultant who will observe for a day or longer (depending on how complex the problem seems to be) in order to determine what needs to be done. An outsider is always more objective and will see more readily any trouble areas that need attention. A medical facility that has a goal of treating ambulatory patients must have an efficient traffic pattern so that there is only a minimal waiting time for each patient.

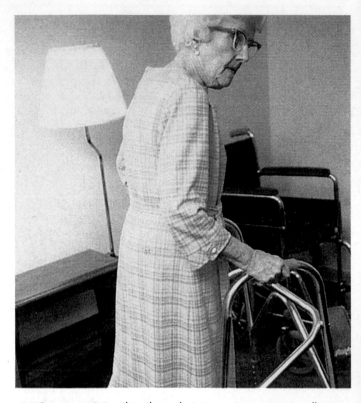

Figure 4–27 This photo shows a patient using a walker.

Another consideration is that the office must be easily accessible to all persons who may visit, Figure 4–27.

CONSIDERATIONS IN MEDICAL FACILITY LAYOUT AND DESIGN

Among the many considerations that need to be studied for an ergonomically sound workplace are:

- original floor plan or blueprint; layout
- connecting hallways/walkways
- actual room space
- environmental factors
- lighting
- acoustics
- decor
- adaptability
- psychology/human factors

This includes a vast array of considerations, of which discussion follows.

Layout

Since the layout of a facility is the basis for the list of complex considerations, its importance cannot be overstated. The layout determines the available space and traffic pattern. Most people—medical personnel in this instance—seem to adapt to just about any situation. Even though space *does* limit work in some ways, there is flexibility with employees. Most people adapt to most situations and do the best they can with what they are given and establish a comfortable routine.

Hallways and Walkways

In any public facility, access for the physically challenged in entering and exiting the premises is a federal mandate. The walkways from the parking lot and hallways into the office must always be clear for safe passage. Ramps for wheelchairs are required wherever necessary. Within the office, aisles must be wide enough to allow a wheelchair clear passage without blocking the path of others. This applies to visitors and employees alike. If there are stairways connecting floors, an elevator must be available for those who are unable to climb stairs. This applies to all patients (and employees) who have various conditions (physical limitations or medical disabilities) which would prevent them from using the stairs. Assistance animals (usually well-trained dogs) must be permitted on the premises to attend to their dependent owners.

Actual Room Space

The actual space of each room should be proportionate to the purpose of the room. In existing buildings, adaptation for the ideal in efficiency is not always possible. The reception area needs to be large enough to accommodate several people at a time. Also, many offices and clinics have many physicians on staff which yields to an increase in the number of people at any given time being present in the reception area. Overcrowded rooms, especially in the medical office setting, can be harmful to those who are not seriously ill when they are exposed unnecessarily to those who are. Having access to a public rest room is a convenience as well as a necessity for patients who are ill. A drinking fountain and a public telephone are also public service **amenities**.

Environmental Factors

The room temperature of a facility is one of the most critical of all environmental factors. This alone can affect work performance and change one's attitude drastically if it is uncomfortably hot or cold. Proper ventilation is also necessary, but drafts should be avoided. The use of window coverings may be necessary to keep out direct sunlight which could also be the cause of overheating.

Another consideration to the environment is the presence of foul odors. Keeping the office clear of trash and other messes will help to control this problem. Daily cleaning and routine "in-depth cleaning" will control odors and eliminate the possibility of potential pests. In the event of an unwanted odor, a room freshener spray may be used. A citrus scent is fresh smelling and will help diminish the offensive odor quickly (avoid spraying directly at persons who are seated). Odors may also signal a problem with overheating of equipment, chemical leaks, or other serious potential health hazards. A quick response to any such odor is critical to the health and safety of all present.

Lighting

The ideal in making a room bright is accomplished with the use of both electrical and natural lighting. Since some facilities have no windows to allow for natural light, this presents a challenge in obtaining an adequate amount of light. Fluorescent lighting is usually the choice because it is the most cost effective, even though natural lighting is the best. In offices where it is possible, skylights are popular. This can improve mood and behavior because it gives one a feeling of being open and light. Many facilities make use of indirect lighting, lamps, and overhead lights in a variety of ways to provide light for a particular need and/or as an aspect of the interior decorating. The avoidance of glare is advised with all lighting as it can impair one's vision and is uncomfortable as well. Mirrors and wall hangings, in addition to wall coverings, must be included in the assessment of lighting and glare capabilities for any room. Reflections from a metallic print wallpaper can be very annoying. NOTE: A safety factor that must have constant attention is the lighting of hallways, doorways, and stairways. The facility should also call attention to all exits. Accidents can be prevented by supplying proper lighting and by regularly checking to assure this is maintained.

Computer Lighting   For those who work with computers on a routine basis, a **glare screen** should be used. The monitor or **video display terminal (VDT)** should be positioned to prevent excess glare, Figure 4–28. The operator must also have eye examinations and vision screening on a regular basis to stay on top of any difficulties that may develop. A frequent exercise for computer operators is to look into the distance away from the computer to prevent **ocular accommodation** which can cause headaches and blurring of vision. Lubricating eye drops may also be helpful to prevent dry, itchy eyes. To prevent conditions of **cumulative trauma disorder (CTD)** and **carpal tunnel syndrome (CTS)**, ergonomists recommend that computer operators work with a

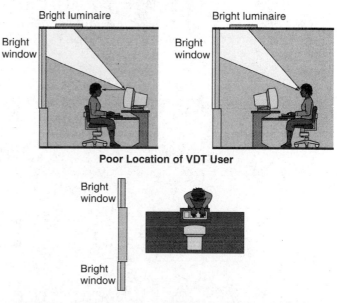

Poor Location of VDT User

Good Location of VDT User (Sight line parallel to window)

Figure 4–28 The positioning of the VDT properly will prevent glare from incoming light from windows and artificial lights in the room.

special keyboard, Figure 4–29. A wrist support for standard keyboards can also prevent these problems, Figure 4–30. Using a vertical document holder that is either free standing or attached to a flexible equipment arm helps to diminish eye strain and promotes good posture, Figure 4–31. Those who must sit for long periods of time should stand, stretch, and move about periodically in order to relax muscles and increase circulation. Planning the work load so that there is a balance of keying, telephone communications, preparing documents, and filing will prevent slumps. This varied schedule of duties also helps to stay mentally alert.

Acoustics

Equally as important for the comfort and well-being of others is attention to the acoustics in a facility. Noise can be kept to a moderate level with the use of fabrics: furniture, carpet, drapes, and other items can absorb sound. A soft, general medley of instrumental-type music can be comforting and relaxing for employees and patients alike. Background music can help eliminate the silence that makes some people uncomfortable. It also can be a deterrent to keep patients in the waiting room from listening to the receptionist's conversations on the phone and with those who speak to him/her at the window. The music selected can be varied but not too loud (under fifty to sixty decibels), as it could be offensive to some patients. Loud noise can be very stressful and can

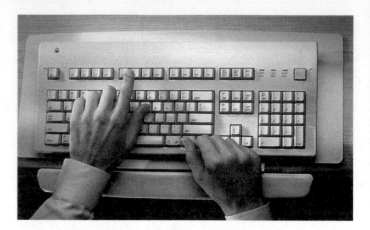

Figure 4–30 Wrist support (Courtesy of Details, a subsidiary of Steelcase, Inc.).

evoke a variety of emotions and possibly hearing loss if it is over ninety decibels for long periods (hours) of time. The same concerns apply to televisions in the reception area. A channel that is positive and uplifting is more acceptable to those waiting. There are some offices that use the television set in the reception area for patient education. Videos that inform patients about the latest in medical news or about diet and exercise, or other valuable information can be very helpful in increasing the knowledge of those in the care of the physician. Educational videos can also be helpful in keeping those waiting from arguing over what to watch. Also, in very large medical centers, there are often water fountains that

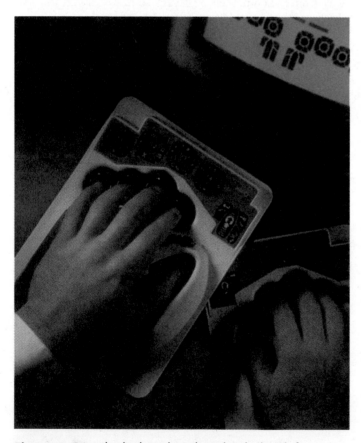

Figure 4–29 This keyboard is adapted to the hands for a natural position that is ergonomically correct (DataHand Systems, Inc.).

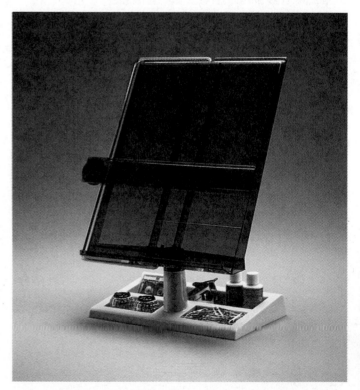

Figure 4–31 Vertical document holder (Courtesy of Eldon-Rubbermaid Office Products).

produce a very favorable sound called "pink noise" from the water falling.

Decor

The decor of the facility is vitally important, as it is the first impression a person processes when entering the office. The environment should be bright and fresh to look at because this subconsciously begins to set the tone of one's attitude. Employees who are in the facility daily should have not only safe but pleasant surroundings for their well-being, too. The decor can have a psychological impact in keeping a positive outlook. In a facility where colors and lighting are dark and sparse, those employed and those who visit may experience a feeling of sadness or depression upon entering and also lose interest in activity. Where light colors are used with soft, but adequate lights, one gets a feeling of comfort and warmth from the surroundings. Everyone feels more positive and energetic in bright and colorful rooms. Use of greenery and plants (either live or artificial) give a nice touch, as do aquariums, remember, though, that they need regular care and/or replacement as necessary for **aesthetic** purposes.

Adaptability

Adaptability of an office is also of critical concern. For employees to efficiently perform their duties, the facility should yield a pattern of fluid workability. This includes adequate space for performing all necessary functions in the most efficient way possible. Figure 4–32 provides an example of a work station for an administrative medical assistant who has a variety of duties to perform daily. Making each job as easy and efficient as possible for optimum use of time and space is the goal of ergonomics. For those who sit most of the day at work, proper seating is necessary in order to avoid back and other work-related conditions. Figure 4–33 shows the effects of one's posture while standing and sitting in two different types of chairs. An adjustable chair is desirable for comfort and support of the back. A footrest may also be helpful in promoting good posture, Figure 4–34.

Patients and other visitors will easily find their way around the facility if thought has been given to their needs regarding the most frequently used areas. This includes rest rooms, a drinking fountain, seating, reading materials, and so on. If those who are providing health care to patients can easily perform their duties, there is a feeling of confidence among those present. Employees who do not constantly have to back-track and bump into others can become efficient and feel good about accomplishments. In a crowded facility where steps are repeated and someone is always in the way, levels of frustration mount quickly.

Psychological/Human Factors

With all considerations for an ergonomically sound workplace, the psychological aspect is by far the most critical. Getting along with others is the single most important factor in employability. Outlining the various areas of concern for the philosophy of ergonomics is the basis for good working relationships. Having one of these areas altered can trigger a potential problem. Careful consideration to all areas is necessary for a smoothly run office and for good public relations to progress.

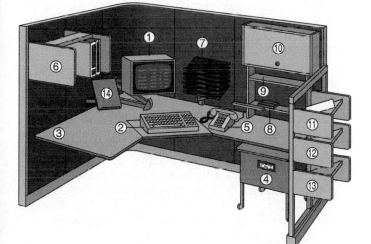

1. Video display terminal
2. Keyboard
3. Primary workstation area
4. Files storage
5. Telephone
6. Storage for procedures manuals and equipment
7. Forms caddy
8. Pens/pencils caddy
9. Additional supplies storage
10. Personal storage
11. In basket
12. Out basket
13. Additional basket
14. Document holder

Figure 4–32 In this workstation, all of the components can be adjusted to fit an individual's needs of safety and comfort to promote productivity.

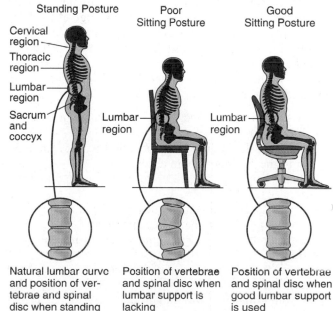

Standing Posture

Cervical region
Thoracic region
Lumbar region
Sacrum and coccyx

Poor Sitting Posture

Lumbar region

Good Sitting Posture

Lumbar region

Natural lumbar curve and position of vertebrae and spinal disc when standing

Position of vertebrae and spinal disc when lumbar support is lacking

Position of vertebrae and spinal disc when good lumbar support is used

Figure 4–33 The illustration shows the effects of improper posture relating to back problems. Proper back support will help to prevent this.

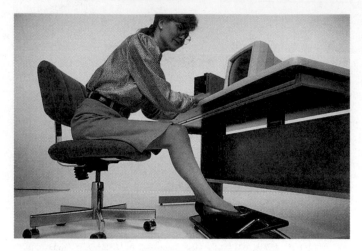

Figure 4–34 Using a footrest may help in avoiding posture problems (Courtesy of Magnuson Group, Inc.).

Complete Chapter 4, Unit 4 in the workbook to help you meet the objectives at the beginning of this unit and therefore achieve competency of this subject matter.

UNIT 5
Preparing for the Day

■ OBJECTIVES

Upon completion of the unit, meet the following terminal performance objectives by verifying knowledge of the facts and principles presented through oral and written communication at a level deemed competent, and demonstrate the specific behaviors as identified in the terminal performance objectives of the procedures, observing safety precautions in accordance with health care standards.

1. List five things to check in a reception room environment.
2. List four tasks to do before opening the office, in addition to the reception room check.
3. Explain why being the receptionist is an important position.
4. List at least five responsibilities of the receptionist.
5. Demonstrate "Open the Office" procedure.
6. Demonstrate "Obtain Preliminary Patient Information" procedure.
7. Identify five pieces of information found on a completed charge slip.
8. List four things you will find inside a new patient's chart folder.
9. List two reasons to use a "check list."
10. Demonstrate "Close the Office" procedure.
11. Spell and define, using the glossary at the back of the text, all the words to know in this unit.

■ WORDS TO KNOW

atmosphere	environment
appointment	insurance
brochure	intervention
communication	preliminary form
confidentiality	receptionist
diversion	schedule

PREPARING FOR THE DAY

There is no set list of things to do in order to prepare for the day. Preparation procedures vary according to the type of practice, number of physicians, weekly schedules, and a lot of other variables. Some doctors may not see patients everyday. Surgeons frequently reserve a day or two a week for surgery and have office hours on the other days. Physicians who are affiliated with university schools of medicine will teach and work with medical students and may see personal patients only one or two days a week. The following content discusses general things that need to be considered when preparing to receive patients in the office.

Opening the Office

The staff should arrive at the office in time to make preparations for receiving patients. If adequate time is not available, it seems like you can never get organized or "caught up." There are several things that need attention before the first patient arrives. Procedure 4–5 "Open the Office" addresses many of these tasks.

1. *Unlock the reception room door.* This refers to the door to the outside hallway or building exterior. The door between the reception room and the interior of the office should probably be locked from the reception room side for safety reasons, as discussed in Chapter 4, Unit 1. Be certain that the lock is set on the outside door so that it does not re-lock itself when it is closed. Check any open/closed sign for proper reading.
2. *Observe the physical environment of the reception room.* Studies have shown that the reception room **atmosphere** can be an **intervention**, or, in other words, a "go between" or mediation to the outcome of the office visit. Atmosphere affects how people experience their environment and may have a relationship to their response to treatment:
   - *Check the temperature.* The room temperature should ensure the patient's comfort.
   - *Look at the room's appearance.* The room should appear pleasant and well maintained. The arrangement of chairs can "say" secluded or sociable, which affects **communication** in the room. The presence of large plants and attractive paintings soften the office **environment**. The choice of color and lighting affects behavior. Soft colors and subdued light tend to calm the hostile person. The use of relaxing background music has become commonplace in medical and dental offices. Aquariums can provide diversion and have an enjoyable bubbling sound. Try standing in the reception room and

PROCEDURE

4-5 Open the Office

PURPOSE: To prepare the office to see patients.

MATERIALS: A simulated office, if available; otherwise, role play explaining the procedure.

TERMINAL PERFORMANCE OBJECTIVE: Following all the steps in the procedure, role play the actions necessary to prepare a medical office to see patients. Actions must be verbally described while performing.

1. Unlock the reception room door.

2. Adjust heat or air conditioning for the comfort of the patients.

3. Check for safety hazards in the office. **NOTE: Check for frayed electric wires, damaged furniture, objects on the carpet which might cause patients to fall.**

4. Check magazines for condition and date. **NOTE: Be sure magazines are current. Torn or damaged magazines should be removed from the waiting room.**

5. Check the telephone answering device or call the answering service for any messages.

6. Pull the charts of patients to be seen. **NOTE: Write or stamp with today's date. Check the patient's previous visit to see if any studies were ordered. Rationale: Results must be filed in the chart before the patient is seen.**

7. Check examination rooms to be sure they are clean and stocked with supplies. **NOTE: This is necessary in case the physician may see a patient after office hours and may not have put things away.**

8. Fill and turn on sterilizer.

9. Prepare hazardous waste disposal containers.

10. If it is the policy of the office, prepare a list of the patients to be seen and the times of their appointments and post and/or place copies in designated areas.

---

looking around. Be conscious of the sights, sounds, and even smells you perceive. Ask yourself, "What does this office 'say' to a me?" Hopefully it is a favorable response.

■ *Perform a safety check.* Review "Safety in the Reception Room" in Chapter 4, Unit 1. Remember to make a daily visual check of electrical devices, furniture, floors, and lighting before any patients arrive. Care should be taken to make the whole office "accident-proof." An incident in the office can result in a patient filing a suit for alleged pain and injury. If anyone should be injured, no matter how insignificant it may seem, the medical assistant must have the individual examined by the physician. If the patient should claim they were not injured and refuse examination, the incident must still be carefully recorded on their chart and the refusal of care noted. Some physicians may require a signed release of responsibility in order to protect against a later claim of injury.

■ *Check the reading material.* Neatly arrange magazines. Make them accessible to several seating areas. Remove torn and very outdated material. Encourage the physician(s) to subscribe to a variety of reading materials appropriate to both males and females of all ages. Many physicians have a prepared **brochure** which describes their practice, discusses the office policies, and provides information regarding appointments, office hours, and other useful details. Often there is a short biographical sketch of the physician(s). The brochure should be given to all new patients and a supply placed in the

reception area for anyone who may be interested. An assortment of informative health-related pamphlets may also be found in a display rack, Figure 4–35. These should be attractively arranged and restocked as needed.

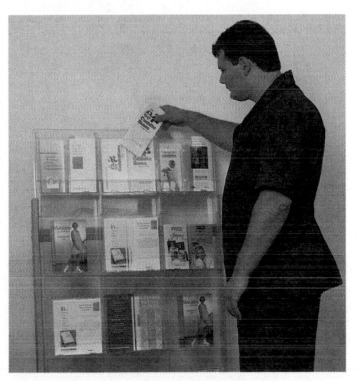

Figure 4–35 Office Practice Brochures and other handouts should be accessible to patients and visitors.

■ *Check the toys and books.* If there are children's toys or books provided, they require constant monitoring. All toys should be washable and of a safe design and material with no sharp edges or parts small enough for a child to swallow. The toys should be cleaned regularly. During daily inspection, remove any broken or visibly soiled toys or books. If at all possible, the children's play area should be situated in a corner or within a half-walled space in order to contain things within a controlled area to reduce the possibility of adults falling over objects on the floor.

■ *Display the smoking policy.* In view of regulations against the use of smoking materials in a public area and the overwhelming evidence of the effects of secondhand smoke, a medical office probably does not permit smoking. Be certain the "No Smoking" sign is displayed and that it is enforced. There should be no ashtrays accessible.

3. *Retrieve telephone messages.* Retrieve and record all messages on the answering machine. If an outside service is used, call and obtain the messages.

4. *Pull charts.* Look at the appointment book or run a hard copy from the computer of all patients who have appointments that day. Pull the charts of previously seen patients. Be certain to attach reports of any previously ordered studies to the chart. Have materials ready for initiating charts for scheduled new patients. This process can often be done the night before to lessen morning preparation duties. Many offices like to post a copy of the day's **schedule** in a common area for reference. Some physicians want a list of patients and appointment times on their desk for their personal use.

5. *Inspect examination rooms.* Visually inspect all rooms for cleanliness. Even if they were cleaned when closed the previous office day, the physician may have seen a patient afterhours. Replace examining paper and be certain waste receptacles are emptied. Observe room temperature and plug in any disconnected electrical equipment. Be certain everything is in working condition. Restock supplies so that needed materials are available.

6. *Check common work areas.* Check for cleanliness and be certain everything is in order. Check the water level in the sterilizer and turn it on. Be sure hazardous waste disposal containers are available for use in all areas where needed.

THE RECEPTIONIST

The medical assistant may fulfill the role of the **receptionist**, whose responsibility it is to greet and receive patients. This is a very significant role. The receptionist is usually the first person a patient encounters in the office. It is extremely important that this initial experience be very positive. Greet the patient promptly and courteously. Make an extra effort to make the patient feel at ease. (Studies have shown that a patient forms their initial impression of the office in the first four minutes of the office visit.)

The receptionist may be perceived as the doorway into the office. A pleasant tone of voice and the maintenance of eye contact is important when talking to patients. Attempt to call them by their full name. Listen intently to the patient's remarks and explain thoroughly any requests you make of them. Take opportunities to show that you care about their concerns and problems. Be especially careful NOT to ask questions or discuss matters that may be personal in a voice that can be heard by others in the reception room. Instead, bring the patient into the office to obtain this information. Respect your patient's right to **confidentiality**.

The receptionist must look and act professionally. Good grooming is essential. When you are neat and clean it conveys the impression of confidence and a business-like manner. Acting professionally is evident in the manner in which you deal with patients, both in the office and over the phone, with visitors, your co-workers, and your employer. It also shows when you perform your duties efficiently and effectively.

The receptionist is usually charged with answering the phone, making routine calls, and scheduling **appointments**. This responsibility requires an understanding of common diseases and disorders and the basic office operational procedures. It often demands tactful dealings with patients. The receptionist must determine when to enlist the assistance of other professionals in dealing with patients' concerns and requests.

The receptionist should be positioned within the office in such a way as to have a clear view of the reception room. If the space is within the office proper, behind a wall with a glass window partition, it may not be easily seen. The area must be observed frequently to monitor the activity and to check for new arrivals who may fail to come to the window. This separated physical arrangement does have the advantage of providing privacy while engaging in a telephone conversation, talking with a patient, or performing duties.

It is important to monitor the social climate of the reception area. Be alert to any annoying behavior which may cause an unfavorable impression of the office. Some people may become involved in a conversation with another patient who eventually becomes overzealous and opinionated. The best solution to the problem is to take the offender into an examination room where he/she can wait to be seen by the physician. Children often become restless, noisy, and irritable while waiting. Occasionally, their parents do not notice the behavior or are unaware that others are being annoyed. They make no attempt to amuse the child. Unless you can tactfully suggest another toy or book as a **diversion**, it may be necessary to move this patient into an examination room as well. Remember: people are affected by their atmosphere.

Be especially alert if a very ill patient enters the office. They should not have to sit and wait in a reception room. As soon as possible, assist them into an examination room where they can be made comfortable until the physician can see them. Remember to ensure the patient's safety. Warn them (and advise their companion) that they must be careful while lying on the narrow examination table.

Charge Slips

The receptionist may also be given the responsibility of preparing the charge slip which accompanies the patient's chart. Medical offices usually have a slip that lists the pro-

PROCEDURE

4-6 Obtain New Patient Information

PURPOSE: To obtain initial information from a new patient.

MATERIALS: An assigned "patient," a patient initial information form, a clipboard, a pen, a mock insurance card, a charge slip, chart folder, tabs, and typewriter.

TERMINAL PERFORMANCE OBJECTIVE: In a simulated situation, clearly communicate instructions and complete the steps in the procedure to obtain patient information and assemble all required materials.

1. Take new patient to private room to ask preliminary questions, or ask new patient to complete a data sheet. **NOTE: Give the patient a clipboard and pen and offer assistance, if needed. Ask the patient to return the form when it is completed. A medical history is a potential legal docu-**

ment. Check to be sure the form is completed accurately and legibly, and signed where appropriate.

2. Prepare a patient folder by typing the patient's name on a label and attaching it to the tab of the folder.

3. Transfer information from the form to the chart sheet.

4. Copy the insurance card, both sides.

5. Insert the chart, sheets, information form, and insurance card copy in folder.

6. Prepare charge slip.

7. Place the folder in the area reserved for charts of patients to be seen. **NOTE: If you have received any referral material on a new patient, be sure to place it with the chart.**

---

cedures, with the respective codes, which are performed in the office. The charge slip has a space for the patient's name and date and may request additional information. Some large clinics prepare "charge cards" which are used to stamp the patient's name and account number on the charge slip. When the physician completes the examination or treatment, the charges are entered on the slip and it is given to the patient with instructions to take it to a designated person on their way out of the office.

Forms will vary from one type of practice to another. Where computers are used, the form will be designed to be compatible with the software program being used. Figure 4–36 is an example of a computerized charge slip specially designed for a medical practice. This form will probably be preprinted with the patient identification information that is stored in the computer.

New Patients

The receptionist is usually responsible for the completion of the new patient information form, Figure 4–37. If this is to be done in an interview format, be sure that others cannot overhear the questioning process. Usually, a new patient is given the form and a clipboard and requested to complete the information. A pen or pencil should be provided. It is important to give clear instructions and ask if there are any questions. Be observant. If the patient seems reluctant to accept the form, appears confused, or is not making progress, they may have a reading problem. Quickly offer to assist. Check to be sure this **preliminary form** is complete and signed by the responsible party.

At this time, it is normally routine to request **insurance** cards from the patient so that they may be copied, on both sides, for the necessary billing information. If necessary, ver-

ification of coverage can be obtained by phoning the insurance company. The copy of the card and the preliminary form are placed in a folder along with chart sheets and any other referral materials received. The patient's name or number, if the filing method is numerical, is typed onto a label which is attached to the tab of the folder. Before the patient is seen, the charge slip is completed and attached to the chart. The chart is then placed in a designated area until the patient is taken to an examination room. Then it is placed in a holder on the door outside the room, ready for the physician when the patient is seen. Procedure 4–6 discusses the steps in obtaining new patient information.

CLOSING THE OFFICE

At the end of the day, the examination rooms should be restocked, cleaned, and discarded material placed for pick-up. This saves time the next morning. Charts must be collected, checked for completeness, and filed in a locked cabinet. If there is not time to file, place in a separate folder of "charts to be filed" and place in the cabinet to be filed the next day. (Some doctors may dictate their notes, which must first be typed onto the chart before it can be filed.) All electrical appliances and the sterilizer must be turned off. Receipts collected during the day can be taken to the bank for deposit or locked in the office safe. If there is time, tidy the reception area and pull the next day's records. Always take a walk through the office to complete your checklist of things to do. Activate your answering system and turn off the lights. Activate the alarm system, if available, and securely lock the door. See Procedure 4–7.

Complete Chapter 4, Unit 5 in the workbook to help you meet the objectives at the beginning of this unit and therefore achieve competency of this subject matter.

PATIENT INFORMATION

PATIENT'S LAST NAME	FIRST	INITIAL	BIRTHDATE		SEX ☐ MALE ☐ FEMALE	TODAY'S DATE

ADDRESS	CITY	STATE	ZIP	RELATIONSHIP TO SUBSCRIBER	INJURY DATE

SUBSCRIBER OR POLICYHOLDER	INSURANCE CARRIER

ADDRESS	CITY	STATE	ZIP	INS. I.D.	COVERAGE CODE	GROUP

ASSIGNMENT AND RELEASE: I HEREBY AUTHORIZE MY INSURANCE BENEFITS TO BE PAID DIRECTLY TO THE UNDERSIGNED PHYSICIAN. I AM FINANCIALLY RESPONSIBLE FOR NON-COVERED SERVICES. I ALSO AUTHORIZE THE PHYSICIAN TO RELEASE ANY INFORMATION REQUIRED.

OTHER HEALTH COVERAGE ☐ YES ☐ NO   IDENTIFY

DISABILITY RELATED TO:
☐ ACCIDENT ☐ INDUSTRIAL ☐ ILLNESS ☐ OTHER

SIGNED
(PATIENT, OR PARENT, IF MINOR) _____ Date _____

DATE SYMPTOMS APPEARED, INCEPTION OF PREGNANCY, OR ACCIDENT OCCURRED:

✓	DESCRIPTION	CPT/MD	FEE	✓	DESCRIPTION	CPT/MD	FEE	✓	DESCRIPTION	CPT/MD	FEE
	OFFICE VISITS	NEW PT			LABORATORY (Cont'd.)				PROCEDURES		
	Moderate Complex	99203			Wet Mount	87210			EKG 93000	93005	
	Moderate/High Comp.	99204			Pap Smear	88150			Resp. Function Test	94010	
	High Complexity	99205			Handling	99000			Ear Lavage	69210	
	OFFICE VISITS	EST. PT			Hemoccult Stool	82270			Injection Inter. Jt.*	20605	
	Minimal	99211			Glucose	82948			Injection Major Jt.*	20610	
	Self Limited Comp.	99212			INJECTIONS				Anoscopy	46600	
	Low/Moderate Comp.	99213			Vitamin B12/B Complex	J3420			Sigmoidoscopy	45355	
	Moderate Complex	99214			ACTH	J0140			I & D*	10060	
	High Complexity	99215			Depo-Estradiol	J1000			Electrocautery*	17200	
	CONSULTATIONS	OFFICE			Depo Testosterone	J1070			Thromb Hemor.*	46320	
	Moderate Complexity	99243			Imferon	J1760			Inj. Tendon*	20550	
	Mod. to High Comp.	99244			Tetanus Toxoid	J3180					
	HOME	EST. PT			Influenza Vaccine - Flu	90724			MISCELLANEOUS		
	Moderate Complexity	99352			Pneumococcal Vaccine	90732			Drugs, Supplies, Materials	99070	
	ER				TB Tine Test	86585			Special Reports	99080	
	Moderate Severity	99283			Aminophyllin	J0280			Services After Hrs.	99050	
	High Severity	99284			Terbutaline Sulf.	J3105			Services 10pm - 8am	99052	
	LABORATORY				Demerol HCL	J0990			Services Sun. & Holidays	99054	
	Urinalysis - Complete	81000			Compazine	J0780			Counseling	99403	
	Hemoglobin	85018			Injection Therapeutic	90782					
	Culture, Strep/Monilia	87081			Estrone Susp.	J1410					

DIAGNOSIS:

☐ Allergic Rhinitis 477.9	☐ Chronic Fatigue Synd. 300.5	☐ Hemorrhoids 455.6
☐ Anemia 280.9	☐ COPD 496	☐ Hiatal Hernia 553.3
☐ Angina Pectoris 413	☐ Costochondritis 733.99	☐ Hiatal Hernia & Reflux 530.1
☐ Anxiety 300.00	☐ CVA 431	☐ HVD 402.10
☐ Aortic Stenosis 424.1	☐ Cystitis 595.9	☐ Hyperlipidemia 272.4
☐ ASCVD 429.2	☐ Deg. Disc. Disease, CX .. 722.4	☐ Hypoestrogenism 256.3
☐ ASHD 414.9	☐ Deg. Disc. Dis., Lumbar . 722.52	☐ Hypothyroidism 244.9
☐ Asthma 493.9	☐ Depression, Endogenous . 296.2	☐ Impacted Cerumen 380.4
☐ Atrial Fibrillation 427.31	☐ Dermatitis 692.9	☐ Influenza, Viral 487.1
☐ Bigeminy 427.89	☐ Diabetes Mellitus, Adult . 250.0	☐ Irritable Bowel Syndrome ... 564.1
☐ BPH 600	☐ Diarrhea 558.9	☐ Laryngitis 464.0
☐ Bronchitis, Acute 466.1	☐ Diverticulitis 562.11	☐ Menopausal Syndrome ... 627.2
☐ Bronchitis, Chronic 491.9	☐ Esophagitis 530.1	☐ Mitral Insufficiency ... 396.2
☐ Bursitis 726	☐ Fibrocystic Breast Disease . 610.11	☐ Moniliasis 112
☐ Cardiomyopathy 425.4	☐ Fissure in Ano 565.0	☐ Myocardial Infarction .. 410.9
☐ Carotid Artery Disease . 433.1	☐ Gastroenteritis 558.9	☐ Neuritis 729.2
☐ Cerebral Vascular Disease . 437.9	☐ Gout 274.9	☐ Osteoarthritis 715.9
☐ CHF 428.0	☐ HCVD 429.2	☐ Osteoporosis 733.0
☐ Cholecystitis 575.1	☐ Headache, Vascular 784.0	☐ Otitis Media 382.9
	☐ Headache, Migraine 346.9	☐ Parkinsonism 332

☐ Peripheral Vascular Dis 443.9
☐ Pharyngitis 462.0
☐ Pneumonia, Bacterial 482.9
☐ Pneumonia, Viral 480.9
☐ Prostatitis, Chronic/Acute .. 601
☐ Rectal Bleeding 569.3
☐ Renal Failure, Chronic .. 585
☐ Rheumatoid Arthritis 714.0
☐ Sinusitis 461.9
☐ Supraventr. Tachycardia . 427.0
☐ T.I.A. 435.9
☐ Tachycardia 426.89
☐ Tendinitis 726.90
☐ Tonsillitis 463
☐ Ulcer Duodenal 532.9
☐ Ulcer Gastric 531.9
☐ URI 465.9
☐ UTI 599.0
☐ Vaginitis 616.10
☐ Vertigo 780.4

DIAGNOSIS: (IF NOT CHECKED ABOVE)   REF. DR. & #

DOCTOR'S SIGNATURE / DATE	NO SERVICES PURCHASED	SERVICE PERFORMED	ACCEPT ASSIGNMENT	TODAY'S FEE

INSTRUCTIONS TO PATIENT FOR FILING INSURANCE CLAIMS

1. MAIL THIS FORM DIRECTLY TO YOUR INSURANCE COMPANY. ATTACH YOUR OWN INSURANCE COMPANY'S FORM.

PLEASE REMEMBER THAT PAYMENT IS YOUR OBLIGATION, REGARDLESS OF INSURANCE OR OTHER THIRD PARTY INVOLVEMENT.

OFFICE ☐   YES ☐   AMT. REC'D TODAY

E.R. ☐   NO ☐

HOME ☐   TOTAL DUE

Figure 4–36 Charge form for medical clinic (Courtesy Bibbero Systems, Inc., Petaluma, CA, 94954).

PATIENT INFORMATION **DATE:**

PATIENT'S NAME	MARITAL STATUS S M W DIV SEP	DATE OF BIRTH	SOCIAL SECURITY NO.	
STREET ADDRESS ☐ PERMANENT ☐ TEMPORARY	CITY AND STATE		ZIP CODE	HOME PHONE NO.
PATIENT'S EMPLOYER	OCCUPATION (INDICATE IF STUDENT)		HOW LONG EMPLOYED?	BUSINESS PHONE NO.
EMPLOYER'S STREET ADDRESS	CITY AND STATE			ZIP CODE
IN CASE OF EMERGENCY CONTACT				DRIVERS LIC. NO.
SPOUSE'S NAME				
SPOUSE'S EMPLOYER	OCCUPATION (INDICATE IF STUDENT)		HOW LONG EMPLOYED?	BUSINESS PHONE NO.
EMPLOYER'S STREET ADDRESS	CITY AND STATE			ZIP CODE
WHO REFERRED YOU TO THIS PRACTICE?				

IF THE PATIENT IS A MINOR OR STUDENT

MOTHER'S NAME	STREET ADDRESS, CITY, STATE AND ZIP CODE		HOME PHONE NO.
MOTHER'S EMPLOYER	OCCUPATION	HOW LONG EMPLOYED?	BUSINESS PHONE NO.
EMPLOYER'S STREET ADDRESS	CITY AND STATE		ZIP CODE
FATHER'S NAME	STREET ADDRESS, CITY, STATE AND ZIP CODE		HOME PHONE NO.
FATHER'S EMPLOYER	OCCUPATION	HOW LONG EMPLOYED?	BUSINESS PHONE NO.
EMPLOYER'S STREET ADDRESS	CITY AND STATE		ZIP CODE

INSURANCE INFORMATION

PERSON RESPONSIBLE FOR PAYMENT, IF NOT ABOVE		STREET ADDRESS, CITY, STATE AND ZIP CODE			HOME PHONE NO.
☐ COMPANY NAME & ADDRESS		NAME OF POLICYHOLDER		CERTIFICATE NO.	GROUP NO.
☐ COMPANY NAME & ADDRESS		NAME OF POLICYHOLDER		POLICY NO.	
☐ COMPANY NAME & ADDRESS		NAME OF POLICYHOLDER		POLICY NO.	
☐ MEDICARE	MEDICARE NO.	☐ MEDICAID	PROGRAM NO.	COUNTY NO.	ACCOUNT NO.

In order to control our cost of billing, we request that office visits be paid at the time service is rendered. We would rather control our billing costs than be forced to raise our fees.

AUTHORIZATION: I hereby authorize the physician indicated above to furnish information to insurance carriers concerning this illness/accident, and I hereby irrevocably assign to the doctor all payments for medical services rendered. I understand that I am financially responsible for all charges whether or not covered by insurance.

Responsible Party Signature

Figure 4–37 New patient information form.

P R O C E D U R E

4-7 Close the Office

PURPOSE: To prepare the office to be closed.

MATERIALS: A simulated office, if available; otherwise, role play explaining the procedure.

TERMINAL PERFORMANCE OBJECTIVE: Following all the steps in the procedure, role play the actions required to close the office. Actions must be verbally described while performing the procedure.

1. Check to see that records are collected and filed in locked cabinets.
2. Place any money received in safe or take to the bank to be deposited.
3. Turn off all electrical appliances. **NOTE: Many offices ask that you unplug electrical appliances. Rationale: Eliminates the chance of electrical fire.**
4. Check that rooms are all cleaned and supplied for the next day.
5. Straighten reception room if time allows.
6. Pull charts for the next day if time allows.
7. Activate answering device on phone or notify answering service and indicate when you will be back in the office.
8. Turn off lights.
9. **NOTE: Activate alarm system, if available.**
10. Set lock and close door.
11. Check to assure that it is locked.

Medical-Legal Ethical Highlights

Consider the following situation: Mrs. Jones is a young woman whose husband recently left her with two small children. Because she was married and began her family soon after graduating from high school, she has not acquired specific employable skills or gained much work experience. She is currently enrolled in a job training program but found it necessary to seek public assistance until she is able to get a good job. She is making her first visit to the physician's office and has just completed the new patient information form and given it to the receptionist.

Ms. Wrong reviews the form for completeness and notices the patient is on welfare. Across the crowded reception room to Mrs. Jones, she calls "I'll need a copy of your Medicaid card so I can bill welfare for this office visit." Mrs. Jones feels embarrassed as she complies with the request. She wonders how many people in the room think she is just too lazy to work. Since the receptionist employee was so inconsiderate she also wonders if the physician will treat her badly.

Fortunately, Ms. Wrong was overheard by the office manager who warned her that her action was very inappropriate and that she was noting this on her performance record. She also told Ms. Wrong that she should apologize to Mrs. Jones for her thoughtlessness.

Employment outlook: Under observation.

Ms. Right reviews the form for completeness and notices the patient is on welfare. She says, "Mrs. Jones, will you please come to the reception window?" After she arrives, Ms. Right asks her to step inside the office where she tells her she will need her Medicaid card so she can make a copy for billing purposes. Mrs. Jones complies with the request and feels Ms. Right is very professional. She thinks the physician must be very competent since his employee is so thoughtful. The office manager saw what Ms. Right had done and commented about the way in which she had respected the patient's right to confidentiality.

Employment outlook: Favorable.

REFERENCES

American Medical Association. *The Physicians' Current Procedural Terminology,* 1995.

Diehl, Marcia, and Fordney, Marilyn. *Medical Typing and Transcribing Techniques and Procedures,* 3rd ed. Philadelphia: W. B. Saunders, 1991.

Fordney, Marilyn. *Insurance Handbook for the Medical Office,* 4th ed. Philadelphia: W. B. Saunders, 1995.

Frew, Mary, and Frew, David. *Comprehensive Medical Assisting, Administrative and Clinical Procedures,* 3rd ed. Philadelphia: F. A. Davis, 1994.

Kinn, Mary E., and Derge, Eleanor. *The Medical Assistant: Administrative and Clinical,* 7th ed. Philadelphia: W. B. Saunders, 1993.

McClung, Christina; Guerrieri, John; and McClung, Kenneth, Jr. *Microcomputers for Medical Professionals.* New York: Wiley, 1984.

Seraydarian, Patricia. *Metroplex Clinic: A Medical Typing Simulation.* Boston: Houghton-Mifflin, 1980.

———. *Word Processing Applications for Electronic Typewriters.* Boston: Houghton-Mifflin, 1980.

Shelly, Gary B. and Cashman, Thomas J. *Computer Fundamentals in an Information Age.* Anaheim, CA: Anaheim Publishing Company, Incorporated, 1984.

Simmers, Louise. *Diversified Health Occupations,* 3rd ed. Albany: Delmar Publishers, 1993.

United States Department of Health and Human Services. *International Classification of Diseases.* 1996.

Vocabulary for Data Processing, Telecommunications, and Office Systems. IBM, 1981.

CHAPTER 5

Interpersonal Communications

One of the most important skills a medical assistant can possess is the art of communicating effectively with others. Both clinical and administrative duties require a constant exchange of written, oral, and nonverbal information.

You must be able to convey messages to many different people and receive vital information in the same manner. You will have daily contact with patients, colleagues, and other professionals, by phone, face to face, or by letter. Telephone and written communications and office mail will be discussed later in this text. This chapter deals with both verbal and nonverbal messages. Understanding how one gives and receives these is vital in the exchange of communication.

UNIT 1
Verbal and Nonverbal Messages

UNIT 2
Behavioral Adjustments

UNIT 3
Patients and Their Families

UNIT 4
Office Interpersonal Relationships

In dealing with patients and their families, learning to listen and to offer advice in a calm, professional manner will help to reduce unnecessary stress for all concerned. Times of sadness and pain can be extremely difficult for those closely involved. You can be instrumental in providing comfort and compassion to those in need.

Since the medical office is usually a very active place, with many people coming and going, asking questions and making payments or appointments, intraoffice communication can become ragged and ineffective. A harmonious team effort makes for an efficient as well as a pleasant work environment. If an atmosphere of accord and cooperation exists among the staff, patients will sense this during their visits. If an uneasy situation exists, with friction evident, this may add to a patient's apprehensions and anxieties. Working together for the single purpose of providing quality health care to patients in a relaxed and friendly manner will help ease the daily pressures for the members of the medical office team and contribute greatly to their collective effectiveness.

UNIT 1

Verbal and Nonverbal Messages

■ **OBJECTIVES**

Upon completion of the unit, meet the following terminal performance objectives by verifying knowledge of the facts and principles presented through oral and written communication at a level deemed competent.

1. Describe the basic pattern of communication.
2. Give examples of nonverbal communication.
3. Explain how verbal and nonverbal communication can sometimes be misinterpreted.
4. Describe ways that tone and speed of speech can affect the message.
5. Discuss the importance of dress in nonverbal communication.
6. Discuss *perception* and state its importance in communication.
7. List and explain the three types of listening and how they effect communication.
8. Spell and define, using the glossary at the back of the text, all the words to know in this unit.

▪ WORDS TO KNOW

active listening	incongruous
articulate	intangible
conceptualize	intuition
contradict	perception
distort	scrupulously
empirically	

To become effective in the art of communication, it may help to **conceptualize** the communication process, Figure 5–1. The message originates with the sender. The encoded message takes form based upon the sender's reference points (or frames of reference), and off it goes. The message is picked up by the intended receiver, who immediately begins to decode it based on his or her reference points (or frames of reference). In responding (or providing feedback) the whole process is reversed: the original receiver becomes the sender, and the original sender becomes the receiver. In receiving this feedback, the original sender (now the receiver) can assess and evaluate how well the original message was received and interpreted and make any necessary adjustments or clarification.

The whole process seems simple enough, and generally it works well. However, many things can happen to affect the quality of the message or even **distort** it. You must be aware of these potential problems.

Foremost is the issue of reference points. For example, the spoken messages may include terminology familiar to you but unknown to the patient. Therefore, though the message will be heard, it may not be understood. Talking to patients on a level that they can easily understand is a skill requiring quick judgment. You will have to adapt to a vast number of different personalities in conveying information.

Some patients may be hearing- or sight-impaired, developmentally disabled, or non-English speaking, and will therefore require extra understanding. If a patient is in some way handicapped, a family member or friend usually accompanies the person, thereby helping with your task of transmitting necessary information. It is important, however, that you speak to the patient directly and acknowledge their presence. It is rude and impolite to discuss their health care with another person and ignore the patient as if he/she was not even present.

Other factors may interfere, such as interruptions or simply the way you feel. These factors must be recognized and dealt with if effective communication is to occur.

The spoken word must be delivered in an **articulate**, clear manner if the intended message is to be received. Correct

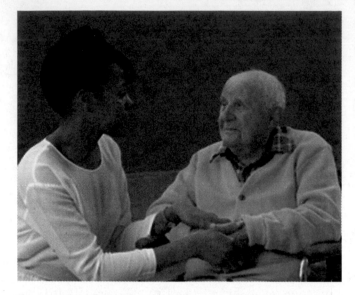

Figure 5–2   The medical assistant stoops down to speak with the patient in the wheelchair for better communication at eye level.

pronunciation and proper grammar help to convey the meaning. You must also be aware of the rate of the spoken word. Patients need to be spoken to in an un-rushed manner so that the information has a chance to register and questions can be asked. Speaking in a pleasant tone of voice is necessary to keep the listener's interest in what you are saying. You must also remember to look the person in the eye while you are conversing. Eye contact makes people pay attention to the words you are saying. It gives the person a feeling of importance and expresses a sincere interest in their well-being, Figure 5–2.

Listening involves giving attention to the person(s) who are trying to communicate with you. **Active listening** is the participation in the conversation with another by means of repeating words and phrases, or in giving approving or disapproving nods. This signals to the message sender that you are hearing and following what is being said. This method of conversation is highly recommended for health care providers and patients in communicating needs, because it requires both parties to interact. The listener must make an effort to pay attention and follow the speaker. Distractions do create problems and interfere with what is being said. It takes concentration and self control to keep focused on a topic when there are many activities and interruptions going on, as often happens in a medical facility. Taking patients into an exam room or to a quiet space away from noise is the most practical way to communicate important information.

Common courtesy is an art which seems to have been lost to some degree. In a professional setting it is essential to be **scrupulously** polite. *Please, Thank you, Excuse me,* and *May I help you?* should be words in frequent use. In this way the entire health care staff will show respect for others and a sense of caring.

PERCEPTION

Perception in the context of communication may be considered as being aware of one's own feelings and the feel-

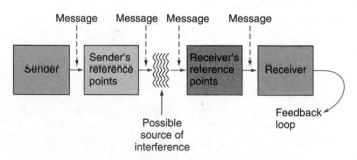

Figure 5–1   A model of the communication process.

ings of others. The feelings you have about other people's moods and the way they act are perceptual, nonspoken communication between you. **Intuition** is another term for perception in this sense. While they cannot be measured **empirically**, these feelings may be strong indeed. Therefore, they must be recognized and reckoned with.

Being perceptive is a skill acquired with experience and practice. Keeping your eyes and ears open to the needs of others and what is going on will help you develop it. Developing the ability to perceive your own needs is a part of perception that will enhance your effectiveness. Planning and thinking ahead will help you develop in this area.

BODY LANGUAGE

The image you project is of utmost importance. Your overall appearance sends out messages to anyone who looks at you. Appropriate dress, uniform, or businesslike attire should be worn. Your professional appearance sends a nonverbal message that you have authority and are in charge.

Proper attire may vary with the medical specialty. For instance, many pediatric practices prefer medical assistants to dress in normal street clothes so as to make young patients feel more at ease. Children sometimes associate a white uniform with an unpleasant hospital visit. Psychiatry and psychology medical office assistants may also be more inclined to wear businesslike dress, for clinical duties are few, if any, and a uniform may not be necessary. However, casual wear is considered unprofessional, and jeans, sandals, and excessive jewelry are out of the question during working hours. Looking like a professional will not only encourage the respect of others for your profession, but it will help you to feel an integral part of the health care team.

Personal hygiene should be impeccable, because setting a good example for others is a part of your responsibility in the care of others. Daily showering, clean attractive hair, and neatly manicured nails shows others that you take pride in yourself and gives them a model to pattern themselves after.

Another part of your appearance, something **intangible** but very real, is your attitude. Your attitude shows *everyone* who sees you or speaks to you (by telephone or in person) how you feel about your work, others, and yourself. You display your attitude in the way you get along with others and interact with them. Body language is a complex communication process. It involves unconscious use of posture, gestures, and other forms of nonverbal communication. It is possible to **contradict** a verbal message by an inappropriate or **incongruous** facial expression. Even when a person says nothing and thinks that the message being sent is positive, body language will send the true message. When a person says for instance, "I'm ok," and you see the person grimacing with pain, the conflicting message shows through the true message. Many of us remember that our parents (or grandparents) could "read us like a book." It seems that body language is nothing new; it was the projection of attitude perceived by those who got to know us well. The importance of a positive attitude cannot be overemphasized. The many hassles and conflicts that can, and do, arise with patients and colleagues during everyday activity in the busy medical office can be handled much more effectively if you possess and project a positive attitude. Constant complaining only makes situations worse and breeds contempt. Having a good outlook on life carries over into every area and promotes well-being. Pleasant, agreeable working conditions increase productivity and efficiency besides giving one a sense of satisfaction on the job.

Facial Expression

Part of perception is being aware of how others think you feel, or see you. You create this impression partly by your facial expression. The most common example of a positive, happy facial expression is a smile, Figure 5–3. This nonverbal signal conveys a positive attitude. Frowning and looking glum only add to other people's troubles. It is especially important to be pleasant and friendly to those seeking medical attention, because their worries concerning their condition are already on their minds. Adding your troubles to theirs is highly inappropriate. A positive attitude and a receptive awareness will show in your facial expression.

Eye contact shows that you are interested in giving and receiving messages of mutual concern and interest. It has been said that the eyes are the windows of the soul. Looking into another's eyes while engaging in conversation permits an open, honest transmission of thoughts and ideas. Looking away while people are talking to you makes them feel that what they are saying is not important. Interest and attention soon disappear and the intent of your message may be distorted or lost.

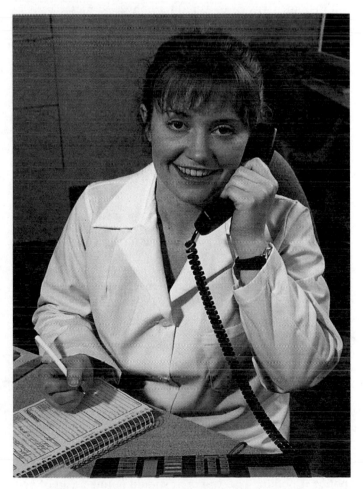

Figure 5–3   A smile conveys a positive attitude.

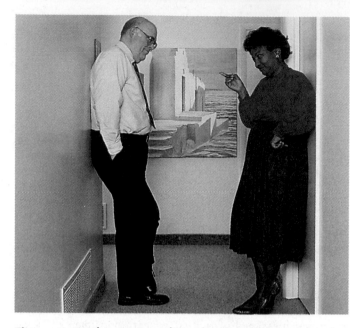

Figure 5–4 The woman is obviously telling the man across from her of some frustration, while he passively listens.

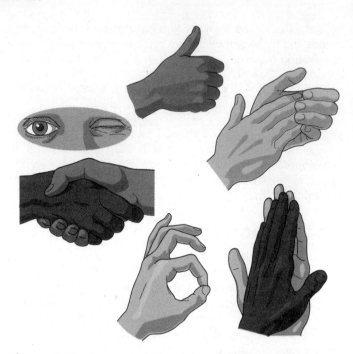

Figure 5–5 Common positive gestures: (clockwise) thumbs up, applause, high five, okay, handshake, winking.

Gestures

Still another way of transmitting nonverbal messages is by gesturing. Gestures are body movements that enhance what is being said. You may know people who seemingly could not talk if they had to sit on their hands. Try to follow their example. Using hand and body gestures to accentuate a point can help the receiver understand your meaning. To emphasize the subject matter in conversation, gestures help to convey the message. In Figure 5–4, a woman's body language shows her feelings of frustration. She is facing her co-worker and making eye contact with him. Her co-worker has his hands in his pockets as he leans against the wall with his legs crossed, thereby looking rather passive. All of this body language (nonverbal communication) is happening while the two are also conversing verbally.

There are many gestures that we use daily that have become such a part of our personalities that we do not even realize we do them anymore. Some of them are positive and some are not. Some that are positive and very popularly known are thumbs up, an okay, a high five, applause, winking, and a handshake. These are all ways of showing signs of acceptance, encouragement, appreciation, and friendliness, Figure 5–5. If you pay attention, the intended message is clearly understood without saying anything at all. Some of the ways of telling if a person is upset or not interested (negative body language) are crossed arms, looking at one's watch, rolling of the eyes, tapping of the foot or fingers, sighing, and talking under one's breath. And there are still other gestures that are very rude and socially unacceptable. Usually it helps to ignore the patient who seeks attention from this type of behavior. If this is not effective, it is necessary to call for assistance from a supervisor, security, or the police if nothing else works. It should not be a part of your job description to put up with verbal or physical abuse of any

kind. If the patient is mentally ill or is under the influence of drugs or alcohol, a certain amount of understanding and tolerance must be employed by all. However, seeking assistance in these situations before a problem begins is always recommended.

A handshake is a sign of friendship. Another meaningful body movement is a hug to convey feelings of warmth and affection. A comforting touch helps patients feel that you care and gives them a sense of security and acceptance. Studies have shown that patients who have been touched, by a hand on the shoulder or a hand held, respond significantly better in treatment than those not touched. Patting someone on the back and saying "Good for you" is a positive reinforcer. You might do that in praise of a patient who followed the prescribed treatment of the physician and lost ten pounds and who needs positive recognition of these achievements to encourage continued compliance. In reinforcing a patient, you should display a positive attitude, facial expression, gestures, and eye contact—all the communication skills so far mentioned. In addition, your tone of voice should be happy and sincere. Patients who believe you are pleased with their progress are more willing to strive to follow future treatment because of the resulting positive feelings.

Another powerful nonverbal communication tool is silence. This method can indeed be most frustrating to the person for whom it is directed. In dealing with patients who exhibit this nonverbal way of communicating, it is best if the inexperienced medical assistant ask for help from a supervisor, a physician, or another staff member who has skill in dealing with this type of situation, Figure 5–6. Patients who exhibit behavior such as this may have serious underlying problems.

Complete Chapter 5, Unit 1 in the workbook to meet the objectives at the beginning of this unit and therefore achieve competency of this subject matter.

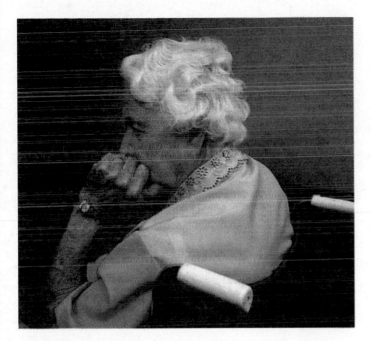

Figure 5–6 The patient is silent and seems to be avoiding eye contact with others. Her nonverbal language could indicate that there is an underlying problem that needs to be addressed.

UNIT 2

Behavioral Adjustments

■ OBJECTIVES

Upon completion of the unit, meet the following terminal performance objectives by verifying knowledge of the facts and principles presented through oral and written communication at a level deemed competent.

1. List the commonly used defense mechanisms and give an example of each.
2. Explain what could happen to a person who habitually uses one or more of the defense mechanisms listed in this unit.
3. Discuss why it is necessary to know yourself before you can relate effectively to others.
4. List problem-solving steps and apply them to a particular problem you may have.
5. Explain the importance of mental and emotional status in regard to overall health.
6. Spell and define, using the glossary at the back of the text, all the words to know in this unit.

■ WORDS TO KNOW

adjustment	projection
analytical	rationalization
ardently	regression
compensation	repression
denial	strategem
displacement	sublimation
intellectualization	suppression
malinger	unobtrusive

We discussed in Unit 1 of this chapter how keeping a positive attitude is of primary importance in our interactions with others. Even though we strive for a good rapport with co-workers, patients, family, and friends, we must realize that we are human beings. Perfection in any relationship, even the best one, is certainly a desirable goal, but rather unrealistic. Understanding ourselves and others is essential in meaningful communications. Often in our daily transactions of conveying and receiving messages, we use certain coping skills to keep ourselves from getting hurt or to protect our image. These complex **strategems** are called defense mechanisms.

DEFENSE MECHANISMS

These defenses are largely unconscious acts we use to help us deal with unpleasant and socially unacceptable circumstances or behaviors. They help us make an emotional **adjustment** in everyday situations. Surely we all use various defense mechanisms from time to time. However, habitual use can cause one to become somewhat out of touch with reality.

Repression

The most commonly used defense mechanism is **repression** which is the forcing of unacceptable or painful ideas, feelings and impulses into the unconscious mind without being aware of it. Certainly, we have all wished something unpleasant would happen to another person when we have experienced feelings of hostility, jealousy, or intense anger from interacting with that person. These feelings do not vanish, but are placed in our unconscious and may surface in dreams or subtle **unobtrusive** behaviors.

Repression, like all of the defense mechanisms, tends to protect us from unwanted messages about ourselves that make us feel bad.

Suppression

Suppression is a term to describe a condition in which the person becomes involved in a project, hobby, or work on purpose so that a painful situation can be avoided. There are those who, rather than face a difficult problem within a relationship, for instance, throw themselves into their work so much that there is little or no time for the relationship. This is a good reason to avoid communication because of the legitimate "work" that has to be done. People only fool themselves for so long until something has to be done to relieve the stress this kind of behavior causes.

Displacement

Displacement is the transfer of emotions about one to another. A typical example of displacement for the medical assistant might be as follows: In the course of the day, the medical assistant has many duties to perform for many others and one patient in particular becomes overly demanding and rude. The medical assistant holds back the strong feelings and deals with the situation professionally. Later in the evening at home, she feels all the pent-up anger and explodes at a family member. This is also done unconsciously, although sometimes, after the fact, we realize our actions have been displaced from the point where they originated to an innocent, unsuspecting target.

Projection

In **projection**, you might blame another unconsciously for your own inadequacies. An extreme form of projection can lead to hostile, even aggressive behavior if you perceive another person to be the cause of the painful feelings. For example, an obese patient may blame a medical assistant for his/her gaining of a few pounds saying that the scales were set up or read incorrectly.

Rationalization

With **rationalization**, you justify behavior with socially acceptable reasons and tend to ignore the real reasons underlying the behavior. This self-discipline unconscious act is relatively harmless. Habitual use of this defense mechanism, as well as all the others discussed in this unit, can become nonproductive or even destructive because they distort reality. A typical rationalization might be, "I dieted very strictly all day; therefore, it's okay to eat a couple of candy bars later in the evening after supper."

Intellectualization

Intellectualization is still another means of denying socially unacceptable feelings or strong feelings that cannot be easily expressed. With this mechanism, you use reasoning to avoid confronting emotional conflicts and stressful situations. You might discuss all the facts and provide endless information about how to begin caring for an elderly relative, elaborating on special diets and home health care in order to avoid dealing with the true feelings of sadness over a relative's illness.

Sublimation

Sublimation is used unconsciously to express socially unacceptable instinctive drives or impulses in approved and acceptable ways. An example of sublimation might be a 30-year-old father and frustrated athlete forcing his child to excel in a sport. Or, an artist may unconsciously direct sexual impulses constructively in the form of writing, sculpture, painting, or photography.

Compensation

Compensation is somewhat similar to sublimation in that it is positive. When you use this defense mechanism, you use a talent or an attribute to the fullest in order to compensate for a realized personal shortcoming. For example, a person who can no longer participate in sports because of an illness or injury may find satisfaction in either writing about the game or helping with coaching.

Temporary Withdrawal

Temporary withdrawal is a defense mechanism in that it is a retreat from facing a painful or difficult situation. This avoidance of something that is unpleasant is another way of protecting ourselves from disagreeable feelings. Watching TV excessively or reading to avoid dealing with an issue are common types of withdrawal.

Putting off issues only makes the situation worse. It produces anxiety and makes the problem more difficult to face the longer the withdrawal goes on.

Daydreaming

A healthy type of temporary withdrawal that all of us do from time to time is daydreaming. This is a way to momentarily escape from reality and relax. At times, you can become very creative and/or return refreshed from daydreams. If, however, this form of escape is done too often and for too long of a time, then it becomes unhealthy and should be of concern to you.

Malingering

Another common defense mechanism is **malingering**. When you malinger, you deliberately pretend to be sick in order to avoid dealing with situations that are unpleasant or that cause anxiety. A malingering individual might stay home sick on a day when he or she was to give a presentation, when in fact, that person is as healthy as always, enjoying the time at home.

Denial

Denial seems to be a commonly used defense mechanism. It is the refusal to admit or acknowledge something so you do not have to deal with a problem or situation. When you are not accepting of the phases of life that may produce anxiety, as an emotional defense you sometimes use denial. It is usually seen only in psychosis in adults who have reacted to a traumatic situation of extreme stress.

When one who has been given the diagnosis of a terminal illness does not accept the reality of it and believes that a recovery is certain, that person is going through the denial stage.

Regression

Regression is behaving in ways that are typically characteristic of an earlier developmental level. This usually happens in times of high stress.

For example, a college student consoles herself during final exam week with eating hot fudge sundaes as she did as a child with her mother whenever problems at school piled up.

Indeed, we all use many, perhaps all of these defense mechanisms from time to time. Since they are mostly used without our conscious awareness, they may be relatively harmless. Again, habitual use of defense mechanisms can veil reality and interfere with facing personal issues and crises, as well as with open and honest communication with others.

PROBLEM SOLVING

In our complex daily lives, we use many coping skills to deal with our difficulties. Defense mechanisms have already been discussed. Another approach to handling interpersonal problems and concerns is to develop problem-solving skills. Taking a step-by-step approach helps one look realistically and logically at a problem. This method encourages **analytical** thinking and confident decision making. Here is an outline of the basic steps in problem solving:

1. Determine just what the problem is and write it down.
   a. Is there a problem chain or a series of events that are contributors?
2. Gather facts and ideas to help you decide what to do about it.
3. Use analytical and creative thinking. (List your decisions and what you think their outcome will be.)
4. Prioritize your decisions and begin testing them one by one until results are satisfactory to you and others concerned.

If results are not pleasing, begin again with step one. Often, step one alone triggers an answer to a problem. Sitting down and writing out what the problem actually is can be most therapeutic. Once you begin to use this skill to think logically about major problems such as changing employment, relocating geographically, or locating a suitable day care facility, you will begin to think more logically in all matters. Making a habit of this skill will increase your peace of mind and reduce stress because you will deal with problems more efficiently and spend less time and energy worrying about what to do. This skill can be a great stride toward eliminating procrastination.

The medical assistant who concentrates on patient education may want to pass this helpful skill on to patients.

MENTAL AND EMOTIONAL STATUS INFLUENCING BEHAVIORS

The medical assistant, in both administrative and clinical capacities, has many opportunities daily to observe patients' mental and emotional states. These observations have a direct influence on the medical assistants' behavior, which in turn directly influences their overall health. We must keep in mind that all medical personnel are patients too. Therefore, all of the information we learn about patients applies to us as well.

The stress in life can lead to ill health. A true understanding of one's self is the primary key to understanding others.

Learning about yourself requires you to take a good hard look at who and what you really are. When assessing your "self," your individual presence may come to mind first. This presence comprises both your physical self (your body) and your self-image (how you view yourself). Another dimension of self, as termed by psychologists, is the "self-as-

process." This refers to the ongoing process inside us that deals with constant changes, or adjustments, in our lives.

Your response to others is dealt with by your social self. You have many different roles with which you identify **ardently**. Finally, you have an "ideal self." This is what you picture yourself to be, the perfect model you have of yourself.

We are, indeed, complex beings, capable of doing just about anything we choose to. Unfortunately, many of us never come close to realizing our true potential. This may be due to never having to look at ourselves squarely. Sometimes it can be quite difficult and even unpleasant to be honest about ourselves.

A good way to begin a basic assessment of yourself is by making a list of all the strengths you have, as well as all your weaknesses. This technique can help point out your abilities and qualities and identify areas that need to be changed. Keeping a journal or a diary, even if only temporarily, is another way to vent feelings, look at problems, and realize and assess your behavior patterns in order to better know your true self.

An ideal time to reevaluate yourself and renew your goals and aspirations is annually on your birthday. Many people prefer the traditional New Year's resolution. Knowing yourself will help you become a more complete person and will help you relate to others more effectively.

COMMUNICATING EMOTIONAL STATES

In Unit 1 of this chapter, we discussed verbal and nonverbal messages. Communication is a complex process in which one must be aware of all facets for complete information exchanges to occur.

The perceptive medical assistant should be able to decide what "feeder questions" to ask a patient to determine whether the look on the patient's face matches the patient's emotional demeanor. The following are feeder questions the medical assistant may use to find out the emotional states of the patients they interview. After greeting the patient with a kind "hello," the assistant may want to ask "What seems to be the problem today?" or "What brings you here to see the doctor today?" or "Can you tell me about the problem you seem to be having?" or "Can we talk about what has been giving you concern that brings you in to see the doctor?"

For a follow-up visit, ask "Are you feeling any better since you were in to see the doctor last?" or "You don't seem to be feeling too well; do you feel any better?" or "Can you tell me how you've been doing since you were here last?"

Hearing patients' answers can provide a general idea of how they feel emotionally. Of course, one can only accomplish this by taking time to find out. That means giving the patients your undivided attention, if only for a few minutes. Unfortunately, many health care professionals lack the skills and perhaps even the concern to establish this rapport, and therefore fail to develop this skill. The medical assistant can be instrumental in pointing out factors that can interfere with a particular treatment approach planned by the physician, Figure 5–7. Patients will likely respond to and comply with the doctor's orders far more readily if the medical assistant imparts a genuine concern for their well-being with each contact.

If a patient seems quieter than usual, for instance, the medical assistant might determine after talking to the patient (with eye contact of course) that he is preoccupied by some problem or matter that he may open up about if interest is shown and the time is taken. Often a statement that begins with "I" can open up a conversation with another person. For instance, you may say to a patient, "I noticed as you were walking in today that you don't seem to be as lively as usual. Is anything in particular bothering you?" This gives patients a feeling that you really pay attention to them and that you care about how they are and you are showing it. This can make the patient feel more at ease and may gain better compliance with the physician's orders. Using the statements that begin with "I" can be of help to the health care team as well. When conversing with co-workers it is important to speak sincerely and to communicate your feelings to each other as professionally as you do with patients. This can prevent a serious situation from happening because the habit of giving and expecting respect and courtesy has been established. If the patient is not allowed to express certain feelings, he may not be attentive enough to listen to the physician's orders, which need to be followed for optimal health benefits. The medical assistant plays an important role in assisting both physician and patient in providing quality health care.

Complete Chapter 5, Unit 2 in the workbook to help you meet the objectives at the beginning of this unit and therefore achieve competency of this subject matter.

UNIT 3
Patients and Their Families

■ OBJECTIVES

Upon completion of the unit, meet the following terminal performance objectives by verifying knowledge of the facts and principles presented through oral and written communication at a level deemed competent.

1. Explain why it is important to develop rapport with patients and their families.
2. Describe means of safeguarding the patient's right to confidentiality.
3. Describe the patient's options in relation to the physician's treatment plan.
4. Describe the stages that follow diagnosis of a terminal illness.
5. Describe your role in dealing with the terminally ill patient.
6. Explain the purpose of the living will.
7. State the purpose of the Hospice movement.
8. List the services of the Hospice movement.
9. Spell and define, using the glossary at the back of the text, all the words to know in this unit.

■ WORDS TO KNOW

absurd	incomprehensible
advance directives	living will
devastate	inevitable
holistic	marginal
Hospice movement	nonchalant
hostility	terminal

The medical profession's first responsibility is to the patient. Thus you must be able to relate to people of all ages, from tiny infants to senior citizens.

The development and growth of your own personality and interests will help you do so. The ability to converse about a variety of subjects shows an interest in people and makes you interesting to be with. Conversation with patients helps to ease their anxieties and encourages a sense of friendship and trust. At times a patient needs to express pent-up feelings, and you will often be the one who provides this necessary listening service. Sincere empathy will often begin to relieve the inner fears and anxieties of a patient who is experiencing an illness for the first time.

Patients and family members may need to discuss the treatment plan the physician has already discussed with them. Often patients do not hear all of what has been said by the physician because they have been preoccupied with worry about their illness. Their questions may sometimes seem trivial, but to the patient they are real and pressing issues that need immediate attention.

This is the reason that giving printed instructions to patients is so important. If the patient is preoccupied at the time the instructions are given, printed material is also given to him so he can at least read over the information later. Usually a phone call will be initiated by the patient at a later time to have questions answered or for clarification or reassurance about something.

Many patients have never before experienced sickness or injury. They may never have set foot in a health care facility. Having to face strange new surroundings, unfamiliar medical language, and possibly puzzling procedures will add to the patient's apprehensions. The way the patient is treated in these new situations will determine how the patient, and

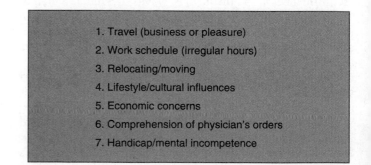

1. Travel (business or pleasure)
2. Work schedule (irregular hours)
3. Relocating/moving
4. Lifestyle/cultural influences
5. Economic concerns
6. Comprehension of physician's orders
7. Handicap/mental incompetence

Figure 5–7 Factors that can interfere with patient compliance in treatment plans.

members of the family, accept the diagnosis and prognosis of the patient's condition. Tact and good communication skills will help to promote rapport with all patients and their family members.

RIGHT TO PRIVACY

As mentioned previously, every patient has a legal right to privacy and confidentiality. Information disclosed to the health care team must be kept in the strictest confidence, and you must be ever mindful of the legal implications in handling patients' records. Information concerning patients may be given to another member of the health care team, such as a laboratory technician or referring physician, only when it pertains directly to the course of treatment. Another medical office may telephone to inquire about a patient's medical history for diagnostic purposes, to confirm symptoms, or to verify a birthdate; patients, in complying with referral appointments or scheduled tests, will have given implied consent for necessary information to be transmitted concerning their condition. In the daily routine, such procedures do not require consent forms to be signed by the patient. If this were not true, very little could be accomplished besides handling forms.

Medical information may be given to parties not concerned in the patient's treatment *only* when the patient has signed a release of information form. Medical insurance forms, for instance, have a section patients must sign to authorize the release of information to insurance companies, Figure 5–8. Only those persons specified by the patient in writing may receive information concerning the patient's condition. Usually the medical facility has a patient information release form, which is completed during the initial visit. Persons to contact in case of emergency are listed

there. Inquiries should be made at this time as to who may be informed about the patient's condition. This document should be filed in the patient's chart for future reference. Those of legal age have the right to privacy in all matters of treatment, and even parents may not be given information about a family member's condition unless specific written permission accompanied by the patient's signature is secured.

In the normal course of conversation you may be told personal information that should be kept to yourself, unless doing so would be harmful to the patient. The patient will usually tell you how far the information should go, or whom to tell or not to tell. Emotional stress and other critical data should be relayed to the physician, for it may have some bearing on the condition of the patient. You must use judgment in this important area. A patient who is experiencing domestic problems, for instance, may be asking for help in telling you about them. Patients usually realize that professional persons can put them in touch with assistance and sometimes expect that it will be forthcoming if they merely suggest that help is needed. Tact is required in handling delicate matters of this nature. Patients trust the medical profession to safeguard matters discussed in the privacy of the medical office. Directly asking each patient who may receive this confidential information and having appropriate release forms signed will ensure that the patient is aware of what has been done and will also protect you from liability.

CHOICE OF TREATMENT

Advising patients of the choices they have in the treatment of their illnesses is often among your responsibilities. A full explanation of the diagnosis, prognosis, and options in treating the condition are given to the patient by the physician. But, some patients have a difficult time in making up their minds and may need additional information and further discussion before deciding to accept a treatment plan, especially when it involves a major event such as elective surgery. There are life-threatening situations in which patients must make these decisions quickly. Often family members must help patients with these difficult decisions.

You play an integral part in reinforcing the physician's orders. You should become proficient in identifying those patients who still seem confused after leaving their conference with the physician. Restating what the physician has already said may be all you need to say to some patients to initiate their compliance. Some patients may have had trouble with the wording used by the physician and look to you to interpret. It is difficult at times to make clear to patients all that is involved in the course of treatment. Great skill in perception is essential for all members of the health care team to ascertain if the approach to treatment is fully understood by the patient. This is a valuable skill which takes time and experience to master.

It is prudent to advise patients to seek a second opinion if they harbor any doubts concerning their condition. It may be that patients disbelieve the diagnosis. Having a second, or even a third, opinion will help them to accept their illness. Many insurance companies encourage patients to seek other opinions before treatment is initiated. This is wise, especially if the patient is troubled about the possible outcome.

RELEASE AND ASSIGNMENT

Date _____

To _____
INSURANCE COMPANY

_____

Group No. _____ Certificate No. _____

I hereby authorize Dr. _____

to release to your company or its representative, any information including the diagnosis and the records of any treatment or examination rendered to me during the period of such Medical or Surgical care.

I also authorize and request your company to pay directly to the above named doctor the amount due me in my pending claim for Basic Medical, Major Medical and/or Surgical treatment or services, by reason of such treatment or services rendered to:

_____
PATIENT

_____
SIGNATURE OF INSURED

_____   _____
WITNESS   ADDRESS

Figure 5–8   Release of information form (Courtesy of Colwell Systems, Inc.).

In more routine matters patients still may have difficulty in complying with physicians' orders, as in weight reduction, exercising, or taking prescribed medicine. Patients must be given sound reasons for following the advice of the physician even though they already know that it is for their own good. The prescribed treatment plan will most likely change the patient's life-style. The patient who has just been diagnosed as hypertensive may have to cope with several lifestyle changes, such as losing weight, following a special diet, and giving up cigarettes. If reinforcement and encouragement are not sufficiently provided to the patient by members of the health care team, cooperation may be **marginal**. The risks of not following the physician's advice should be outlined in the simplest terms. Acting **nonchalant** or showing no interest in the patient will not be much help in prompting a patient to follow orders.

The final choice is always the patient's, to accept and follow the outlined plan of treatment or not. Knowing what is best does not always dictate compliance. Motivation is the key. Giving patients realistic suggestions can help them accept a treatment plan that may initially have seemed impossible to follow. Changing behavior will probably be resisted. The patient who experiences setbacks, who does not remember to take medication, who breaks away from the prescribed diet, and the like, will need additional encouragement to get back on track. You can be of particular value in this type of situation. You must always be reinforcing with your remarks made to patients concerning the intended goals of treatment. Furthermore, by being a good role model, you subtly reinforce the physician's advice. An assistant who should be, but is not, following a weight-reduction plan will give a negative impression to a patient who has just been told to do so by the physician. A patient who has been instructed by the physician in personal hygiene will be less likely to follow advice if the medical assistant does not also heed the advice.

In conversing with patients you will find that their areas of interest will prompt ideas for encouraging compliance with treatment. One good motivator is the physician's fee for services. Many patients quickly realize that they should follow the physician's advice, for it will certainly be more costly in the long run if they do not.

TERMINAL ILLNESS

Dealing with patients who have been diagnosed as having a **terminal** illness will be a challenging and rewarding experience: challenging because of its difficulty and rewarding because of the knowledge that you are giving supportive care when patients and their families need it most.

Many patients have a hard time accepting the diagnosis. Their initial reaction is to deny it. Indeed, knowing that one's life is about to end is an almost **incomprehensible** fact. Patients wrestling with this new reality claim that the diagnosis is **absurd**. But ignoring the problem cannot provide solace.

As frustration mounts and anger becomes apparent, patients feel isolated, for they see others as the picture of health. Feelings of **hostility** are natural and **inevitable**. Patients in this plight may lash out at anyone with whom they come in contact. Blaming themselves and others becomes a means of dealing with their anger for a time. Questioning becomes a way of venting anger for some. "Why does this have to be?" is the most troublesome question. Following this stage of anger is a period of depression. This is the reaction to the final realization of the course of their illness. Patients in this stage are usually ready to talk about their illness, hoping someone will understand. It is a difficult subject to talk about, but you may be influential in helping them to respond and talk about their fears. Eventually the patient attempts to accept the terminal illness by bargaining, or seeking ways of "buying" more time. This sometimes gives them inner strength to stay a while longer, holding on to see someone be married, wanting to hold the new grandchild, waiting for someone to return from the service. In this stage of bargaining, patients may look for spiritual inspiration. The zest for life is strong and the fight is one not easily given up.

In the final stages of terminal disease, patients come closer to accepting the course of their disease. This is truly a sad time for patients and their families. To know that one may not see the next spring, to know that one will no longer experience the joys and pleasures of loved ones, is **devastating** to the patient. Empathy and genuine compassion may be offered to a patient who is reaching out for comfort. You will be touched deeply, and your fortitude will be challenged to the maximum in interacting with the patient and family members during this most stressful time, Figure 5–9.

Finally, patients resign themselves to impending death. An inner peace is often evident in patients in this final stage of their illness and they are willing to make plans for their final days.

Some patients prefer to spare family members the ordeal of prolonging treatment when their physicians reach the decision that death is likely to occur in the near future. Late in 1991 a law was passed in the United States that requires all health care providers to inform and advise patients and their families of **advance directives**. The **living will** is a legal document that allows patients to terminate medical procedures that would sustain their lives if they became unconscious or unable to make further decisions, Figure 3–1 (pg. 45). This document is not recognized in all states in the United States, but is fast becoming a more acceptable way to eliminate continued life-support treatment of the terminally ill patient. The phrase advance directives also refers to the living will as it gives direction to those who will be following the wishes of the patient who prepared the legal document. With this legal

---

The stages of terminal illness:

1. Denial

2. Anger

3. Bargaining

4. Depression

5. Acceptance

Figure 5–9 The stages of terminal illness.

form the patient and family are able to avoid an agonizingly long period in waiting for the inevitable and also keep the cost of health care to a more realistic and reasonable amount.

The patient signs this document and a copy is filed with the physician, the attorney, and the family. In assisting patients with this procedure, it would be helpful if you would remind them to make sure that all details have been worked out and that the family has been properly informed and who is responsible for honoring the document. Patients now know that they have a right to die with dignity and that they have a choice in making their last days of life more meaningful.

For many years a concerned group of individuals has recognized and commiserated with this grief-stricken group of people. These people have formed the **Hospice movement** to provide some health care to those with terminal illness. In recent years the Hospice movement has gained strength. Instead of the tiring and impersonal surroundings that are sometimes associated with hospital care, the Hospice movement helps the family provide care so that patients can remain in their comfortable, familiar home surroundings during the last days of their lives and be among their family members and friends more conveniently. Support and caring assistance is given to help the family learn to cope with the turbulence of the patients and their illness. Efforts are coordinated with physicians and hospital staffs when necessary to give patients the best possible care.

Patients and their families in this stage of the patient's illness may need more spiritual guidance. The counsel of a minister, priest, or rabbi, may also be found through the Hospice movement. **Holistic** care is their purpose. You should refer patients with life-threatening illness to the local Hospice movement for consultation.

Society is returning to the idea that there is a human need to share the experiences of birth and death with loved ones. These natural parts of life have been largely removed from our experience for some time now. We have even become uneasy in talking about them. The need for human love in these significant times in our lives is evident in the return to the practice of entering and leaving this world at home.

Complete Chapter 5, Unit 3 in the workbook to help you meet the objectives at the beginning of this unit and therefore achieve competency of this subject matter.

UNIT 4
Office Interpersonal Relationships

■ OBJECTIVES

Upon completion of the unit, meet the following terminal performance objectives by verifying knowledge of the facts and principles presented through oral and written communication at a level deemed competent.

1. Describe relationships between the medical assistant, the employer, and co-workers.

2. List positive methods for dealing with stress.
3. Describe the reasons for staff meetings.
4. Explain methods of intraoffice communication.
5. State the purpose of an employee evaluation.
6. Discuss the obligations of the employer and the new employee in providing a smooth transition in the workplace.
7. Spell and define, using the glossary at the end of the text, all the words to know in this unit.

■ WORDS TO KNOW

description	perplexing
evaluation	petty
externship	transition
obligation	

The medical assistant employed in a medical office or clinic must learn to relate well not only to patients but to other members of the health care team as well. Dealing with the needs of patients on a day-to-day basis can sometimes become an overwhelming task. Schedules in most medical practices can easily become overbooked; sometimes it seems everyone has an emergency and must be seen by the physician today! Health care employees should be able to shift gears and handle these situations gracefully as well as efficiently. The essential ingredient in running a medical office smoothly is cooperation. When each employee contributes, a good team that works together for quality patient care results.

The field of medicine is by its nature stress-filled. Patients are troubled by an abnormal state of health and are naturally anxious and on edge. Commonly they exhibit their feelings by acting irritable and uncooperative at times. They not only expect but demand patience and understanding from medical personnel.

STAFF ARRANGEMENTS

Picture the ideal medical office where patients and medical staff are going about the business at hand in a pleasant, efficient manner. Everyone gets along well with everyone else, patients are smiling and friendly, and every interchange is courteous. The schedule is kept down to the minute, all the filing is caught up, the phone rings only when there is nothing else pressing at the moment, referral reports are all back, and everything runs like clockwork. This picture is unreal. This ideal situation is what every medical practice hopes to achieve. But to bring this model practice into existence would require the perfection of all persons involved. This is, of course, impossible. Nevertheless, each member of the staff has a unique set of values, principles, and standards and each must respect the others to ensure compatible relationships.

The number of employees varies in the many types of medical practices. Some physicians in private practice employ only one medical assistant to perform both administrative and clinical duties. This is a tremendous responsibility and requires a highly motivated and mature personality. Medical assistants must realize that sometimes long hours and limited benefits may be the result. A good rapport with the employer is necessary to accomplish the objectives of daily patient care. Usually a good friendship develops between physician and medical assistant over a period of time, and working together is an enjoyable learning experience for both. Interest in each patient is easy to cultivate since individual contact is made at each office visit. You may get to know patients even better than the physician because of frequent phone conversation. You will soon become the physician's right hand by supplying important patient information obtained in this manner.

Communication lines must remain open with this one-to-one relationship, as in all employer-employee relationships. If misunderstandings occur, they must be rectified as soon as possible. More complex problems can mushroom if incidental misunderstandings are not cleared up. Solutions to these problems must be worked out together. You will have to be assertive in decisions concerning administrative, clinical, and personal employment matters. Being on one's own as a medical assistant in a private practice has its rewards as well as its disadvantages.

Many physicians in both private and group practices find it necessary to employ several medical assistants. Although this can be an enjoyable experience for all members of the staff, a great deal of cooperation and respect for one another is necessary for a harmonious relationship among the staff members to be maintained. Specific job **descriptions** encourage each employee to remain in a particular area and promote efficiency. Overstepping boundaries may cause friction and misunderstandings. At the same time all staff members must be willing to pitch in where help is needed. Again, a positive attitude is needed to create a pleasant work environment.

The physician usually delegates responsibility for office management to one of the employees, most often the one with greatest seniority, qualifications, or both. This frees the physician to attend to patients and also relieves the physician of personnel management. This is a major area of concern, especially in large clinics with many employees, and, as a rule, is an area physicians are not trained to handle. Many of these supervisory or personnel management positions are filled by registered nurses, but they also have little or no specific training in medical office management. Their training centers primarily around the hospital model and direct patient care. Since a trained medical assistant can, in most states, perform most of the procedures that a nurse can, under the supervision of a physician, resentment may arise. You must come to grips with this reality before accepting a position where it may be a source of irritation and discontent.

Physicians and office managers appreciate the versatility of the medical assistant, respect their initiative and industriousness, and employ them with pride and satisfaction. However, each medical practice has its own unique office policy regarding employees. There are still some physicians who would rather take charge of their own office business affairs.

Working closely with others can have both positive and negative effects. In a large office practice or clinic, when there are many employees, a certain amount of give and take must prevail. Completing assigned tasks is expected so that the work is shared equitably. **Petty** differences should be settled with tact. Sharing enlightening experiences and significant events with other employees is a natural inclination. This is fine if it does not interfere with patient care. A certain amount of self-discipline and self-control is necessary in a professional setting. Remaining aware of the situation at hand will help you perceive what is appropriate.

INTRAOFFICE COMMUNICATION

Many physicians hold regular staff meetings that all employees are expected to attend. They are usually held in the medical office either before or after patients have been seen and are announced far enough in advance so that arrangements can be made to attend. Many staff meetings are scheduled at regular times, i.e., the second Friday of each month, a meet-and-eat meeting at noon every other Wednesday, and so on. At these meetings decisions concerning office policy changes are reached and problems are discussed. This is a time for new ideas to be expressed and exchanged. It also allows all members of the staff to get to know each other.

Some situations between employees may be impossible to iron out. These are usually personality conflicts, and the usual course of action if the situation does not improve is termination of one of the employees, usually the one who is more troublesome or less valuable to the practice. This kind of **perplexing** problem may be discussed during a staff meeting. Personnel managers are often aware of these problems before they are reported, and they are usually handled privately.

Employers sometimes use office meeting time for in-service programs, such as training in cardiopulmonary resuscitation. Some employers encourage holiday celebrations on occasion to promote better working relationships.

An intraoffice memo is a means of communicating important information to members of the staff, especially between regularly scheduled staff meetings. Each employee is instructed to read the memo and initial it, indicating that the information has been received, and then pass it on to another employee. This helps ensure that all employees are informed. Word of mouth is not a sure way to relay an important announcement for it may get distorted en route.

Some offices and clinics use a bulletin board as a means of intraoffice communication, Figure 5–10. Notices of educational programs, seminars, or meetings are posted for all members of the staff to read, in an area such as the staff room or eating area. Meetings of the American Registry of Medical Assistants and the AAMA should be posted there.

CAREER ENTRY

According to recent statistics, there is an increasing need for qualified medical assistants across the nation. Employers in the health care field are recognizing the benefits of employing medical assistants who have had specific training in this most versatile field. This, of course, eliminates the need for extensive and expensive additional training on the job. **Externship** plans are very successful in cooperative programs that provide soon-to-graduate medical assistant students. These students are somtimes hired at a part-time rate, and the supervisor agrees to allow the instructor to periodically visit the facility and observe the student's performance. (Many programs do not allow the students to be paid.) Other

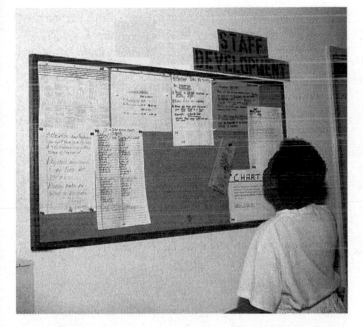

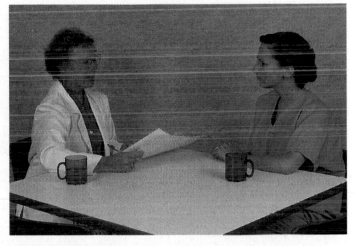

Figure 5-11 This supervisor and medical assistant have established a good rapport through open communication during the evaluation process.

Figure 5-10 Checking the bulletin board daily is a good idea and a valuable resource for current information about AAMA and ARMA meetings, seminars, staff activities, in-service programs.

training programs require only that students observe for a certain number of hours to fulfill the program's standards. In either case, the trend is most welcomed after the past practice of hiring assistants without any training in the field, who sought either full-time or part-time employment in the physicians' offices or clinics.

The **transition** from student to medical assistant, at any age, poses certain adjustment considerations to all concerned in the health care setting. Employers have an **obligation** to assist the new employee in feeling accepted in the profession and to give helpful advice with patience. The new employee is obligated to strive to perform skills with both proficiency and efficiency. An effort to get along with others is required of each member of the health care team. A smooth transition by the new member of the team is possible if each employee recognizes the individual worth of each person and the value of each position in fulfilling the health care needs of the patients they serve.

EMPLOYEE EVALUATION

In most employment situations, an **evaluation** of work performance is made on an annual basis. This is filed in your record. The initial employment review is usually held after a probationary period of thirty, sixty, or ninety days. In this meeting, you and your employer will discuss your job performance. Evaluation forms outline the most important qualities and abilities needed for the job and include a section for strengths and weaknesses to be listed. An example of an employee evaluation form can be found in Chapter 21, Unit 2 with further discussion on securing employment. Employers are always aware of an employee's behavior. Little goes unnoticed when you share a daily routine. Your attitude shows at all times. Even though the word *attitude* may not be a part of the evaluation, the other categories cover it comprehensively.

Initiative is an important factor. Demonstrating resourcefulness will help you advance in your career. Following office policy is also important. Being on time and being dependable on the job are always pleasing to employers. Absences and tardiness are difficult to tolerate from employees who make it a habit. Another area of extreme importance to employers is the quality and quantity of your work. Performing assigned tasks in a reasonable amount of time, without needing to be reminded, is a valuable trait.

The employee evaluation need not be a threat to the conscientious medical assistant. It is a time when questions about advancement and salary may be openly discussed. If you have lived up to the standards of the job, your performance should receive a favorable review.

Some employers find that annual evaluations motivate employees and keep communication lines open, Figure 5-11. Others choose not to have official evaluations, but wish employees to discuss whatever is on their mind at any time. For some office personnel this works quite well. For the private practice physician with one or two medical assistants this is usually the case.

Complete Chapter 5, Unit 4 in the workbook to help you meet the objectives at the beginning of this unit and therefore achieve competency of this subject matter.

Medical-Legal Ethical Highlights

Throughout this chapter you should be mindful of all medical-legal/ethical implications. Listed below are a few important reminders.

1. Be constantly aware of how you project yourself, verbal and nonverbal messages.
2. Develop and maintain good personal health habits to be alert on the job.
3. Respect the rights of all individuals.
4. Attend all in-service and staff meetings.
5. Follow office policy where employed.

Ms. Right attends the monthly staff meeting where office policy is reviewed. She is considerate of all co-workers and patients by addressing them with their appropriate titles courteously in a pleasant tone of voice. Her body language exhibits professionalism as her appearance is consistently fresh, neat, and clean without excessive use of makeup, perfume, or jewelry. Patients sense her sincerity because she makes eye contact while speaking to them and she listens carefully when spoken to. She never talks about patients where other patients may overhear her.

Employment outlook: Continuous.

Ms. Wrong rudely calls patients by their first names regardless of their age or status. She does so while alternating cracking her gum, blowing bubbles, sneezing, and coughing. She missed the staff meeting because she was sick, again. Her appearance is untidy, her uniform and "jogging" shoes are obviously dirty. She complains to patients that she's the one who should be seeing the doctor and ignores the patients' questions. She pays no attention to reminders regarding office policy. She talks and laughs about patients where other patients can hear her.

Employment outlook: Termination.

REFERENCES

Bates, Richard C. *The Fine Art of Understanding Patients,* 2d ed. Oradell, NJ: Medical Economics, 1972.

Calhoun, James F., and Acocella, Joan Ross, *Psychology of Adjustment and Human Relationships,* 2d ed. New York: Random House, 1983.

Kinn, Mary E., and Derge, Eleanor. *The Medical Assistant: Administrative and Clinical,* 7th ed. Philadelphia: W. B. Saunders, 1993.

Milliken, Mary Elizabeth. *Understanding Human Behavior,* 5th ed. Albany: Delmar, 1993.

Physician's Desk Reference. Oradell, NJ: Medical Economics, updated annually.

Purtilo, Ruth. *Health Professional/Patient Interaction,* 4th ed. Philadelphia: W. B. Saunders, 1990.

Riker, Audrey Palm, and Riker, Charles. *Me: Understanding Myself and Others,* rev. ed. Peoria, IL: Bennett, 1982.

Sehnert, Keith W., M.D. *Stress/Unstress.* Augsburg Publishing House, 1981.

U.S. Department of Health and Human Services. *Saying No.* 1981. Alcohol, Drug Abuse, and Mental Health Administration, 5600 Fishers Lane, Rockville, MD 20857.

Wright, H. Norman. *How to Have a Creative Crisis,* Berkley ed. New York: Berkley Publishing Group, 1987.

The Administrative Medical Assistant

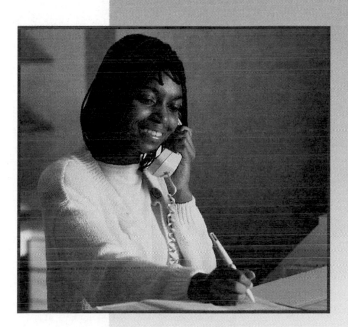

Oral and Written Communications

The office assistant must have sufficient knowledge of medical terminology to deal efficiently with the unending variety of telephone calls received daily. A pleasant voice and good listening skills are essential. Practicing patience and demonstrating compassion to those in need of such attention are important. The medical assistant needs to have legible handwriting for recording appointments and messages. Typing or keyboarding skills are necessary if appointments are to be made on a computer. The student who enjoys keyboarding or working on a computer has an opportunity to develop this skill as an administrative medical assistant. You will have an opportunity to demonstrate your knowledge of anatomy, medical terminology, spelling, grammar, and punctuation as you complete progress notes on charts. You will use these skills also in the completion of correspondence. You may have the responsibility of processing incoming and outgoing mail. Written communication skills must be as flawless as possible. A number of people may view the letters or forms you send out and each will receive a mental picture of you and your office—good if the work is neat and correct, and definitely questionable if it is inaccurate or messy.

UNIT 1
Telephone Communications

UNIT 2
Schedule Appointments

UNIT 3
Written Communications

UNIT 4
Receiving and Sending Office Communications

UNIT 1

Telephone Communications

OBJECTIVES

Upon completion of the unit, meet the following terminal performance objectives by verifying knowledge of the facts and principles presented through oral and written communication at a level deemed competent, and demonstrate the specific behaviors as identified in the terminal performance objectives of the procedures, observing safety precautions in accordance with health care standards.

1. Organize desk space for efficient use of the telephone.
2. Demonstrate a professional method of holding and answering the phone.
3. Describe methods of screening incoming calls.
4. Locate information in a telephone directory.
5. Demonstrate a procedure for referring a patient to another health facility.
6. Spell and define, using the glossary at the back of the text, all the words to know in this unit.

WORDS TO KNOW

colleague	personality
confirmed	pertinent
empathy	rely
etiquette	screening
expressed	verify

ANSWERING THE TELEPHONE

The telephone is the center of all activity in the medical office just as it is with any business. The professional attitude conveyed is critical to the success of the business of practicing medicine. The medical assistant who handles phone calls must be courteous, articulate, and a careful and active listener. The rapport established by the assistant will contribute to successful communication with patients. Most medical facilities have telephones with two or more phone lines. This means that someone should answer each line as soon as possible or at least by the third ring. It seems that on some days all lines ring continually and there is no letup. Because of this situation, an automatic answering device is available that will come on with a recording that asks the caller to please hold and explains that the call will be taken as soon as possible in order of the calls. The responsibility of responding to calls takes a great deal of maturity and patience. Knowing what to ask and when to ask it in order to determine how serious a situation or condition is, is a skill that one develops over time.

Telephone Triage

An established phone triage manual should be kept near the phone for reference so that each assistant who answers the phone will ask the same standard questions and give the same standard advice which the physician has pre-authorized. The assistant must learn how to logically proceed through a set of questions that will reveal the caller's condition and help to determine, if necessary, how soon the patient should be seen by a physician. This process is telephone triage. The assistant must stay alert and ask questions of co-workers and supervisors as they come up to learn how to best deal with problems. If the assistant does not know how to handle a patient, or if the questions have not been addressed in the manual, referring the problem to one who is more experienced is necessary and appropriate. Never guess in response to a patient's questions and do not treat any question lightly. If there is a serious telephone emergency that cannot be handled in the facility, it is best to refer the patient to an emergency medical service (give the phone number to the person if they do not know it) and explain that they will send someone as soon as possible to help. It may be best to direct the person to an emergency room of the nearest hospital. It is a sensible practice to have all emergency phone numbers listed by each phone in the office. In stressful times, this will be helpful in giving the patient phone numbers they might need quickly or in calling an emergency service for the patient. If you are speaking to a patient face to face at the office and you must answer the phone, say to the patient, "Excuse me for a moment, please," answer the phone call, and then continue with what you were doing. Every emergency call must be handled immediately.

Non-emergency Calls

If the person on the phone needs additional information, or if the call is going to take a while, excuse yourself from the phone call by saying, "Would you mind being put on hold for a moment?" However, if it will be more than one minute the caller should not be put on hold; in this case say, "May I call you back with that information?" and find out when a good time is to call back. There may be times when the patient has to wait to speak to the physician. In this case, you should check back each minute until the doctor answers to let the patient know that he or she has not been forgotten. During the time the caller waits, many medical facilities provide the caller with a pleasant recording with reminders of immunization updates, the services and procedures offered by the staff, when routine office hours are, what to do and

who to call in an emergency, and other relevant information. This gives the person who is waiting helpful information while the time passes. The assistant must beware of leaving callers on hold for too long. You can be sure that callers will let you know how long they had to wait and how many times they heard the entire recording.

If you need to transfer a patient's call to another department or office, first give the caller the phone number, extension number, and the person's name you are transferring them to in case there is a disconnection. You should signal the person (or page them) and when they answer, explain who is waiting to speak to them and give a brief summary of what it is regarding. You may say, for example, "Excuse me, Ms. Winters. Mr. Robert James is on line three with a question about his insurance." Ms. Winters should respond with, "Yes, I can talk to him." You should then say, "Thank you, I'll transfer him now. Go ahead please, Mr. James." Then listen to make sure the call was transferred before you hang up. All of this needs to be done quickly and efficiently with a pleasant tone and a polite attitude. This process is much more polite and acceptable than yelling across the room or down the hall for another member of the staff to pick up the phone to speak to someone, or worse, asking the caller to hold while you "find" the person requested, regardless of whether the person is a patient or not. When a patient is calling for information, remember to pull the file and have it ready for the physician along with any test/lab reports that may be the reason for the call. If you have a public address system where everyone can hear the page, be very careful with confidentiality and merely say, for instance, "Dr. Smith, you have a call on line two." You may have to repeat the page if the call is not answered within one minute. Make sure you tell the caller that the person they wish to speak with has been paged and will be with them as soon as possible. If there is no way to announce a call over a loud speaker, simply use a small note to confidentially let the doctor know who is waiting to speak to him or her on the phone and which line the patient is on. There may be times when the physician is close to the phone; simply ask the doctor to take the call and tell him or her who is calling and what the call is regarding. Remember to say please, thank you, excuse me, and so on when appropriate. Establishing good communication, especially over the phone, is essential to building good rapport. It is important to make a list or a log of all phone calls and note who the person is that you should call back. You should also ask when it is best for a return call, repeat the number to ensure that you wrote the correct number down, and follow through with their request as close to the time as possible. This considerate practice should almost eliminate the frustration of playing "phone tag" which is repeatedly calling back and forth and never getting to speak to the intended party.

DOCUMENTING TELEPHONE MESSAGES

Documenting telephone messages is of vital importance and should be treated likewise. Of primary concern is the issue of confidentiality. Data regarding patients may not be given out over the telephone to anyone unless the patient has given written permission for the release of specific information with his or her signature. It is equally important that the date, time, a brief message regarding the call, and the initials of the person who responded to the call be recorded. Then any questions concerning a call may be further explained by the person whose initials are on the message. All calls, regardless of what you may think about their importance, should be documented in the same manner. All messages that are urgent should be given priority and handled as soon as possible to prevent further discomfort, pain, and anxiety for patients.

There are commercial answering services available which provide physicians with a practical way to handle all calls during lunch breaks, evenings, weekends, vacations, and any other time necessary. This can be a convenient service for the physician and office staff. There seems to be a greater acceptance of this type of answering assistance because the caller gets to speak to a live person instead of listening to a recording. In an emergency situation, people are more easily comforted by another human voice even if the doctor is not available. However, problems can arise with these systems because the business employing the service is unable to know all of the persons who answer the phone lines. There is the risk that someone who is not adequately trained may be too abrupt or possibly rude to a patient. Yet, keeping the human element integrated within professional boundaries is the most desirable way to build rapport when communicating with patients.

Voice mail, pagers, and other answering service devices make communications much more accessible than ever before. Answering machines are especially good to use for short time blocks such as during lunch time. If the standard in your medical office is an answering machine that records messages whenever the physician is not in the office, it should tell the caller how to contact the physician or how to leave a message. This must be done day and night, 365 days a year. Messages need to be played back and recorded as soon as possible. Then, all of the calls need to be returned in the order of their importance within an appropriate and reasonable time period. Some physicians prefer to have patients call them at their home, while others employ an answering service to screen calls and take only urgent cases at home. In this instance, the one who screens the calls will contact the doctor at home (or wherever, usually by pager) and have the doctor return the patient's call.

A telephone message pad and pen should be placed by each office telephone. You cannot **rely** on memory in a busy office where there are constant interruptions. Individual offices have a variety of methods for recording telephone messages. You may use a preprinted duplicate message pad; the top sheet is removed and the carbon remains as a permanent record of calls received. The office may use a secretarial notebook that is dated each day; calls are recorded and checked off when returned. You need to develop a follow-up method to be sure calls have been returned. The call pad or messages should not be filed until the requests have been given a response. Some offices have a stamp made up to indicate in the patient chart a telephone communication and a brief note with the date the patient was contacted. It is not advisable to have loose slips of paper in the file as they are too easily lost. If it is desired to keep these in the chart, they should be filed shingle fashion on a sheet of bond paper with the latest call on top. The slips should be fastened with a piece of transparent tape horizontally across the top of the

slip. A vertical piece of tape along the side allows curling of the edges of the slip, resulting in a messy record that is difficult to read.

Self-stick telephone message forms are helpful in establishing effective control of patient calls. One form comes in a single looseleaf style with a stub (like that of a checkbook or loan payment book) which remains in a binder for future reference. Another style has a duplicate copy which remains in a spiral binder and provides a master reference for future review. When a call is received from a patient, the message form is completed. After completing the form, tear it at the perforation and attach the form to the patient's chart by removing the adhesive protection strips at each end on the back of the form. If a patient call requires a return call from the physician, the form is stuck to the front of the patient's chart and given to the physician. When the physician completes the call and records the message, the form is simply removed from the front of the chart and restuck on the inside of the chart for future reference, Figure 6–1. Another telephone message form is a log sheet and message slip with carbon. The benefits of this system are that you do not have to rewrite the message in the patient's chart, use a telephone stamp, or be concerned about loose slips of paper falling out of the chart. The carbon copy is a permanent record of calls for reference. Examples of telephone message forms are shown in Figures 6–1 and 6–2.

The important items of a telephone message are:

- Caller's full name, spelled correctly
- Brief note indicating the nature of the call
- Action required
- Date, time of call, initials of person receiving call
- Phone number of caller. Include the area code if this is a long distance call.

If the telephone has a speaker phone or a headset, your hands will be free to use a pen to either write a message

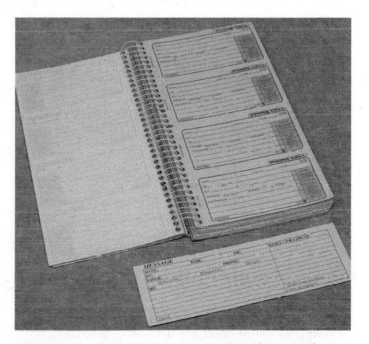

FIGURE 6–1 These telephone message forms have a carbon copy that stays intact for a permanent record of each call.

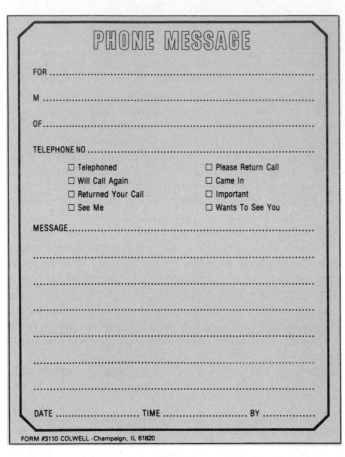

FIGURE 6–2 Telephone message forms (Courtesy of Colwell Systems).

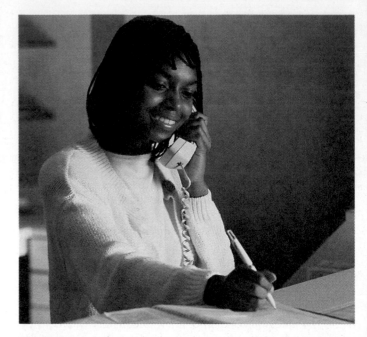

FIGURE 6–4 The medical assistant in this picture shows the proper distance in holding the phone receiver. Even though the caller cannot see this receptionist, her pleasant attitude is evident.

or use the keyboard to log in the patient's call, retrieve the patient's file, or schedule an appointment. Figure 6–3 shows the medical assistant using the headset in phone conversation. The proper position of a phone with a receiver is shown in Figure 6–4. When you hold the receiver of the

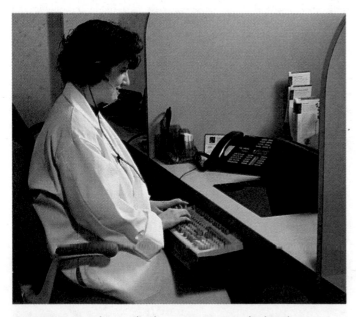

FIGURE 6–3 This medical assistant is using the headset in answering calls to free her hands to use the keyboard, take messages, open mail, and so on.

telephone, it should be 2 to 3″ in front of your mouth so that the caller may clearly hear your voice. Many professional offices have cordless phones, speaker phones, or phones with long cords on the receiver part of the phone for ease in accessing files as needed. The hold (relief) button, transfer extension dialing, conference calling, and other various features may vary from office to office. You should be honest about your knowledge and experience with phone systems. You must ask to have a certain feature explained and demonstrated to you if you do not know how to use it. You must use proper technique with a telephone system or the caller may be rudely interrupted or accidentally disconnected during a call. Since you never know who is on the other end of the phone, always answer as promptly as possible in a professional manner. Emergencies can happen at any time and your efficiency on the phone could affect the outcome.

The following example highlights the proper manner of a polite and efficient way to answer a call: "Good morning, Central Medical Center, Ellen speaking, how may I help you?" The caller usually is prompted to give you his or her name after saying hello to you and explains the reason for the call. Your response should be appropriate and spoken in a pleasant tone of voice to each caller. Make sure that you get the complete name and phone number of the patient in case your call is interrupted. This is a safe practice to follow in case the call is an emergency and you get cut off. If the information that the patient gives you is not clear, you must say, for example, "Could you please repeat that for me?" or, "Would you spell your name for me again, please?" It is better to ask someone to repeat what was said initially than to have to go back over the whole conversation and redo all of it—the patient may wonder if you paid attention to *anything* that was said. You should convey confidence rather than insecurity. If you cannot understand someone because their voice is too soft, ask them to speak a little louder. If the person talks too loud, ask if they could speak a little softer, faster, slower, and so on, as indicated by the way the caller sounds to you. It is also a good practice to ask patients each time you speak to them (over the phone or in person) if there is any change in their address, phone, and so on, to keep files current.

When you are finished with the conversation, it is best to allow the caller to hang up first. If you hang up first you might miss something the patient wanted to add. It is not considered professional to say "Bye-bye" when you finish the call. You should say "Goodbye."

When you have more than one telephone line coming in to the office, never answer the second line with "Hold the line, please," and then go back to your first call. You need to place the first call on hold and find out who is on the second line. Then you can determine whether or not it is an emergency and if it is not, ask the second caller to hold for you to finish the first call. Make all calls as brief as possible. You should keep any personal calls to a minimum.

Your voice is an important part of your **personality** at any time, but over the telephone, your voice *is* you. Callers form a picture of you as they listen to your voice. Does your telephone personality reveal a confident, courteous, friendly, and efficient medical assistant? It is equally easy to be heard as uncertain, irritated, abrupt, or inefficient.

Since the phone call is often the first contact a patient has with the office, your manner of speaking and the **empathy** you convey are critical to your success as a receptionist.

COMMON TYPES OF PHONE CALLS

The process of **screening** calls requires you to be aware of the most frequent types of phone calls that will be received in the medical office. They are:

- Referrals
- Patients who are calling for appointments, prescriptions, or the results of tests
- Emergency calls
- Other physicians, hospitals, or laboratories
- Personal calls and general business calls

A workbook and cassette titled *Handling Patients' Telephone Calls Effectively,* used in the Department of Practice Management as a guideline for workshops on this important aspect of the management of a medical office, is available from The American Medical Association.

Appointments, Prescriptions, and Test Results

Patients who phone for appointments should be given a choice of two appointment times. Usually one of the times will be satisfactory and this will eliminate the patient asking for multiple dates and times that are not available. Do not say "When would you like to come in?" It is better to say "Do you prefer mornings or afternoons?" Do not say "Are you a patient here?" It is better to say "When did we last see you?" Do not say "What's the problem?" It is better to say "Can you tell me what seems to be the problem, so that we can schedule you properly?" The appointment should be con-

firmed by reading the scheduled time back to the patient after it has been recorded in the appointment book.

You will find that patients will frequently ask to speak with the physician. Never say "The doctor is busy," as this may give the impression that the doctor does not want to be bothered by the caller. Be aware of the statements you make in reporting why the physician cannot speak on the telephone. It would be much better to state "The doctor is with a patient now. May I take a message and we will return the call as soon as possible?" The caller will usually respect the right of others to have the full attention of the physician and will not expect to interrupt the doctor except for an emergency.

Prescriptions

Each office will have its own rules for giving information to patients regarding tests or for calling pharmacies for prescription refills. It is important that you learn the rules for the office you work in and follow them without exception. The general rule is that a medical assistant does not give out information or call in a prescription without the **expressed** direction of the physician.

Write messages requesting prescriptions or test results in legible handwriting. If a patient requests a prescription refill, you need to know the name and phone number of the pharmacy as well as the name of the medication, strength, and prescription number. You also should record a telephone number where the patient can be reached in case the physician needs to talk with the patient before prescribing the medication. The physician may need to examine the patient first and you would need to call and schedule an appointment.

Professional Calls

When a physician telephones to speak to your employer, politely ask the caller for his or her name and inform the physician. Professional **etiquette** dictates that a physician will not keep a **colleague** waiting unless the physician is involved with an emergency or a surgical procedure.

Any calls that come into your office for the purpose of giving x-ray or laboratory results need to be recorded accurately. Always record the name of the person making the report. It is best to read back everything you have written down to be sure it is correct and complete before allowing the caller to leave the line.

The physician should review and initial all reports the day they arrive at the office. Pull the patient chart and attach the report. Never file a report that the physician has not seen and initialed. The patient or referring physician may need to be notified of the results by your physician employer. After this is completed, the report will be ready to file.

Some physicians also dictate reports, which you will be required to transcribe and mail. Always be sure to make a copy of any correspondence mailed out so you have a copy to file in the patient chart. This is always filed with the most recent correspondence on top when the folder is opened.

When a patient calls for test results, you should never give them without receiving the physician's instructions on what to report. You would never give information to other people

PROCEDURE

6-1 Answer the Office Phone

PURPOSE: Answer the office telephone promptly and efficiently in a professional manner.

EQUIPMENT AND SUPPLIES: Telephone, paper, pen, computer—if available.

TERMINAL PERFORMANCE OBJECTIVE: In a simulated (or actual) situation, using proper grammar, answer the telephone by the third ring identifying the office and yourself.

1. Answer the phone promptly (by the third ring) in a polite and pleasant manner.

2. Identify the office and yourself by name.

   NOTE: Your voice must be clear, distinct. Speak at a moderate rate, expressing consideration for the needs of the caller.

3. Listen to and record the name of the caller, the reason for the call, and the date and time of the call.

NOTE: ■ Obtain the correct spelling of the name.
■ Process emergency calls immediately.
■ Before placing a caller on hold, wait for a response.
■ If you must place the caller on hold, check each minute to let him know you remember he is waiting (a patient should never wait longer than three minutes).
■ Complete all calls that were interrupted and/or were placed on hold.

4. Screen and complete as many calls as possible before adding names to the physician's call back list.

5. Respond to an untimely request to speak to the physician by taking a message for the physician to return the call or having advice relayed by you.

about a patient without the written permission of the patient and the approval of the physician. Procedures 6–1 through 6–4 outline steps of answering the office phone.

Business and Personal Calls

Your employer should let you know how to handle calls from family members, business associates, and salespeople. Calls from attorneys requesting information about a patient must be handled with great caution. Attorneys know the patient must give written permission to divulge information to anyone regarding their health, yet attorneys will call and ask for information. Pull the patient chart and look for authorization listing the name of the attorney and the signature of the patient. If you find it, you may answer questions about the patient. If you do not find authorization listing the name of the attorney, you must tell the caller to send an authorization signed by the patient and then you will be able to release information. It is advisable to return a call from an attorney even if you have authorization so you can be sure whom you are talking to. Anyone can call and claim to be a patient's attorney. Unless you know the caller, you cannot be sure you are talking to the correct individual.

Only information that has been authorized by the patient in writing, with the patient's signature, may be given to another party. Otherwise, the patient record is considered confidential information.

Angry Calls

You may receive calls from patients regarding their statement or their insurance. If you are very careful in your accounting and billing, these should be infrequent calls. If you do receive a call from a patient who is angry, be sure you listen attentively, then tell the patient "Please hold so I can get your record." If you have made an error, be sure you admit it, apologize, and offer to send a revised statement. Never raise your voice or allow yourself to blame someone else for a mistake you have made. Sometimes it is best to say you will check the records and call back. Always keep your word and follow up with the promised action. Patients will soon learn to trust you if you gain a reputation for careful follow-up of promises. Frequently patients need to know if insurance has paid the bill or how much was paid by insurance. You can quickly check the record and answer the questions.

Reports from Patients

When the physician routinely tells patients, "Call me and let me know how you are getting along," you can expect to receive calls to report how the patient is feeling or to report reactions to medications. These reports should be carefully recorded and given to the physician. You need to determine whether or not the physician is expected to respond to the call.

Physician Visits Outside the Office

When a patient calls and requests a house call, be sure you check with your physician employer before you schedule one. If your employer makes house calls, you should have a city map or county map to help locate any new patient scheduled.

Many physicians visit patients in hospitals and nursing homes on a regular basis. You need to establish a method of recording these visits and hospital calls. The physician should have a list of calls to be made each day along with a checklist of needed follow-up and charges for services.

Long Distance Calls

You may need to place long distance calls. If you are calling an area outside of your time zone, you should consult the telephone directory for the map Figure 6–5 of time zones so you can establish the appropriate time to call. Take into consideration when it is lunch break in a different time zone so that you will not waste time trying to phone an office when the staff is not available to take your call. Be sure you know the code number needed to dial for your long distance service, in addition to the telephone numbers of the persons you need to call. A record book should be kept on all long distance calls made.

Call Monitoring

When your employer asks you to monitor a call either by an extension phone or speakerphone, listen quietly and take notes of the conversation. It is important to make certain the caller agrees to your listening and taking notes. It is illegal for you to do this without the consent of the caller. Another type of monitoring is to record the phone call so that it may be played back if necessary at a later time. This, also, is illegal to do without the party's written consent.

Refusal and/or Inability to Identify

Your office may have a specific method of handling individuals who call and refuse to identify themselves. A good general rule is to suggest that the individual write a letter to the physician and mark it *personal*, in which case the physician will receive it unopened. Most physicians do not wish to talk to unidentified callers during busy office hours.

The rules for handling the physician's telephone can be summarized as follows:

1. Answer the telephone as promptly as possible.
2. Keep a pad and pen next to the telephone at all times.
3. Verify the caller's name and correct spelling. If an adult calls about a child, make sure you have the correct last name. Do not assume the child's last name is the same as the caller's name.
4. Determine the reason for the call.
5. Handle as many telephone calls as you possibly can without disturbing the physician.
6. If the physician prefers to speak to patients, call physician to the telephone after asking who is calling. Pull patient's chart and give it to the physician.
7. Whenever possible, if you cannot handle the call alone, take a message for the physician. The physician will tell you what to do or call the patient back as time allows. (Figure 6–6)
8. Make a memorandum for the physician of every telephone call. Use printed telephone memorandum pads that show date of call, time of call, name of caller, telephone number, and message.
9. Always know where to reach the physician. If the message is urgent and the physician is not in the office, telephone at once and relay the message.
10. If the physician cannot be reached, have the message by your phone. When your employer checks in, you may relay the message.
11. Learn how much medical information the physician wishes you to give over the telephone. Patients frequently call the office because they have forgotten the physician's instructions about treatments or medications. If these instructions are clearly stated in the chart, or in a pre-approved triage manual, it may be possible for the assistant to repeat them to the patient.
12. When answering a second line, determine if it is an emergency or another physician before placing the caller on hold and returning to finish the first call.
13. End all telephone conversations on a friendly note. In general, let the caller be the first one to hang up or say "good bye."
14. *Never* promise a cure over the telephone or in person. Never say "I am sure the physician can help you."

If you have answered the phone and no one answers you back after trying twice to converse with them, simply hang up. Some phone systems may have caller ID, which may help in this type of situation. Immediately returning the call in this case may link you to a person in distress. However, it could be a prank call or possibly an obscene call, which should be ignored. Of course, if it persists, it should be reported to the police and to the phone company. Many times the phone directory has a section which outlines the steps that should be taken in situations such as harassing phone calls. Simply telling the caller that you have reported the problem may be enough to make it stop. Taking action as soon as the situation begins is the most sensible course to take. **CAUTION:** Never tell anyone over the phone (or in person) that you are alone (even if you are) as this could possibly be an invitation for undesirable behaviors. For your safety, it is not wise to work alone when there is no one near for assistance. If you must, and only if it is absolutely necessary for you to complete your

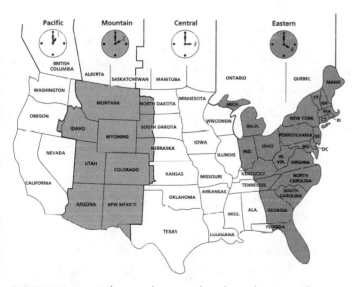

FIGURE 6–5 Make sure that you place long distance calls within regular business hours by referring to a time zone map such as this.

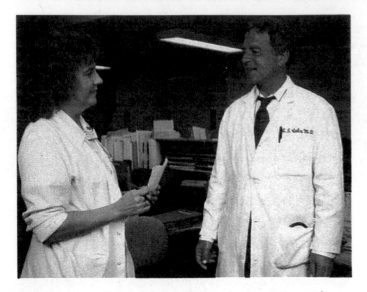

FIGURE 6–6 Phone messages that you cannot answer without the physician's advice should be done as soon as possible between seeing patients.

responsibilities, a neighboring office staff or someone you trust should be informed of your being alone.

FINDING PHONE NUMBERS

You can save a great deal of time by keeping an up-to-date index of your most frequently called numbers by the telephone. In addition, when you need to use the telephone directory, it is helpful to know how it is organized.

The introductory section usually contains:

- Emergency numbers
- Community service numbers
- General telephone information
- Directory assistance information
- Rates for telephone calls
- Out-of-city area codes and time zones
- Money-saving tips on use of the telephone
- Directions for making international calls
- Rights and responsibilities
- Directory listings

You will find an alphabetic listing of individuals in the white pages. There may be separate listing of business and professional organizations in a second section of the white pages. An index of city, county, state, and United States government offices may be found in a separate section of pages. Local zip code numbers by street address are usually in the introduction or a separate section of the telephone book. This section can be taken out of the large phone book and kept on the top of the desk in a stand-up organizer for easy access. This makes your job less taxing and eliminates the need to lift a heavy book many times each day. There are also books of complete listings of all zip codes in the country available. This is a necessary reference to have in the office as it saves you from making frequent calls to the post office for information. Within the "rights and responsibilities" section of a telephone directory, you will find very helpful information regarding phone service and safety.

The contents section should be reviewed with each new updated directory as it will contain information which may have changed from the last edition. Another feature that most telephone companies now have are specialized services and

PROCEDURE

6-2 Process Phone Message

PURPOSE: Process a phone message properly.

EQUIPMENT AND SUPPLIES: Telephone, pen, paper/phone message log or computer, calendar, timepiece.

TERMINAL PERFORMANCE OBJECTIVE: In a simulated situation (or actual situation) receive, evaluate, and document a phone message.

1. Answer the phone properly (refer to steps in Procedure 6-1).

2. Listen carefully to the caller and determine the caller's needs (refer to triage manual, page 136).
   NOTE: Scheduling a routine appointment may be all that is necessary.

3. Document information regarding the message, including date and time of call, on a message pad or phone call log. You must remember to include:
   - who the request is for.
   - what it is concerning.
   - when the information is needed.
   - where to return the call.

4. Repeat the message to the caller to **verify** the contents. **Rationale: This practice helps to avoid errors.**

5. End the conversation with the caller politely.
   NOTE: It is a good practice to allow the caller to hang up first.

6. Sign your initials after the message.

7. Pull the patient's chart and record/attach the message.

P R O C E D U R E

6-3   Record Telephone Message on Recording Device

PURPOSE: To provide a clear and precise message with all necessary information to the caller in a pleasant tone of voice when you (and other staff members) are unavailable to answer the office phone.

EQUIPMENT AND SUPPLIES: Telephone message device, pen, paper/phone message log or computer, calendar, timepiece.

TERMINAL PERFORMANCE OBJECTIVE: In a simulated situation (or actual situation) produce, with all necessary information in a pleasant tone of voice, a clear, accurate, and precise phone message on the telephone message device.

1. Assemble all necessary items in an area away from noise and distractions.

   NOTE: Determine the amount of time allowed on the recording device for the message before you begin.

2. Write out the appropriate message, check for completeness and accuracy, and read and determine the length of the message.

3. Record the message according to the directions of the answering device.
   - Speak in a pleasant, clear, and articulate tone of voice.
   - Sit up straight and project your voice into the speaker.
   - Identify the office.
   - Avoid being too wordy and overly friendly.
   - Be complete and accurate with information, Figure 6–7 on the following page.

4. Play the message back and evaluate the quality of the message. Listen and determine if the message is of good quality and is appropriate for all callers who are trying to contact your medical facility.

5. Set the device to play the recorded message when you are unavailable to answer the phone.

equipment for the deaf. You may have an opportunity to pass this information on to patients who may need these services and not be aware of them. The yellow pages (or classified directory) list the name, address, and phone number of every business subscriber, grouped under product and service headings. The classified directory also contains an index that can help you determine the headings under which a specific type of product or service may be listed.

Complete Chapter 6, Unit 1 in the workbook to help you meet the objectives at the beginning of this unit and therefore achieve competency of this subject matter.

P R O C E D U R E

6-4   Obtain Telephone Message from Phone Recording Device

PURPOSE: To obtain accurate message(s) from the recording with all necessary information from the caller in order to correctly process requests.

EQUIPMENT AND SUPPLIES: Telephone message device, pen, paper/phone message log or computer, appropriate patients' charts.

TERMINAL PERFORMANCE OBJECTIVE: In a simulated situation (or actual situation), obtain all necessary and **pertinent** information from the phone message recording device.

1. Assemble all necessary items in an area away from noise and distractions.

2. Listen to the recordings and write out each message accurately.

   NOTE: You may have to listen to the recording more than one time in order to obtain complete information, as some

voices may be difficult to understand. It is a good practice to ask another staff member to listen if you have difficulty.

3. Sign your initials after the message. The date and time of the message must also be written.

4. List all patients who leave messages so you can pull their charts.

5. Prioritize messages according to the nature of their seriousness and distribute to the appropriate staff member/department to be processed.

   NOTE: If you are to obtain messages from an answering service, call the service and obtain the messages from a customer service representative. Obtain messages from various answering services offered by phone companies by following the instructions for specialized features. Then, follow the steps as outlined above.

Thank you for calling the Central Park Medical Center. [(Optional) It is: day of the week, month and day, year, time of day.] No one is available to answer your call at this time. If this is an emergency, please call either 555-0000 **immediately** or phone the emergency medical service in your area, or go directly to the nearest hospital emergency room. If this is a non-emergency, and you wish to speak to a member of our staff, please call us between the hours of 8:00 A.M. and 4:30 P.M., Monday through Friday. We will be glad to help you in any way we can. After the tone sounds, please leave your name, phone number, a brief message, and when you may be reached. Your call will be returned as soon as possible. Have a pleasant day.

FIGURE 6–7 Example of phone recorder message.

UNIT 2
Schedule Appointments

◼ OBJECTIVES

Upon completion of the unit, meet the following terminal performance objectives by verifying knowledge of the facts and principles presented through oral and written communication at a level deemed competent, and demonstrate the specific behaviors as identified in the terminal performance objectives of the procedures, observing safety precautions in accordance with health care standards.

1. List and discuss ways that an office staff can establish the most desirable method of scheduling for their individual needs.
2. Discuss what is meant by "establishing a matrix" and explain why it is important.
3. List and explain the various methods of scheduling.
4. Discuss the advantages and disadvantages of each method of scheduling.
5. List and discuss the most important points to consider in determining appointment scheduling when someone calls the office.
6. Discuss the importance of a triage manual for handling telephone calls.
7. Discuss the most practical way to schedule a patient who is always late.
8. Explain and discuss the purpose of the rules for handling a canceled appointment.
9. List and discuss the goals of the physician, the medical assistant, and the patient regarding the appointment schedule.
10. List common abbreviations and their meanings used in making appointments.
11. Discuss various ways of recording appointment schedules and give advantages and disadvantages of each.

12. State what information should be included in a procedure manual to help the medical assistant with making referral appointments.
13. Explain and demonstrate the procedures for making various appointments.
14. Spell and define, using the glossary in the back of this text, all the words to know in this unit.

◼ WORDS TO KNOW

angina	myocardial
chemotherapy	obliterate
commonality	precertification
criterion	ramification
downtime	remote
flex time	sequentially
gatekeeper	sigmoidoscopy
geriatrics	unstructured
guarantor	utilization
increments	work-in
matrix	

APPOINTMENT STRATEGIES

One of the most primary and vital functions in the course of managed care is the scheduling of appointments, Procedure 6–5. Managing time well for the physician and support staff will help keep patient flow at a satisfactory pace and promote a good professional working relationship. This may seem like an ideal situation that is unattainable. However, if there is genuine cooperation among all staff members, the schedule should flow well with some understandable exceptions due to emergencies and other unpredictable situations from time to time. Office hours may be scheduled with appointments made during specific times, or left as an open, **unstructured** block of time.

First, the entire staff must be made aware of the intended schedule of the physician(s) in the medical facility. An in-service or an orientation, whichever the case may be, is a practical way to inform employees about the schedule and enforce the established guidelines for "office hours." An organized routine helps the office staff as well as the patients with intended goals. In addition to providing the public with the routine hours when services are provided in printed form, the information should be posted at the entrance of the medical facility, on appointment cards, and on other printed materials. This information should also be placed in phone directories and wherever may be applicable. This way, everyone will know when the doctor is in and at what time business calls and appointments are taken. More discussion about an office policy manual is provided in Chapter 10.

After the office hours have been determined, the appointment schedule must be fashioned to meet the specific goals of the physician(s) and staff. Figure 6–8 outlines the goals that must continually be considered when scheduling.

Several styles of appointment books are available to schedule an entire year or more. A standard type of appointment book contains each day of the year printed with hours ranging from 8:00 A.M. to 5:00 P.M., as shown in Figure 6–9.

The goals of the patient, the physician, and the medical assistant need to be considered. In general, the *goals of patients* are:

1. a minimum wait for an appointment.
2. a minimum wait in the office.
3. maximum time with the physician.

The general *goals of physicians* are:

1. cost-effective use of time.
2. to spend needed time with the patients.
3. uninterrupted time.
4. time for referrals, emergencies, and so on.

The general *goals of the medical assistant* are:

1. a smooth-running office.
2. to close the office on time.
3. a lunch hour and breaks.
4. patient and physician goals.

FIGURE 6–8 Goals of the patient, the medical assistant, and the physician must be considered when preparing an appointment schedule.

Individual medical facilities can have appointment books custom made for their needs. Where several physicians' schedules are kept, the computer is the most desirable log of appointments as it eliminates the awkward use of several appointment books.

When you use computerized appointment scheduling, you totally replace the paper appointment book. You should certainly have an accounts receivable system well estab-

lished before converting to appointment scheduling. This feature should not be added if you have a single terminal, but can be effective if you have several terminals. You also must consider how you would handle **downtime**, when, for whatever reason, the computer is not functional. This is a reality you need to plan for before it takes place so the office will run as smoothly as possible through the downtime. Downtime in this context refers to the time when the computer is basically not working and you are unable to enter or obtain information.

A computerized appointment system locates automatically the next available time, gives you a record of all appointments already made, allows you to locate a specific date and time, and prints copies of the daily schedule. These printed copies should be filed with the accounting records of the day as a legal document that you could be called on to produce in the event of an IRS audit of the office practice. Some computer systems can be used to print charge slips for the patients as they are seen. It is not recommended to try to add an appointment scheduling procedure to the computer until you have a smooth operation under the handwritten system.

ESTABLISHING A MATRIX

The appointment book or computer program schedule must have a fixed **matrix**, which means that wherever there is a section of a page crossed out or a full page (or pages) crossed out with an "X," such as is shown in Figure 6–10, nothing should be scheduled. In a medical practice schedule, this usually means that in these spaces, services by the physician(s) will not be performed during this time. For instance, nothing should be scheduled between the hours of 8:00 A.M. and noon on Thursdays, and nothing scheduled before 9:00 A.M. and after 4:45 P.M. on Fridays because the

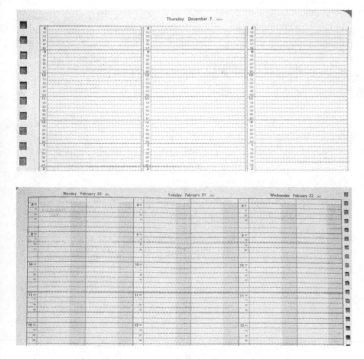

FIGURE 6–9 Appointment scheduling styles.

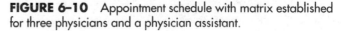

FIGURE 6–10 Appointment schedule with matrix established for three physicians and a physician assistant.

physician(s) will not be in to see patients. It can also mean simply that no one should be scheduled in this time slot because it is reserved specifically for urgent conditions and **work-ins**. All staff members need to be aware of the exact meaning of this practice for consistency in scheduling, i.e., an entire day with an X through it means that the doctor is out, an X through the afternoon means that the doctor is out only in the afternoon, and an X from 11:00 A.M. to 11:45 A.M. or 2:45 to 3:15 usually means that this time is reserved for catch-up and for work-ins (whichever is needed). It may also referred to as **flex time** and can also be useful for time to return phone calls to patients during the day as necessary. If there is an established "lunch" time each day from 12:00 to 1:00 P.M., it should be crossed out also. Toward the end of the scheduled day, from 4:40 to 5:00 P.M., for instance, time is saved so that there will be room to take work-ins, if needed. Whether the physician is away for a medical meeting, on vacation, performing surgery, involved in a community service, or whatever else, as soon as the doctor informs the staff, the entire time that is needed should be blocked out so that no one will be scheduled by mistake during this period. To be practical and efficient, time should be blocked out for the entire year ahead if it is regarding a routine day off, or at least as soon as possible as dates of activities are made known to you by the physician.

When scheduling appointments on the computer, it is an efficient and practical habit to make a hard copy of each of the scheduled appointments for the day for pulling patient charts. It also is a good practice to do this the day before to get ready for the arrival of patients for the next morning. It is not good to pull medical records too far in advance as it makes files difficult to find when so many are out without guides. It is not practical to place a guide card in place of every record when pulling them for the daily schedule. As patients come in for appointments, the receptionist can cross through their names as they report in for their appointments and their records are pulled, or as they are taken in to be prepared to see the physician. An additional hard copy of the daily schedule can make it easier for all to work from so that the staff can keep track of patient flow and anticipate the needs of patients.

Another practice which may be helpful is to highlight in a color (or several) for specific types of appointments, i.e., yellow is urgent, green is re-check, blue is injection, and so on. A separate schedule, or section of the master schedule, for those professionals in your facility (physician assistant, medical assistant, insurance secretary, and so on) who take appointments for various services, apart from the physician's appointment schedule, should also be kept. Figure 6–10 gives an example of a multiple appointment schedule. Patients who only need to be given immunizations, have weight and blood pressure checked, urinalysis re-checks, and so on, do not need to be seen by the doctor unless there is a problem. This should be done to avoid having all patients show up at the same time. In many cases the assistant, who reports the findings to the physician, is given instructions from the doctor and will then report back to the patient. This can save the physician valuable time that may be spent in providing managed care to others. This schedule should also have an established matrix. This is a sensible practice which helps to avoid possibly having to reschedule patients because of unplanned meetings, vacations, lectures, and so on. Clear communication among the entire staff must be ongoing to prevent confusion, mistakes, and misunderstandings.

In cases where patients have a set, or a standing, appointment, rescheduling should be done only when emergencies arise and it is absolutely necessary. The process of rescheduling involves calling each scheduled patient and offering an

P R O C E D U R E

6-5 Schedule Appointments

PURPOSE: Schedule appointments appropriately in a professional manner.

EQUIPMENT AND SUPPLIES: Appointment book and pen, and appointment cards.

TERMINAL PERFORMANCE OBJECTIVE: In a simulated situation, schedule an appointment for a patient according to accepted medical standards with consideration for the physician, staff, and needs of the patient.

1. Determine the means of scheduling: appointment book or computer entry.

2. Mark off the hours when the physician will be unable to see patients. Include daily hospital rounds, lunch hour, meetings, vacation, and so on.

3. Attempt to give patients two choices of times for the appointment.
   NOTE: In black ink, record patients' names as well as phone number(s) so that you can easily and quickly get in touch with them if necessary.

4. Ask patients to schedule their next appointment before leaving the office.

5. Write patients' names in the schedule book.

6. Complete an appointment card and give it to the patient. Be sure to record the appointment first in the appointment book and then on the appointment card.

7. Avoid over-scheduling and leave sufficient time for work-ins.

8. Allow time for the doctor to return phone calls. Patient charts should be pulled and given to the doctor for these calls.

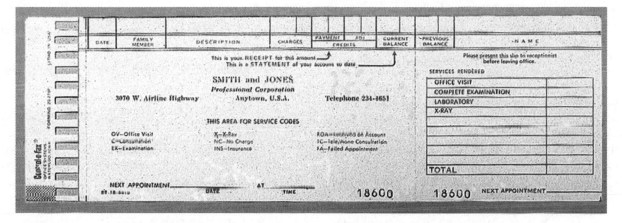

FIGURE 6–11 As shown on this pegboard system form, the receipt given to the patient has a space for recording the next scheduled appointment.

alternative appointment time as close to the original one as possible. This, of course, may crowd an already full schedule for a few days—or weeks—depending on the extent of the downtime created by the emergency. Downtime in this context refers to the time when the physician is called away from the routine schedule because of an emergency outside the office, usually with a hospital patient, or a personal emergency. The office staff may proceed with duties such as processing records, filing, inventory, and so on, that can be performed without the physician's presence.

Once the matrix has been established, the style of scheduling must be decided. There are several different ways to schedule. The preferred method of scheduling that is adopted for a particular medical practice is up to the physician and the staff. The choice should be determined only after creatively planning and carefully reviewing all of the options. In order for a schedule to run smoothly, many points must be taken into consideration. The medical assistant (receptionist or telephone secretary) must have excellent communication skills, a solid knowledge of the signs and symptoms of diseases and disorders, and an understanding of medical terminology and anatomy in order to proficiently perform telephone triage and prepare an efficient schedule. Obtaining the most precise assessment of a patient's condition by speaking calmly and empathically to the patient over the phone and actively listening to what is being said is referred to as phone triage. Using this type of assessment technique should result in obtaining accurate information and yield in appropriate and complete care. When patients phone the medical facility with the request to see the doctor, the medical assistant must find out who the caller is (ask the correct spelling of the caller's name and address, and so on) and determine whether the person has previously seen the doctor. Refer to the procedures in this unit that will help you follow a pattern of order with this detailed task.

Patients who either stop at the desk after seeing the doctor or who stop in to make an appointment should be given the same courtesy that patients receive over the phone. Offer the person a choice between two dates and times, allow sufficient time for the person to decide, and then confirm it by repeating it to the person before writing (printing) it in the appointment book. Remember to write the phone number(s) of the patient in the schedule book next to the name (so that you can call the patient quickly, if necessary, without pulling the chart) and note briefly (using abbreviations) the nature of the office visit. Write the time and date on an appointment card and politely hand it to the patient. If the pegboard system is used to record all patient transactions in the "write it once" fashion, you may record the next appointment in the space provided on the receipt section of the form. You should call attention to the space where the appointment is on the form when you hand the receipt to the patient. Figure 6–11 shows an example of the pegboard system form. At this time you should also provide the patient with any appropriate printed instructions or educational materials regarding the patient's condition, further treatment, or scheduled studies. Keep in mind that all appointment cards or forms that are used for this purpose should have the full name of the physician, complete address, phone number, and type of practice printed clearly on them. If the practice is new or in a new location, it is a convenience to the patient to have a small map or instructions of how to get to the office. If there are other office locations, they should also be listed with complete information. Many appointment cards for professional services state that the patient must give the staff a 24-hour notice if a change in the scheduled appointment must be made. A verbal reminder to patients also helps to reinforce this policy. This can be very helpful in maintaining a smooth schedule.

A new patient must provide you with complete information not only so that you can prepare a chart for the initial appointment, but also in case it becomes necessary to reach the patient before the scheduled appointment. If data is on the computer, the needed information can also be called up immediately.

APPOINTMENT-MAKING SUGGESTIONS

As you gain experience in listening to patients' complaints over the phone, you will become more keen in assessing problems. Using a pre-approved phone triage manual or a medical office handbook is a wise practice, as it reinforces continuity among staff members. All employees must be instructed to use the same format and ask the same questions every time of every patient who complains of similar symptoms. Following these pre-set guidelines that have been approved by the physician will help uncover serious conditions and lead to more efficient care of patients. Overlooking any of the questions or leaving out any part of a patient's symptoms is potentially a serious risk to both the patient and the medical practice. Also, you must be careful not to put words in the caller's mouth. Asking precise questions and waiting for a response from the patient is recommended. The medical assistant should not offer to speak for the patient, but tactfully encourage the patient to tell in their own words what the problem seems to be, and how long it has been going on. Next, the caller needs to let you know what has been done to relieve the problem, if anything. When writing down the information, be exact in how much and how often regarding medications, home remedies, and other treatments. Never leave out information that the patient tells you no matter how minor it may seem to you. The information disclosed to you by the patient should provide you with sufficient information necessary to determine how soon the appointment should be made. A sample phone call between the medical assistant and a patient is offered in Figure 6–12.

If the physician(s) in your medical facility cannot take new patients, as a courtesy, be prepared to suggest a physician in the area who may be able to take the caller. Ask the physician periodically who may be taking new patients in the area so that you may send them referrals as necessary. This service is a professional courtesy also in cases where the physician cannot take any more patients because of a full capacity. Often a person's doctor is determined by the patient's insurance company or health maintenance organization (HMO) for full coverage of medical services. If the provider is not a member of a patient's medical insurance program, the patient must seek a physician who *is* in order for medical care expenses to be covered. All information must be determined before the appointment is made. This procedure is called **precertification**. This "pre-cert" must be done before certain procedures and treatments are performed to confirm that these services are, in fact, approved for guaranteed coverage and to determine what the percentage is. If a person has no medical insurance and wants to see the physician, the patient must understand that all expenses incurred must be paid for in cash at the time of service, or agree in writing as to the method of payment. If a patient is receiving government assistance for medical treatment, this also must be docmented.

All staff members must be willing to work cooperatively and efficiently in order to provide quality care to patients. Included in the many choices for scheduling appointments are the following methods: clustering, double-booking, open hours, single-booking, streaming, wave, and modified wave. Figure 6–13 lists these methods of scheduling with a description of the purpose of each. Any one of these methods can be used exclusively by itself or in combination with one or more to fit the specific individual needs of the practice. Even when appointment times have been assigned to patients, it is a good policy to have the patients sign in with their name, address, phone number, the time of arrival, if a

Medical Assistant: Good afternoon, Dr. Michael's office, this is Marla, how may I help you?

Caller: Hello, this is Mrs. Evans. I need to bring Kelvin in to see the doctor.

Medical Assistant: What seems to be the problem, Mrs. Evans?

Mrs. Evans: Well, I just got off work and I'm at the day care center to pick up the kids, and Kelvin feels feverish and has a runny nose.

Medical Assistant: Have you or anyone at the day care center taken his temperature?

Mrs. Evans: No, he just feels hot to me and he looks flushed.

Medical Assistant: Has he been sick or are there any other problems that you think seem to be bothering Kelvin?

Mrs. Evans: Kelvin gets an earache every time he gets a cold. He is telling me that his left ear hurts as we speak. I just wanted to see what you thought before we go home.

Medical Assistant: How long has Kelvin had a cold?

Mrs. Evans: For a few days I guess, but he hasn't had a fever until now.

Medical Assistant: Have you given Kelvin any medication for his cold?

Mrs. Evans: Just some decongestant cough formula twice a day.

Medical Assistant: Can you be here in a half hour, Mrs. Evans? We will work Kelvin in to see Dr. Michael as soon as possible.

Mrs. Evans: Oh, thank you, we will be right there!

Medical Assistant: You're welcome, Mrs. Evans, we'll see you soon.

FIGURE 6–12 A sample phone conversation between caller and medical assistant.

new patient, and if seeing the doctor for the first time. This way, current patient information is obtained as well as the order in which the patient should be taken in. It also is a more fool-proof method of keeping track of patients so that no one is overlooked. A sign should be posted giving instructions for patients to "sign in" as they arrive. Periodic checking of waiting patients will help in case a new patient has not signed in and registered with you. It must be stated that leaving the sign in sheet out for all to read is a risk, as it allows all patients to read everyone's personal information. You know that you would not leave the appointment book open for the general public to read because it would break the confidentiality of patients. The ideal way to keep this from being a potential problem is to write the information down your-

Methods of Scheduling

Clustering—This scheduling technique is frequently exercised in specialty practices as well as in the General and Family practice office. A cluster, or group, of patients who have the same complaint, diagnosis, or other **commonality** are scheduled **sequentially** every ten minutes throughout the morning or afternoon, or throughout a particular day of the week. Some specialists, such as pediatricians, prefer to use this method as a routine standard. Many patients can be provided with the necessary preparations, be examined by the physician, and have appointments completed quickly when clustering is used in scheduling.

Double-booking—Appointment times are given to two or more patients for the same time slot in this method of scheduling. Since most people have varying degrees of the concept of and the respect for time, the possibility of all patients entering the reception room at the same time for an appointment for instance at 2:00 P.M. are **remote**. The usual course of events is that one of three will arrive at 1:40 to 1:45 P.M., another at 2:00, and the third, a little past 2:00. This is precisely the reason that double-booking works out so well. For services that take a small amount of time, this is the ideal way to schedule. It is also a great help if there are patients who are "no shows" (those who do not come in for appointments with no courtesy call).

Open hours—For a very active practice, such as general and family practices, clinic settings, student health centers and so on, this method of scheduling is usually the most practical. Patients sign in, noting the time they arrive, and they are seen by the doctor in that order. Emergencies and urgent conditions must be given priority attention. However, as this is being completed, there is usually a back up with patient flow. There may be procedures and treatments that are not anticipated when the patient first arrives. After the physician talks with the patient and performs the appropriate exam, further testing or treatment may be necessary. This process utilizes a considerable amount of time. There is no way to regulate the order of the seriousness of patients' problems. Whenever possible, the urgent medical problems are sent to the emergency room of the local hospital or an emergency medical service is called to provide immediate care.

Single-booking—This method is used when the appointment for the patient will take a considerable amount of time, as in consultations, counseling, patient education, or other types of therapy. The medical practices that would be more likely to use this method of scheduling are psychiatry, physical or occupational therapy, and other specialty services. Usually when there is only one patient or family scheduled each hour, the appointment is made for only forty-five to fifty minutes of the hour. This allows for

the session to wind down comfortably as well as for the possibility of the session going overtime a few minutes. It also gives the professional conducting the services a short break in between patient care and to prepare for the next appointment.

Streaming—The focus of this method of scheduling is, as the word suggests, to keep a continuous flow of patients coming in through the facility and to avoid having alternating periods of idleness and crowding. Since most standard appointment books have a printed schedule of a twelve hour day in fifteen minute **increments**, appointments are made to accommodate the specific needs of patients. New patients and those needing complete physical examinations, for example, require a long appointment in order to perform all the necessary preparations, examinations, and any diagnostic tests that may result. Specific medical problems, such as a child with an ear ache, a blood pressure recheck, or a dressing change, will routinely take no more than a maximum of ten to fifteen minutes. In some instances, some of the scheduled appointments that are allowed fifteen minutes may in reality take only five minutes. This is the reason that scheduling by the streaming method seems to work out well most of the time.

Wave—This method of scheduling is used in many large medical clinics, family and general practice, and group practices because it runs most efficiently in a facility where there are several medical service departments and qualified personnel to provide managed care of patients. Appointments are made during the first thirty minutes of each hour. The number of patients that are scheduled depends on the type of practice and the amount of time needed for services. The remainder of the hour may be used for those patients who phone the same day and need to be checked by the physician. Since many patients are already scheduled in this type of scheduling, the times in the schedule are most likely filled. If there is a cancellation or a patient "forgets" to come in, the entire schedule is not ruined. Most often the staff is grateful for a little extra time to catch up on other duties.

Modified Wave—The modified wave method of scheduling is the same as the wave method plus scheduling patients in the last half hour of each hour in ten and twenty minute intervals according to the medical problems. For those patients that you know will need the most time with the doctor, the beginning of the hour is the logical choice of time. For patients who will most likely take only a few minutes, the last half hour seems to work best. Scheduling in this manner yields some flexibility so that patients who have urgent health problems or injuries can be worked in between already scheduled patients.

Figure 6-13   Methods of scheduling.

self as patients arrive, or enter it into the computer, keeping the screen from the view of others. This should be discussed by the staff and an agreement made to determine how this is to be handled.

MAINTAINING THE SCHEDULE

After a period of time, through trial and error, each medical practice staff arrives at a schedule that works best for them.

An assessment should be made of the efficiency of the schedule and appropriate changes should be made to better serve expedient patient flow. Management consultants suggest an evaluation of old appointment sheets for a twelve to fifteen week period. The number of work-ins, cancellations, and no shows, and the time spent with specific exams and complaints of patients will help determine the course of the revision of scheduling techniques. The time slots needed for various procedures, exams, and consultations can then be handled in short, medium, long, and extended appointment times. Often, a patient needs to have several procedures performed or must see one or more doctors in an office or a medical center. Coordinating all of these appointments for the patient on the same day is most thoughtful and will save the person from having to repeat unnecessary expense and travel which can be very tiring, especially to the elderly patient. The medical assistant may be expected to provide an explanation of different medical specialties, medical terms, instructions for procedures, exams, or treatments for patients who are unfamiliar with such matters. Sending the patient printed instructions regarding procedures and exams along with an appointment card prior to the scheduled appointment helps patients get prepared and reduces their anxiety. Further discussion and helpful information about diagnostic examinations is provided in Chapters 15 and 16. Another thoughtful service to patients is to give simple but precise directions of how to get to your location. A map or printed instructions mailed to the patient before their appointment is appreciated by persons who are not familiar with your geographical area. An office brochure is a way to give new patients a brief explanation of your facility's policies and procedures regarding office hours, location and directions, when to call, who to speak to for administrative business, the procedure for medication refills, and so on, and the philosophy of the practice. This way, all information is in one neat package. Educating the patients in these areas is most helpful in the elimination of repeat calls asking the same information.

Remember that patients who have to wait a long time before being seen by the physician become impatient and eventually angry, especially if the patient had a scheduled appointment. Understandably, this patient may wonder why an appointment was even made. Surveys have shown that patients usually do not mind as much as a half-hour wait, but tend to become angry if it is any longer. This could lead to medical-legal **ramifications** if it is not handled properly. Patients' time is as valuable to them as it is to you and the physician. Delays should be made known to patients tactfully as soon as they are realized. Patients need to be given the choice of waiting for as long as it may be, or rescheduling for another appointment time altogether. This is a considerate way to treat patients and prevents problems from starting. Announcing that there will be a delay as soon as you have been given the information for instance, that the doctor is caring for a patient with an emergency at the hospital, is something that patients will understand and appreciate. It is far better to be honest with patients and let them know what the situation is from the start than to be silent. Patients appreciate your letting them know so that they can make a choice about waiting or returning at another time. A periodic announcement should be made to those patients who are waiting as to how much longer it may be before the doctor is able to see them.

Handling Patients Without Appointments

There may be a time when a patient who has an appointment brings along a family member or a friend to be seen. This complicates the schedule and presents a challenge in tact and diplomacy to the staff. When a patient arrives who has no ap-

pointment in a practice where it *is* necessary to have an appointment to see the physician, you need to explain this to the person as tactfully and as politely as possible. When the patient realizes that the doctor can spend a sufficient amount of time only with those patients who are scheduled, cooperation is usually attained. Patients who are persistent because of the nature of their problems should be referred to the physician. If a patient walks in to your office with no appointment, the person should be referred to an appropriate medical facility according to the person's symptoms, if there is no way your schedule can accommodate him. The physician should be made aware of the situation before any definitive action is taken. The nature of the patient's problem will determine how quickly you should act. Often, the physician will make an exception and reinforce the policy for future appointment scheduling. If it is a serious emergency, you should automatically call for emergency medical service. In some cases, the physician may agree to take care of the emergency and then refer the patient to another physician for continuous managed care.

Canceled or Missed Appointments (No Shows)

If a patient cancels or does not show up for the scheduled appointment, it should be noted in the person's chart and the appointment time given to another patient as soon as possible. The physician should be notified about the patient's cancellation or "no show." He will advise you about further action as warranted by the patient's condition. For example, if a patient is being treated for a wound that requires follow-up care and a dressing change, the patient may cancel (or just not come) and the wound area could become infected. The patient might decide to sue the doctor for inadequate care. The record of the canceled appointment or no show is important in proving that the patient had an appointment but failed to follow the physician's instructions. The patient's name should be left in the appointment book with a single line drawn through it. It is also wise to phone the patient at home (and leave a message with someone or on the recorder if the patient cannot be reached) about the missed appointment. If patients cannot be reached by phone, mailing them a letter noting the missed appointment with a request that another appointment be arranged by calling the office. This procedure provides legal protection if a lawsuit is filed against the physician for failure to provide care for the patient. Having this process documented will show concern for the patient. It is difficult to prove negligence when such efforts to offer medical help have been made.

Appointment Book Maintenance

You should never erase a name or use liquid paper to **obliterate** a name in the book. Do not use pencil. There are those who, even though it not a suggested practice, use pencil in their appointment books. If this is the case, the entries should be written over at the end of the day in black ink. Having used pencil and possibly erasing from time to time during the course of the day may make the appointment book look messy, besides raising questions as to what names were erased and why it was done. Having a patient's name in the

1.	NP	new patient
2.	CPE (CPX)	complete physical examination
3.	FU	follow-up examination
4.	NS	no show
5.	RS	reschedule
6.	C&C	called and canceled
	C	canceled
7.	Ref	referral
8.	Re✓	re-check
9.	PT	physical therapy
10.	Cons	consultation
11.	Inj	injection
12.	ECG	electrocardiogram
13.	Sig	**sigmoidoscopy**
14.	Surg	surgery
15.	Lab	laboratory studies
16.	BP✓	blood pressure check

FIGURE 6–14 The entire office staff must know abbreviations (specific to the practice) and their meanings and use them consistently. Here is a sample list.

schedule book even though the appointment may not have been kept will help defend efforts of providing the patient with the opportunity for medical care if ever the need arises. If there is no name on the appointment schedule because it has been erased, it is very difficult to prove that care was offered to the person. Management consultants advise that no altering of the schedule be done, as it may look as if one was trying to conceal information or fraudulently add it in at a later date. The appointment schedule is an official legal document and must be legible. For a cancellation, place a large letter "C" at the beginning of the person's name to indicate a cancellation, or C&C to indicate that the patient did call to tell you the reason the appointment had to be canceled. Some office personnel find it helpful to use a stamp to record in the chart the fact that the patient did not keep the appointment. The date, time, and reason (if known) for the missed appointment would be all that you would need to write, plus your initials. All staff members should be given a copy of the abbreviations common to your facility so that there is consistency with their use and the meanings are clear. A list of some common abbreviations that can be used in the appointment schedule is shown in Figure 6–14. A more extensive list of abbreviations is in the appendix of this text.

For legal concerns, all appointment schedule books must be kept for three years. It should be positioned out of the reach and eyesight of other patients and unauthorized persons.

MISCELLANEOUS APPOINTMENT SCHEDULING

In addition to routine scheduled appointments, emergency situations, and unexpected disruptions, there are other ancillary health professionals who may stop in to give the physician new information regarding medications, office equipment, medical supplies, and so on. A smart way to deal with this before it becomes a routine disruption is to offer a regular appointment to the sales person or pharmaceutical representative (or detail person). Having a standing appointment (meaning at the same time and occurring regularly) for sales reps will give the physician the opportunity to acquire the most current information on products and have any questions answered immediately by the professional sales person. Many reps bring in a variety of complimentary items on occasion, including lunch and other treats for the office staff. Leaving brochures and sample medications is another common practice of sales reps. You will have to organize and file or store all of the items which are left after the physician sees them. There is no need to schedule an extended amount of time for these individuals. Often the doctor chats briefly in the hallway and only a portion of the time blocked out for the appointment is actually used. Many physicians prefer not to see these sales people and ask that they talk to the office manager or medical assistant or just send information by mail only. If any new items are of particular use to the practice, information and samples may be left for the physician's perusal. If another doctor or a family member stops in to see the physician, you should politely interrupt and let the physician know so that the guest does not have to wait. A reminder to the physician-employer that the reception room has x number of patients waiting is a good idea before the meeting ensues. If this practice of surprise visits becomes a habit, it should be addressed in a staff meeting or in a private conference with the physician.

The medical assistant should note trouble spots in the schedule and report them to the physician or office manager periodically. This subject can be presented at staff meetings so that, with sharing ideas and suggestions, a better schedule may result. If the problem is that patients have had to wait far too long to see the doctor over a period of time (that is more often than not), then it is possible that there are more appointments made than the doctor can see in the set "office hours" and the simple remedy is that fewer appointments should be scheduled. It is vital to the success of a schedule that the medical assistant maintain open communication with the physician and staff regarding patient flow. The development of a team feeling should allow staff to be honest, consistent, loyal, considerate, and by all means to avoid gossip. A professional image is reflected through attitude, abilities, appearance, and ethics. When these characteristics are evident in a team spirit, cooperation and success will be obvious.

In certain situations where it seems that all efforts to improve scheduling have failed, it is smart to enlist an efficiency expert for an objective viewpoint. One who is not involved daily is better able to observe many points that could be changed for the better. Their expertise can make all staff members more aware of how the schedule affects everyone throughout the office. The ideal schedule should provide a comfortable pace for the staff without making the patients feel rushed or slighted. *The importance of building good rapport with patients is invaluable; scheduling is where it begins.*

SETTING AND KEEPING REALISTIC SCHEDULES

Since the physician generally expects the medical assistant who schedules appointments to do so in time slots that are realistic for presenting complaints of the patients, a sample guideline for some typical office visits is presented in Figure 6–15. This is just a sample of the amount of time that may be spent with procedures and other services. The actual amount of time spent with patients will depend on the speed of the staff, the patient, and the physician, as well as how talkative all concerned are before, during, and after the service rendered. A good rapport is built with patients when the service is achieved, pleasantries are exchanged, and the time seems to pass quickly. Variations and rearranging of appointments may be necessary according to the way the course of events unfolds during any given day in the medical practice. Experience will be the best teacher in arriving at a successful schedule.

Helping to Maintain the Physician's Schedule

In addition to scheduling patients appropriately, the medical assistant has the responsibility to help the physician keep on time. If it looks as though the doctor is working faster than usual, calling in patients to be seen earlier to keep the patient flow moving at a steady pace is a sensible idea. On the other hand, if there is an obvious slowing down on the part of the physician or other staff members, and the schedule is getting backed up, the medical assistant should call patients and either delay their arrival time or reschedule them for another day if the physician agrees that catching up is nearly impossible. Studies have shown that while a ten hour day is 25% longer than an eight hour day, the increase in productivity only rises 6% because of the increased likelihood of making errors. Therefore, overworking could prove hazardous to patients as well as to yourself and co-workers. The medical assistant may also want to work out a signal with the physician for those times when the patient gets too talkative and is taking more time than was allotted for the appointment. A suggestion is to interrupt either by a signal over the speaker, such as "excuse me doctor, you have a call on line five (and there are only four phone lines). You may decide that a simple knock on the door, or a particular signal on his or her pager can help the physician stay on task and help avoid getting further behind in schedule.

Handling Late Patients

There may be a few patients who seem to be late for every appointment they make. In this situation, you may schedule them just after you come back from a lunch time and just work in the appointment when they arrive, or you may decide to schedule them at the end of the day. If the person does not arrive for the appointment at the time it was scheduled, a reasonable time of waiting was documented, and attempts were made to reach the patient by phone to determine if he or she was still coming, the patient will find no one at the site and may think twice before being late again. You should pre-determine a reasonable amount of time that you will wait for a patient, possibly up to fifteen minutes for unexpected and reasonable delays, to avoid problems that could stem from leaving the premises before all patients have been seen, even if the patient is late. Providing printed information regarding office hours as well as posting them will help to avoid such situations from happening.

At certain times of the year there seems to be expected conditions that play havoc with a schedule, such as colds and flu in the winter months, injuries during winter and spring breaks from school, rashes and other ailments related to summer, and so on. These problems must be taken into account when preparing the daily schedule, especially the types of problems specific to the particular practice where you are employed. A pause of a few minutes between patient exams is acceptable. However, if there is too much slack time and more than a few minutes between patients happens too often, scheduling techniques need to be reviewed. Figure 6–16 offers a list of some helpful points to keep in mind when scheduling appointments. The saying "time is money" is a good thought to consider. It should remind us to use time well and for the purpose intended. Efficient use of the physician's time and the entire staff's as well in treating patients is the main purpose of a schedule. Again, cooperation among the staff is required for a successful outcome.

APPOINTMENTS OUTSIDE THE MEDICAL OFFICE

When a patient develops a condition or requires an examination that your office cannot take care of, your employer will refer the patient to an appropriate colleague or facility. The office should have a page in the office procedures manual listing the names, addresses, and phone numbers of physicians your employer wishes to refer patients to in the different specialty areas. You should give at least two names. Have the

12	Lunch
12.15	
12.30	Carol Wang-Sig 555-0050
12.45	↓
1	Kenneth Franks BP✓ Lab
1.15	↓ 555-8846
1.30	Susan Steele-ECG
1.45	↓ 555-4495
2	Arnold Wing-CPE
2.15	
2.30	555-6483
2.45	↓
3	Work ins
3.15	Peggy Watters Inj 555-9913
3.30	Walter Matthews PT
3.45	↓ 555-2237
4	Latasha Peters Cons
4.15	↓ 555-7702
4.30	Work ins
4.45	Robert James BP✓ 555-4951

FIGURE 6–15 Sample time blocks for commonly scheduled appointments in a medical office.

The main points to remember in making appointments are:

1. Have the name exactly right.
2. Make the appointment for the next hour available.
3. Be sure the date and time are clearly understood.
4. Allow enough time for each appointment.
5. Check to see that no one else is scheduled at the same time for the same service.
6. Try to remember the time of day each patient prefers for an appointment.
7. When scheduling a series of appointments for the same patient, try to use the same day and time to make it easier for the patient to remember.
8. Offer a choice: "Would you like to come today at 3:00 or tomorrow at 9:00?"
9. If you have to refuse a request for an appointment at a certain time, explain why this is necessary and try to find another time that is convenient for the patient.
10. Enter the appointment in your appointment book or computer.
11. Complete an appointment card and hand it to the patient.
12. Try to allow extra time for emergencies each day.

FIGURE 6–16

name, address, and phone number of facilities where you might refer patients, i.e., laboratories, x-ray facilities, and community clinics, handy for use. Keep in mind that certain managed care plans require referrals (Procedure 6–6) to specialists within the plan with the approval of the primary care physician (**gatekeeper**). A list of these plans and participating physicians for handy referral is an excellent time saver.

When a patient is to be admitted to the hospital, it is important to know what admission information the hospital will require. Be prepared when you call to give the necessary information regarding the patient.

Hospitals have established guidelines for admitting patients. The purpose of these guidelines is to cut the cost of hospital care. If the care needed by the patient can be given in an outpatient facility, this must be the method used. Many insurance companies and government sponsored programs require a preadmission evaluation of the need for hospitalization of a patient. To determine the need for admission, a **criterion** statement would need to be composed by the admitting physician using specific terminology as to severity of the illness and an assessment of need. Definitions that may be given for these terms are:

acute onset—symptoms occurred within last six hours.

sudden onset—symptoms occurred within last twenty four hours.

recent onset—symptoms occurred within past week.

recently or newly discovered—symptoms not present on previous examination.

P R O C E D U R E

6-6 Arrange Referral Appointment

PURPOSE: Schedule a referral appointment for a patient in a professional manner.

EQUIPMENT AND SUPPLIES: Patient's chart with referral request, phone directory, phone, pen, and paper.

TERMINAL PERFORMANCE OBJECTIVE: In a simulated situation, schedule a referral appointment for a patient by phoning the requested medical facility according to accepted medical standards with consideration for the physician, staff, and needs of the patient.

1. Obtain patient's chart with request for referral to other facility.
2. Use phone directory to obtain phone number and address of the referral office.
3. Place the call to the referral office and provide the receptionist with:
   ■ your name and physician's name and address
   ■ patient's name, address, and so on, and reason for the appointment

NOTE: It is a courtesy to also write the person's name down who schedules the referral appointment for the patient for any further questions the patient may have and for directions on how to get there.
   ■ indicate if you will send a confirmation letter of the referral request by mail or fax.
   ■ record appointment information on the patient's chart; also write the time, day and date, name, address, and so on, on paper for the patient to keep.

NOTE: If the patient is standing before you while you make the referral appointment call, be sure to ask if the date is okay before you finalize the conversation. (If the patient is not present, you must phone the patient to confirm the appointment.)

4. Give the patient printed instructions regarding the appointment as appropriate.
5. Initial the patient's chart, signifying the completion of the request.

In some cases, in addition to terms describing the severity of the illness, the vital signs (temperature, pulse, respiration, and blood pressure), laboratory workup, any functional impairment, the physical findings, the need for monitoring, the medications needed, and the procedures, along with criteria for discharge, must be considered as part of the determination for need of admission.

In scheduling an admission, you may be asked to identify the attending physician for the admission, the service admitting under (i.e., whether medical, surgical, obstetrical, and so on), the admission date requested, and the type of reservation. The type of reservation might be: Inpatient, admitting day surgery (ADS), ambulatory surgery (ASU), or patients who walk in, have surgery and go home, or outpatient. Some hospitals furnish nearby hotel rooms for **chemotherapy** patients or other patients who need daily treatment for several hours but do not need to be admitted to a hospital room. Other information needed is listed here:

1. Full name of the patient (include maiden name of married female patient)
2. Age and date of birth
3. Sex of patient
4. Marital status
5. Social security number
6. Address (including zip code)
7. Telephone numbers (home and work) of patient and closest relative
8. Primary insurance **guarantor** and Social Security number of this individual
9. Employer of guarantor and work telephone number
10. Hospital insurance coverage along with verification if prior authorization granted
11. Name and address of referring physician
12. The physician needs to furnish the diagnosis and plan of care needs for the **utilization** committee review.
13. If surgery is to be scheduled, you need to give the date of surgery, expected length of procedure in hours, name of procedure, type of anesthesia, units of blood needed, and whether x-rays will be taken.
14. When preadmission testing is to be carried out, you need to know the date, time, and names of tests, x-rays, ECG, etc. If a generally required test is not ordered, you need to explain why it was not ordered.

The following conditions will generally justify inpatient hospital care for an otherwise outpatient procedure if the severity of the illness or intensity of service needed warrant it:

1. Severe **myocardial** insufficiency (with or without **angina**)
2. Chronic congestive heart failure
3. Chronic obstructive lung disease
4. Bronchial asthma
5. Diabetes
6. Thyroid disease
7. Hypertension

Guidelines are generally established with a detailed listing by ICDA–9–CM codes (International Classification of Diseases, 9th revision, Clinical Modification) for elective outpatient procedures, for elective procedures that might require a preoperative length of stay, and for those procedures to be done on admission day.

FOLLOW-UP APPOINTMENTS

It is the medical assistant's responsibility to assist patients with their payments and any necessary follow-up or referral appointments after the physician has seen them.

The need for a follow-up appointment may be marked by the physician on the charge slip, or the patient may be told to inform you of this need. The patient should be given the choice of two appointment times, and only after the entry is made in the appointment book should an appointment card be prepared and given to the patient. This practice will prevent the possibility of forgetting to enter the patient's name in the book.

Physicians who treat patients who need regular follow-up but do not make appointments for six months or a year in advance may choose to send a recall notice. This notice could be a preprinted card sent to the patient as a reminder to call or write for an appointment. An example would be a reminder for an annual Pap test. Some offices find it helpful to send a reminder notice of appointments that were made far in advance. You might even ask the patient to address such a card at the time the appointment is made. The patient is handed an appointment card which he or she may lose, and at the same time addresses a card with the appointment time marked on it. You place this in a file under the date when it should be mailed. This practice might be helpful for the forgetful **geriatric** patient, or the busy executive who may forget to put the appointment in the date book along with business appointments.

Complete Chapter 6, Unit 2 in the workbook to help you meet the objectives at the beginning of this unit and therefore achieve competency of this subject matter.

UNIT 3
Written Communications

▌ OBJECTIVES

Upon completion of the unit, meet the following terminal performance objectives by verifying knowledge of the facts and principles presented through oral and written communication at a level deemed competent, and demonstrate the specific behaviors as identified in the terminal performance objectives of the procedures, observing safety precautions in accordance with health care standards.

1. List seven types of correspondence medical assistants may need to prepare.
2. Name instances when form letters may be indicated.
3. Produce a memo.
4. Demonstrate correct grammar, spelling, punctuation, and sentence structure to compose original letters.
5. Name six specific criteria for written communications.
6. Name and give examples of the eight parts of speech.

7. Identify the nine standards for producing a mailable business letter.
8. Explain the characteristics of business letter styles.
9. Use the formatting standards to prepare a business letter.
10. Correct a typewritten copy.
11. Use standard proofreading marks.
12. Discuss eleven problem areas in written communications.
13. Spell and define, using the glossary at the back of the text, all the words to know in this unit.

■ WORDS TO KNOW

adjective	interjection
adverb	mailable
apostrophe	misspelled
clause	modifies
communication	noun
compose	postscript
congratulations	preposition
conjunction	pronoun
context	proofread
contraction	punctuation
correspondence	signature
critique	stationery
denote	thesaurus
ellipses	verb
galley proofs	watermark
hyphen	

WRITTEN COMMUNICATION

What is **communication**? Webster defines it as "the giving or receiving of information; a system for sending and receiving messages." You can communicate in many ways such as talking, gesturing, or writing. Written communication is often called **correspondence**. Again Webster says correspondence is "communication by the exchange of letters." An individual who is hired by a newspaper or magazine to furnish news regularly from a certain place is called a correspondent. There are schools which you can receive instruction in a particular subject, by mail. They are known as correspondence schools. But in its broader sense, correspondence can be thought of as any exchange of information between persons. With this interpretation, correspondence or written communication could include the sending of notes, inneroffice communications (IOCs), form letters, information sheets, and business, professional and personal letters.

In a physician's office, written communication may be necessary:

- to officially inform the staff of a policy or decision.
- to contact professional colleagues.
- to correspond with professional associations.
- to request or respond to a medical consultation.
- to engage in business communications with medical suppliers, financial consultants, attorneys, and insurance companies.
- to send personal messages.

Inneroffice Communication (IOC)

This is an informal memo style communication that is usually specific to one concern. It is an effective way of being certain that everyone is aware of some event, policy, concern, and so on. If you want to ensure that everyone reads the memo, a copy must be given to each person or one can be posted or circulated with an attached list of all people involved, who then must enter their initials next to their name to indicate they have read the IOC. An example might look something like Figure 6–17 (a) and (b).

SAMUEL E. MATTHEWS, MD
100 EAST MAIN STREET, SUITE 120
YOURTOWN, US 98765-4321

DATE: April 3, 19--
FROM: Office staff
TO: Doctor Sam
SUBJECT: New office computer system

Representatives from ABC Electronics will be at our office on April 10 and 11 to provide instruction on the use of our new equipment. Please see Joyce and schedule yourself into one of the four orientation sessions. After you have selected your time, enter your initials next to your name on the sheet at her desk to verify you have responded to this memo.

Thank you for your cooperation in this matter.

(A)

SAMUEL E. MATTHEWS, MD
100 EAST MAIN STREET, SUITE 120
YOURTOWN, US 98765-4321

After you have read the memo and selected a time for your orientation, please initial below on the line by your name. Your initials verify your response to the memo to attend one session presented by ABC Electronics on April 10 or 11.

_____	Amy Austin	_____	Gerri Gore
_____	Betty Barry	_____	Harry Hart
_____	Chuck Coates	_____	Inez Immel
_____	Diane Delong	_____	Jacki James
_____	Emily Everett	_____	Kelly Kraft
_____	Frank Farber	_____	Lisa Long

(B)

FIGURE 6–17   (A) Inneroffice communication (IOC). (B) IOC circulation sheet.

Informal Notes

This type of correspondence is also informal in nature and would be indicated for times when "thank you's," **congratulations**, or similar expressions are desired. Usually, these are personal in nature. Often, these are written on a first name basis.

Personal Letters

The physician may ask for assistance with personal correspondence. It is common for medical assistants to correspond with travel agencies, mail order catalogs, perhaps clothing suppliers, and specialty shops. A competent medical assistant should be able to **compose**, or write, the necessary letter given the specific information desired, so all the physician has to do is sign his **signature**.

Professional Letters

Physicians may need to write to their professional associations, licensing boards, and other physicians regarding some issue or concern affecting personal medical activities or their professional practice. Perhaps your employer holds an office in a medical society which requires communicating with the members or issuing the group's opinion on a particular subject to the community or media. Some physicians hold office on a hospital medical board which might necessitate issuing of written communication. Physicians who participate in research do a great deal of professional correspondence in regard to the experimental studies being conducted. Some physicians enjoy writing professional journal articles about a unique patient or explaining a procedure they have developed. Obviously, these specific writings require detailed dictating and perfect transcription.

Business Letters

The greatest amount of correspondence however, is of the business type required to manage the affairs of the practice. This would include the referrals, consulting, annual examination reminders, collection letters, school and work releases, suppliers of equipment and materials, and other correspondence necessary to the office operation. These types of letters can be individually composed or a type of form letter. Pre-written form letters can be developed and stored electronically on disks of computers or word processors. When needed, the letter is pulled up, the appropriate date, name, address, amount due, and so on, is added, and it is sent without the need to prepare the total letter. Form letters are especially well suited for:

- return to work or school approvals (following surgery or illness).
- annual diagnostic examination reminders (eye examinations, Pap tests, mammogram, sigmoidoscopy).
- delinquent account reminders, usually in about three increasing levels of request intensity.
- office visit verifications (for work or school absence).

- athletic participation approvals.
- providing information to referred patients regarding appointment confirmation, office location, information needed, approximate time required for appointment, payment policy, and so on.

Several businesses offer prepared medical forms both in hard copy for completion or as software packages for computer use. If your office is not yet computerized, it is possible to draft the necessary letters on a typewriter leaving adequate spaces to insert the appropriate information specific for each patient. The "master" of each form letter is stored in a file and copies to be filled in are made as needed. This method requires a little practice to line up margins and the typing line so that it matches the rest of the letter.

Information Sheets

Specific written instructions regarding the examinations and diagnostic tests performed in your office are very beneficial to patients. They help to reinforce what you have explained and serve as a reminder after they leave the office. They typically explain to patients how to prepare themselves for a particular test or what to expect when the test is performed. Usually there is a place on the form to enter the date and time the examination is scheduled. These information sheets can be prepared and stored in the files to be used as needed.

PREPARING WRITTEN COMMUNICATION

Almost every day, when the mail carrier arrives, there will be something received which requires a response. Your employer may want to review all the mail personally and request that you only open the envelopes and arrange everything neatly on the desk. Some physicians allow the mail to be opened and sorted, referring to only professional or personal material which requires their response; anything pertaining to the practice operation is handled by the office manager.

After a few days, the physician will need to devote some time to drafting responses to inquiries or responding to referrals. Some may use a dictating machine while others may prefer to dictate in person. Surgeons and other specialists who have a large number of referral patients will have the greatest amount of responses to compose. Usually a type of form letter is developed with the opening and closing paragraphs being a standard format and the middle of the letter specific to the patient. This format only requires minimal dictation, after the opening "Thank you for referring . . ." and the closing "If I can be of any additional assistance . . ." Of course, occasionally, written communication is required that is specific to a request or concern so the total correspondence is individualized.

Probably the most important criteria about any communication is that it be written using proper grammar and punctuation and have no **misspelled** words. It also must be spaced on the page properly and be neat and clean. Try to not use the same major word twice in the same or even consecutive sentence. The following information will assist you in producing attractive, error free communications.

Spelling

Spelling is difficult for some people. If you are one of them you will have to try exceptionally hard until you master certain rules and habits. Here are some ideas that might help.

- If you have certain words that you cannot seem to spell correctly, try making a list of them to use as a quick reference.
- Make a mental picture of the word correctly spelled.
- Pronounce the word correctly several times.
- Write the word, dividing it into syllables and inserting accent marks.
- Write or type the word several times.
- Learn to use a dictionary when you are in doubt.
- If you use a word processor or computer software to compose correspondence, be sure to run your document on the spellchecker. It will catch most errors. (Unfortunately you cannot rely on the checker completely because it is possible that the word is spelled correctly but you have entered the wrong word, a word "out of **context.**" Examples of this are using "their" for "there," "cite" for "sight," "rite" for "right," "your" for "you're," and several others.)

There are 14 rules about spelling which are very helpful once you understand how to use them. Refer to Figure 6–18.

Parts of Speech

To compose effective, well written communications, you need to be aware of the eight parts of speech and how they are used.

1. A **noun** is the name of anything. It may be a person, a place, an object, an occurrence, a quality, a measure, or a state. Examples of words that may be used as nouns are *assistant, laboratory, instruments, office, empathy, manners, kindness,* and *attention.*
   Examples:
   The *assistant* draws *blood* and takes it to the *laboratory.*
   The *assistant* shows *kindness, empathy,* and *attentiveness* to all *patients* in the *office.*
2. A **pronoun** is a word that is used as a noun substitute. The most often used pronouns are *I, me, she, her, you, he, him, who, which, that, one, all, some, everyone, it, their, they, any* and *nobody.*
3. A **verb** is a word (or word group) that expresses action or state of being. Every sentence must have a verb. Examples of words which may be action verbs are *do, write, speak, hesitate, educate, perform, assist, obtain,* and *attend.* Examples of verbs that may express state of being are *am, are, is, will be, have been, feel, seem,* and *appear.*
4. An **adjective** is a word that describes, limits, or restricts a noun or pronoun.
   Examples:
   The *conscientious* medical assistant reports for work on time.
   She is an *energetic, efficient,* and *dedicated* employee.

5. An **adverb** is a word that **modifies** a verb form, an adjective, or another adverb. The most common ending for adverbs is *ly.* Adverbs should be used to answer questions such as: How? When? Where? How often? To what degree? It is incorrect to say "I did real good on the terminology test." You should say, "I did very well on the terminology test."
   Examples:
   Sometimes the assistant reports *early* at the office and stays *late.*
   Usually when a patient *angrily* confronts an assistant, she should answer *calmly* and *quietly* after the patient has finished talking.
6. A **preposition** shows the relationship of an object to some other word in the sentence. Prepositions *must* have an object. If a pronoun is the object of a preposition, it must be in the objective case.
   Examples:
   Medical supplies arrived *for* the doctor, the nurse and *me.*
   Between you and *me* that physician's handwriting is most difficult to read.
   Some common prepositions include: *with, without, for, against, above, below, on, under, through, between, by, during, among, concerning, in, from, to,* and *of.*
7. **Conjunctions** are connectives that join words, phrases, and clauses. Examples are *and, but, or, nor, for, yet, because, if,* and *since.*
8. An **interjection** is a word used to express strong feeling or emotion. Examples are *ouch, hurray, well,* and *oh.* These words are usually followed by an exclamation point or a comma. Examples of sentences containing all eight parts of speech:
   Yes! A busy medical practice like theirs always employs efficient and energetic medical assistants.
   Well, a conscientious medical assistant like you will sit confidently for the certification examination and pass it!
   Oh, that emergency patient canceled after he had rested and settled down.

Once you have the spelling and the parts of speech under control, it is time to put the words together in sentences. Written material should be composed of sentences of differing lengths and complexity to appropriately match the type of written matter being prepared. Patient referral or business letters require concise material while personal correspondence or medical articles can contain more variety. Be careful not to make run-on sentences containing too many clauses. The following information outlines sentence construction.

Sentence Structure When writing letters, write in complete thoughts. A *simple sentence* consists of only one complete thought, that is, one independent clause with a subject and a verb.
   Examples:
   Physicians examine patients.
   Physicians prescribe medication.
   The receptionist scheduled appointments.
A *compound sentence* contains two or more independent clauses.

Rule 1. Write *ie* when the sound is *ee*, as in:

achieve	piece
field	shield
grief	yield

EXCEPT after *c*, as in:

conceive
deceive
perceive
receive

EXCEPTIONS:

leisure
neither
seize
weird

Rule 2. Write *ei* when the sound is not long *e*, especially when the sound is long *a*, as in:

freight	veil
height	vein
sleigh	weigh

EXCEPTIONS:

friend
mischief

Rule 3. The prefixes *mis, il, in, im* and *dis* do not change the spelling of the root word:

mis + spell = misspell
il + legal = illegal
il + literate = illiterate
in + audible = inaudible
im + mature = immature
dis + appear = disappear

Rule 4. Only one word in English ends in *sede:* supersede. Only three words end in *ceed:* exceed, proceed, and succeed. All other words of similar sound end in *cede,* as in:

concede
recede
precede

Rule 5. The suffixes *ly* and *ness* do not change the spelling of the root word:

sudden + ness = suddenness
final + ly = finally
truthful + ly = truthfully
lean + ness = leanness

EXCEPTIONS: Words ending in *y* preceded by a consonant change *y* to *i* before any suffix not beginning with *i:*

kindly + ness = kindliness
happy + ly = happily
happy + ness = happiness

Words ending in *y* preceded by a vowel also follow this rule.

Rule 6. Drop the *e* from the end of a word before adding the suffixes *al, ed, ing,* and *able:*

complete—completed—completing
care—caring
fine—final
love—lovable
observe—observable

EXCEPTIONS: Words ending in *ce* and *ge* usually keep the silent *e* when the suffix begins with *a* or *o* in order to preserve the soft sound of the final consonant:

notice + able = noticeable
change + able = changeable

Rule 7. Keep the final *e* before a suffix beginning with a consonant:

large + ly = largely
care + ful = careful
care + less = careless
state + ment = statement

EXCEPTIONS:

argue + ment = argument
true + ly = truly

Rule 8. With words of one syllable ending in a single consonant preceded by a single vowel, double the consonant before adding *ing, ed,* or *er:*

sit + ing = sitting
hop + ed = hopped
dip + er = dipper
run + ing = running
swim + ing = swimming

Rule 9. If a one-syllable word ends in a single consonant not preceded by a single vowel, do not double the consonant before adding *ing, ed,* or *er:*

reap + ed = reaped
heat + ing = heating

Rule 10. To make a word ending in *y* plural, check the letter before the *y*. If it is a vowel, just add *s:*

birthday—birthdays
day—days
ray—rays
toy—toys

If it is any other letter, change the *y* to *i* and add es:

city—cities
lady—ladies
study—studies
guppy—guppies
fly—flies

Rule 11. Most nouns (names of people, places, things, ideas) become plural by adding *s:*

boy—boys
dog—dogs
desk—desks
window—windows

Rule 12. The plural of nouns ending in *s, x, z, ch,* or *sh* is formed by adding *es.*

wax—waxes
dish—dishes
waltz—waltzes

Rule 13. The plural of most nouns ending in *f* is formed by adding *s.* The plural of some nouns ending in *fo* or *fe* is formed by changing the *f* to *v* and adding *s* or *es:*

gulf—gulfs
belief—beliefs
knifes—knives
life—lives

Rule 14. The plural of nouns ending in *o* preceded by a vowel is formed by adding *s.* The plural of nouns ending in *o* preceded by a consonant is formed by adding *es.*

patio—patios
ratio—ratios
tornado—tornados
hero—heroes

EXCEPTIONS:

eskimo—eskimos
silo—silos

FIGURE 6–18 Spelling reference rules.

Examples:

The physician dictates letters and the medical assistant transcribes them.

Administrative medical assistants perform clerical duties and clinical medical assistants perform nursing skills.

Laboratory technicians analyze specimens and medical assistants assist with physical examinations.

A *complex sentence* contains one independent clause and one or more dependent clauses. A dependent clause cannot stand alone as a sentence.

Examples:

The doctor, who is off on Thursdays, sees allergy patients in the morning. (an adjective clause)

Patients are sometimes quite apprehensive when they come to the office for diagnostic examination. (an adverb clause)

Physicians require that patients receive proper instructions for diagnostic procedures. (noun clause)

A *compound–complex sentence* contains two or more independent clauses plus one or more dependent clauses.

Example:

Medical assistants should seek continuing education because medical technology is constantly changing, and the medical assistant must keep current with new procedures.

Punctuation Marks

In order to make sentences easier to read, and to tell a reader when you come to the end of a thought, a variety of markings called **punctuation** are used. The most common are the comma, period, apostrophe, hyphen, and ellipsis. The following information describes the correct usage of these marks.

- A *period* is placed at the end of each sentence.
- A comma or period should appear in front of an ending quotation mark, i.e., "or."

There are four general rules for the use of a comma:

1. Use between main **clauses** connected by *and, but, so, for, or, nor,* and *yet.* If main clauses are short, no comma is needed.
2. Use following long introductory phrases or clauses that may begin with words such as *after, whenever, if, until, since,* and *once.*
3. Use to separate items in a series.
4. Use to set off nonrestrictive modifiers. A *nonrestrictive phrase* or clause is a nonessential phrase or clause. It just adds descriptive or explanatory detail. A *restrictive modifier* restricts or limits the noun it modifies.

Example:

The medical assistant, being dedicated to her profession, helps the doctor in countless ways.

The medical assistant, who is a part of the medical team, needs to be especially careful in attending to details.

An **apostrophe** is used in **contractions** to signify that one or more letters have been left out. Be sure if you use *it's* that you mean *it is. Who's,* meaning *who is,* should not be confused with *whose,* and *there's,* meaning *there is,* is not to be confused with *theirs.*

An apostrophe is also used to signify possession in a noun.

Example:

The medical assistant's pen, pencil, and note pad are always beside the office telephone.

The assistant's stethoscope hangs in the examination room.

Carefully check all **hyphens** at the end of a line to be sure the word is divided correctly. Check your dictionary if you are in doubt about the end of a syllable.

Two forms of **ellipses** may be used—three and four dots. The three-dot ellipsis is used with spaces at each end, and between the dots, to signify an omission of words.

Example:

"They come in two varieties—the three-dot variety . . . and the four-dot variety."

The four-dot ellipsis signifies an omission of words and the end of a sentence with no space between the last letter and the first dot.

Example:

"The four-dot. . . ."

Use a *semicolon* between two clauses of a compound sentence when they are not joined by a conjunction, unless they are very short and are used informally. Samples of conjunctions are: therefore, however, then, nevertheless. The semicolon can also be used for clarity.

A *colon* is used to formally introduce a word, a list, a statement or question, a series of statements, or a long quotation. It is used after the salutation of a business letter and between numbers denoting time.

Quotation marks are used to enclose a direct quote. They are also used with titles of articles, chapters of books, and titles of short poems and stories. Spoken words in written narrative are also placed in quotes. A *question mark* or an *exclamation mark* is placed inside the quotation marks *if it is a part of the quotation; outside* if it applies to the main clause. Question marks are placed after every direct question. The exclamation mark is used after words, expressions, or sentences to show strong feeling.

Parenthesis may be used to enclose matter apart from the main thought; even though it contains a complete sentence, it does not have to start with a capital or end with a period; however, if it is an interrogative statement (question), it ends with a question mark.

Capitalization Capitalize names of persons and places, the first word in a sentence, names of holidays, principal words in titles of major works, and any product or title that might be trademarked. Many medical terms begin with a capital letter because they are names of the physicians who named them. Medications are usually trademarked. Again, use your dictionary when in doubt.

Be especially careful to check every word in a heading or title for correct spelling. Use your medical dictionary or a good general dictionary. Always have these reference books in the office.

Numbers The use of numbers must be consistent. If you follow a specific reference style book (e.g., *The Chicago*

Manual of Style, CBE Style Manual, AMA Manual of Style), you should follow its instructions for using numerals or spelling out the numbers. Also, follow the rules your employer wishes to be used for your office.

In the absence of other references and if the physician's preference is unknown, usually any number under 100 is spelled out while those above are used in numeric form. A partially contradicting general rule says to spell out the number if it can be done in one or two words. A number at the beginning of a sentence must be spelled out. A person's age and the time of day is also usually written out. Dates, street numbers, and page numbers are written in figures. When several numbers are mentioned within a short space, figures should be used for all of them.

COMPOSING A BUSINESS LETTER

With all the previous information, you are now ready to compose a business letter. There are certain steps in the process to consider in order to produce a final copy without errors.

- Determine what information needs to be included (a) to answer a letter, (b) to respond to a verbal request, (c) to request information, (d) to obtain a specific response.
- Determine the style for the letter and set margins and tabs for appropriate spacing on the page.
- If using a computer or word processor, select the type font (if appropriate).
- Type a rough draft using concise, easy to understand sentences. Use the words "I" and "we" as infrequently as possible, especially to begin sentences. Remember it is awkward to use the same word twice in one sentence or even in two consecutive sentences. The use of a **thesaurus** to increase the usage of different words makes the content more interesting.
- Proofread the draft and make changes. Eliminate redundant (extra, unnecessary) phrases.
- Type the final copy and sign it or give it to the sender to sign.

In a specialists office one of the most common letters received which will require a response is a request from another physician for a consult of a patient, Figure 6–19. Before a response can be sent, the patient must be seen. You will often find it necessary to correspond with the patient if you need to send any special instructions, directions to your office and other information. Be certain the material has ample time to arrive at the patient's home before they are due in for their examination.

- the reason for the appointment.
- the date and time of the appointment (it should request notification if the appointment cannot be kept).
- a statement saying that if there are any questions, please feel free to call your office. Be sure to include your office's phone number.

The office visit will require a follow-up letter from your employer to the referring physician, identifying the findings, diagnosis, and recommended course of treatment.

Samuel E. Matthews, MD
100 East Main Street, Suite 120
Yourtown, US 98765-4321

October 7, 19--

Robert Smith, M.D.
50 North Broad Street
Mytown, US 43200

Dear Dr. Smith:

I am referring Susan B. James to your office for evaluation of severe headaches of approximately six months duration. She was treated initially at a pain clinic in Yourtown. Susan will be calling your office for an appointment. I am sure you will find her to be a most cooperative patient.

I would appreciate a report of your diagnosis and recommended course of treatment.

Sincerely,

Samuel E. Matthews, M.D.

lk

FIGURE 6–19 Sample referral letter.

MAILABLE STANDARDS

All communications leaving your office should meet the standards for a **mailable** letter. These include:

- if typewritten, use clean, crisp type and a well inked ribbon; no smudges should appear on the paper.
- attractive letter placement on page, Figure 6–20 (A).
- all parts ("enclosures") of the letter are included.
- the right margin is fairly even; other margins are generous.
- punctuation and spacing that follows acceptable business practice.
- if typewritten, no errors or strikeovers should show.
- divided words at end of line are done correctly.
- letter content is accurate as dictated.
- no spelling errors.

SELECTING A LETTER STYLE

Letter styles vary in the location of some of the parts. Compare Figures 6–20 (B), (C), and (D). They are samples of the full block letter, the modified block letter, and the modified block letter with indented paragraphs. Notice the different placement of the parts of the letter with each style. Your employer may have a preference so be sure you know which one is to be used. In full block style, the dateline, address, salutation, body of letter, complimentary close,

SAMUEL E. MATTHEWS, MD
100 EAST MAIN STREET, SUITE 120
YOURTOWN, US 98765-4321

SHORT LETTER — 2 inch margins

MEDIUM LETTER — 1¼ inch margins

LONG LETTER — 1 inch margins

FIGURE 6–20 (A) Spacing of letter.

Samuel E. Matthews, MD
100 East Main Street-Suite 120
Yourtown, US 98765-4321

August 15, 19--   **(DATELINE)**

Robert Smith, M.D.
50 North Broad Street
Mytown, US 43200   **(INSIDE ADDRESS)**

Dear Dr. Smith: **(SALUTATION)**

RE: Amy D. James   **(REFERENCE)**

I am referring Amy James to your office for an eye
examination. She is complaining of some difficulty with
reading. She will be returning to school soon and her parents
wish to ensure that her vision is properly corrected.

Mrs. James will call your office for an appointment. I would
appreciate a report of your findings.

Sincerely yours,   **(COMPLIMENTARY CLOSE)**

        (SIGNATURE OF SENDER)

Samuel E. Matthews, MD   **(NAME TYPED)**

lk   **(REFERENCE INITIALS)**

(ENCLOSURE IF ANY)

FIGURE 6–20 (B) Sample full block letter.

Samuel E. Matthews, MD
100 East Main Street-Suite 120
Yourtown, US 98765-4321

August 15, 19-- **(DATELINE)**

Robert Smith, M.D.
50 North Broad Street
Mytown, US 43200   **(INSIDE ADDRESS)**

        RE: Amy D. James **(REFER-
ENCE)**

Dear Dr. Smith.   **(SALUTATION)**

I am referring Amy James to your office for an eye examination. She is complaining of some difficulty with reading. She
will be returning to school soon and her parents wish to ensure that her vision is properly corrected.

Mrs. James will call your office for an appointment. I would
appreciate a report of your findings.

(COMPLIMENTARY CLOSE)   Sincerely yours,
        (SIGNATURE OF SENDER)

(NAME TYPED)   Samuel E. Matthews, MD
(TITLE IF NEEDED)

lk   **(REFERENCE INITIALS)**
(ENCLOSURE IF ANY)

FIGURE 6–20 (C) Sample modified block letter.

Samuel E. Matthews, MD
100 East Main Street, Suite 120
Yourtown, US 98765-4321

August 15, 19-- **(DATELINE)**

Robert Smith, M.D.
50 North Broad Street
Mytown, US 43200   **(INSIDE ADDRESS)**

        RE: Amy D. James **(REFERENCE)**

Dear Dr. Smith: **(SALUTATION)**

I am referring Amy James to your office for an eye examination. She is complaining of some difficulty with reading. She
will be returning to school soon and her parents wish to ensure that her vision is properly corrected.

Mrs. James will call your office for an appointment. I
would appreciate a report of your findings.

(COMPLIMENTARY CLOSE)   Sincerely yours,
        (SIGNATURE OF SENDER)

(NAME TYPED)   Samuel E. Matthews, MD
(TITLE IF NEEDED)

lk   **(REFERENCE INITIALS)**
(ENCLOSURE IF ANY)

FIGURE 6–20 (D) Sample modified block letter with indented
paragraphs.

typed signature, and initials of typist are flush with the left margin. This is a popular style because no tab stops are needed. The most popular style is the modified block with the dateline, complimentary close, and typed signature beginning a bit right of center. This style is compatible with most letterheads. The dateline sets the style. If you place the date at the right, you must follow with modified block style, lining up the complimentary close and typed signature with the date. The least popular of the three styles customarily used in the medical office is the modified block with indented paragraphs.

Stationery

The type and quality of **stationery** is a statement about the physician's office. If it becomes your responsibility to select the stationery, be sure to inspect any anticipated choice carefully. The letterhead is usually the choice of the physician. Letterhead stationery and matching envelopes are usually 16-, 20-, or 24-pound weight. The larger the number, the heavier the paper. It is usually ordered by the ream, which

consists of 500 sheets of paper. Continuation pages are plain bond and should match the weight of the letterhead.

A **watermark** appears on bond paper and should read across the paper in the same direction as the typing. You can determine the correct watermark side by holding the paper to the light. If you type on the wrong side of erasable paper you will lose the erasable quality.

Be certain to make a copy of every business letter or report to be sent from the office. Copies of correspondence regarding patients need to be filed in the patient's chart. Correspondence in answer to business letters need to be copied and placed in the appropriate file. If your office still uses carbon paper for copies of correspondence, be sure the copies are also corrected whenever corrections are made on the original. (See Procedure 6–7, "Make Corrections on Typewritten Copy.")

TYPING A BUSINESS LETTER

A letter can be typed from dictated notes, from a dictation machine tape or composed by you at the keyboard (refer to

---

PROCEDURE

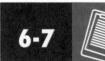
6-7 Make Corrections on Typewritten Copy

PURPOSE: To correct errors on a copy which has been typewritten so that they are not noticeable.

EQUIPMENT AND SUPPLIES: Typewriter, copy with errors, eraser, soft brush, correction paper in white or a color to match paper used, correction fluid in white or appropriate color, and correction tape (use only if making a master copy that will be reproduced).

TERMINAL PERFORMANCE OBJECTIVE: Given access to all equipment and supplies, make neat, acceptable corrections using the various methods described in the procedure. The corrected copy must be without error and corrections should be difficult to identify.

1. Proofread copy before removing paper from the typewriter. **Rationale: It is easier to correct errors because copy remains "lined up."**

2. Make corrections using typewriter correcting ribbon, if available.
   NOTE: (a) Position over character next to error
   (b) Press correction key
   (c) Retype error
   (d) Type correct letter

3. When using a non-correcting typewriter, with erasable paper, use a pencil eraser to remove the error ONLY.
   ■ When using Selectric model, move the typing element so it is out of the way and eraser crumbs will not fall on it.
   ■ Carefully erase only the error.
   ■ Brush any eraser crumbs away.

■ When using carbon paper, place a guard between the paper and carbon while erasing. Erase both pages. Remove the guard before resuming typing.

4. Use correction paper.
   NOTE: (a) Use color to match paper.
   (b) Insert over error.
   (c) Retype error.
   (d) Remove paper and type correct letter.

5. Use correction fluid.
   NOTE: (a) Shake bottle.
   (b) Apply sparingly and smoothly.
   (c) Discard thick fluid.

6. When paper has been removed before an error is found, realign the line of typing so the correction will blend in.
   NOTE: (a) Study the relationship of letters on the page to lines on the paper guide.
   (b) Insert scratch paper in typewriter.
   (c) Set typewriter to stencil.
   (d) Clean keys by striking scratch paper several times.
   (e) Reinsert letter. With ribbon still on stencil, strike missing letters.
   (f) When alignment is good, strike missing letter; if in alignment, set ribbon on print and make the correction.

7. Use correction tape (only when producing copy).
   NOTE: (a) Cut tape and carefully cover error.
   (b) Make correction.

Chapter 4, Unit 3). There are certain formatting standards which result in a mailable letter. The following are points to remember as you perform Procedure 6–8, "Type a Business Letter."

- The date typed indicates when the content of the letter was dictated.
- The month is spelled out in full (traditional style is month/day/year; military style is day/month/year).
- The inside address should be copied exactly from the correspondence to be answered or as printed in the phone book or medical society directory.
- A courtesy title is used (Mr., Mrs., Miss, or Ms. If gender unknown, use Mr.).
- Do not use Dr. before the physician's name if MD follows.

- If a street address and box number are given, use the box number.
- The words North, South, East, and West preceding street names and Road, Street, Avenue, and Boulevard are NOT abbreviated.
- The words Apartment and Suite are typed on the same line as the address and are separated by a comma.
- Apartment may be abbreviated if the line is long.
- The name of the city is spelled out and is separated from the state by a comma.
- The state name can be spelled out or abbreviated (see Unit 4 for list of abbreviations) and is separated from the zip code by one space; there is no punctuation between the state and the zip code.
- A proper salutation is Dear followed by the person's last name. If the correspondence is to a colleague or friend,

P R O C E D U R E

6-8 Type Business Letter

PURPOSE: To prepare a mailable business letter.

EQUIPMENT AND SUPPLIES: Typewriter, word processor or computer, paper, appropriate correction materials, dictation or dictation tape, and transcriber.

TERMINAL PERFORMANCE OBJECTIVE: Given access to equipment and supplies, complete a mailable letter following the steps in the procedure within the number of attempts and time frame specified by the instructor. The number of attempts is to be specified. The final copy must meet mailable standards described in this text.

1. Move type down at least three lines below letterhead.
2. Type the date. **NOTE: Be sure that the location is appropriate for the chosen style.**
3. Move to the fifth line below the date.
4. Type the inside address.
   NOTE: Be sure the address is in the appropriate location for the style of letter. Use the appropriate courtesy title and type the name exactly as printed on the received letterhead or as is in the phone or medical society directory.
5. Double space after the last line of the address.
6. Type the appropriate salutation followed by a colon.
7. Double space.
8. Enter the reference line in the location appropriate for letter style. Type RE: Enter patient's name or person about whom the letter is written.
9. Double space.
10. Type the body (content) of the letter.
    - Be sure the paragraph style is appropriate to the style of the letter.

- Always double space between paragraphs.
- If a second page is necessary, (A) when using a typewriter proofread page one and make corrections before removing it from the typewriter and (B) type at least two lines of the paragraph on the first page. Do not divide the last word.

11. If a second page is necessary, type the second page heading in vertical or horizontal format.
    NOTE: Includes name, page number, and date.
12. Continue body of letter.
13. Type a complimentary closing in letter style format.
14. Go down four spaces.
15. Type the sender's name in letter style format exactly as printed on letterhead.
    NOTE: An official title follows the name on the same line separated by a comma, or directly below with no comma required.
16. Double space.
17. Type reference initials to indicate the typist.
18. Single or double space if enclosing materials.
19. Type preferred style enclosure.
    NOTE: Number and identify if there is more than one enclosure.
20. Single or double space if copies will be sent.
21. Type cc and the recipient(s) name(s).
    NOTE: Enter bcc on file copy if sending a blind copy.
22. Double space.
23. Type PS for postscript, if desired.

a first name is appropriate (ask the physician). When writing to a business, use Gentlemen, Dear Sir, or Dear Madam.

- To use a reference line, type RE: then the patient's full name. This line goes two spaces *below* the salutation, flush with the left margin in block style. It may be lined up with the date and follow the address in the modified block style. (This is a common error because the dictator usually names the person before the salutation.)

- Always double space between paragraphs, flush left with block style and indented five spaces with modified block.

- If a second page is necessary, stop the first page at the end of paragraph, if possible. If not, type at least two lines from the paragraph on the bottom of the first page.

- The bottom margin must measure at least one inch.

- The last word on a page cannot be divided.

- Always proofread typewritten page BEFORE removing the paper from the typewriter so that corrections can be made more easily (refer to Procedure 6–8, "Make Corrections on Typewritten Copy"). If word processed or computer generated, print the copy and proof it. Proofing on screen is difficult because you cannot view the total letter at one time. Make corrections on the stored copy and print.

- Capitalize only the first word of a complimentary closing; follow with a comma.

- The formality of the letter determines the closing: Cordially or Sincerely is considered informal while Very truly yours is more formal.

- The sender's name is typed four spaces below the closing exactly as on the letterhead; an official title follows on the same line, separated by a comma, or it can be typed on the next line with no comma.

- The typist's initials, in lower case, are placed two spaces below the sender's name. When the sender will not be signing the letter, both dictator's (in upper case) and typist's initials are used. Typists do not use their reference initials on letters they sign.

- When items will be enclosed with the letter, type Enclosure or Enc. one or two lines below reference initials; number and identify if more than one enclosure is included.

- If copies are sent to others, type cc (for carbon copy) and the other receiver's name one or two spaces below initials or last notation. When more than one individual is carbon copied, list their names alphabetically or by rank. When a copy is sent to another person without the knowledge of the recipient, it is known as a *blind copy.* No notation is placed on the recipient's letter but *bcc* is placed on the file copy to **denote** it was sent.

- A **postscript** (PS) is typed two spaces below the last notation.

- When using a second page, a heading of the patient's name, page number and date, is typed either vertically or horizontally, one inch from the top. If the letter does not concern a patient, the receiver is listed.

- The letter continues on the third line after the heading; the page should contain at least two lines of a paragraph.

Type a business letter following the steps in Procedure 6–8 and the points to remember.

Proofreading

All written communication must be **proofread** before it is sent. This is a process of carefully reading printed material and marking errors for correction. There are certain problem areas to watch such as; (1) words ending in "s", (2) apostrophes, (3) combinations of punctuation, (4) period, (5) commas, (6) double letters in words, (7) capital letters, (8) two-letter words, (9) hyphens, (10) numbers, and (11) dashes. Proofreading requires concentration and attention to details in a step-by-step process. Career proofreaders use at least a three read system. First they read through the material to make sure it makes sense and to check for errors in composition such as a misaligned margin, paragraph indents, spacing on the page, etc. Then they read for content, to make certain correct words, punctuation, and grammar are used. And last, a check of spelling. Because we can be fooled by what we think we see when we read normally, spelling is checked by reading the content *backwards,* checking each word, one word at a time. Going through these steps should ensure an error-free communication. If possible, as a final precaution, have someone else **critique** the letter.

When you proofread a draft copy, you should use standard proofreader's marks to indicate changes that need to be made. Knowledge of these marks is very helpful if your employer writes for professional journals or other publications, since materials which are submitted may be returned by the publisher with these markings and any other clarifications or charges they may desire. The final draft, called **galley proofs**, will require very careful proofreading for any remaining errors before the material goes to print. The most common marks are shown in Figure 6–21.

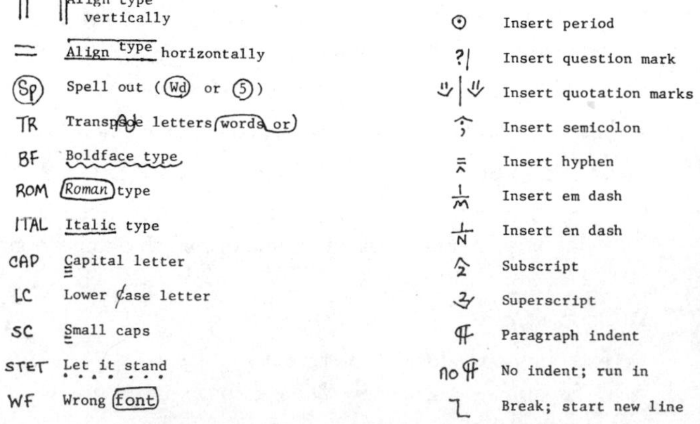

FIGURE 6–21 Proofreader's marks.

Developing good transcription and typing skills and the ability to produce error-free communications are very desirable traits. It can make you a real asset to the physician's practice. If you enjoy this type of work, it will probably be possible for you to specialize in communication preparation.

Complete Chapter 6, Unit 3 in the workbook to help you meet the objectives at the beginning of this unit and therefore achieve competency of this subject matter.

UNIT 4
Receiving and Sending Office Communications

■ OBJECTIVES

Upon completion of the unit, meet the following terminal performance objectives by verifying knowledge of the facts and principles presented through oral and written communication at a level deemed competent.

1. Sort, open, and annotate incoming mail.
2. Describe how vacation mail might be handled.
3. Identify postal services that may be required by an office.
4. List points to remember in processing metered mail.
5. List eight classifications of mail.
6. List three examples of first class mail.
7. List an example of second class mail.
8. List four examples of third class mail.
9. List four examples of fourth class mail.
10. Describe at least four of the specifications of express mail service.
11. Describe two reasons to use certificate of mailing.
12. Explain why you might use certified mail.
13. Describe purpose for use of registered mail.
14. Name six means of communication other than by mail.
15. Name six uses for a FAX machine.
16. Spell and define, using the glossary at the back of the text, all the words to know in this unit.

■ WORDS TO KNOW

abbreviations
annotating
cancellation
certified
confirmation
consecutively
domestic
envelope
facsimile
foreign

guarantees
judgement
polling
postmark
priority
recipient
teleconference
thermally
transmitted

INCOMING MAIL

The amount of mail coming into the physician's office depends on the number of physicians. In smaller offices the task is manageable but in large clinics it may be necessary to have a mail clerk who is responsible for sorting and delivering the mail within the clinic.

The office policy manual should give instructions regarding the handling of mail. If no manual is available, the office manager or the physician should be consulted. Following are some generally accepted practices.

SORTING MAIL

Incoming mail should first be sorted. Any mail marked *personal* should be placed on the physician's desk unopened. Special delivery mail, mailgrams, or special messenger mail should be opened immediately. (The mailgram is a postal service offered jointly by the USPS and Western Union). Mailgrams are transmitted over Western Union's communication network to printers located in over 140 post offices, then placed in special envelopes carrying the postal service emblem and delivered the next day by regular carrier.

First class mail may consist of:

Special delivery mail

Mailgrams

Special messenger mail

Correspondence from patients

Payments from patients

Payments from insurance companies

Insurance forms to be completed

General correspondence
a. referral letters or reports from physicians
b. laboratory reports
c. hospital reports
d. professional organization mail
e. miscellaneous mail

Second, third, and fourth class mail consists of:

Professional journals

Magazines

Newspapers

Advertisements

Promotional literature and samples from pharmaceutical companies

First class mail may be sorted into mail from patients, from physicians, from insurance companies, and miscellaneous. Other classes of mail, such as magazines, professional journals, and newspapers, should be separated from drug samples and advertisements.

OPENING MAIL

When opening mail, you will need a letter opener, paper clips, a stapler, and a date stamp. It is more efficient to stack all envelopes so that they are facing in the same direction. A quick tap on the desk will move contents away from the flap side of the **envelope**. Open all letters along the flap edge being careful to remove all contents from each envelope. As the mail is removed be sure the contents contain the same name and return address shown on the envelope. Some offices want you to keep the envelope with the mail received, and certainly you should if it is needed to help identify the contents. Otherwise you may discard the envelopes.

Date-stamp the correspondence and attach any enclosures. If an enclosure is indicated on the letter but is missing, it is necessary to write "none" after the "Encl." notation and circle it to indicate need for follow-up.

PROCESSING INCOMING MAIL

Exercise your best **judgment** to determine which mail can be handled without the aid of the physician. This type of mail would include routine office expense bills, insurance forms, and checks for deposit. If cash is received in the mail, you should always seek a witness to verify the amount of money and have that person sign a receipt along with you to be sent to the patient. This helps avoid the possibility of the patient saying that more was sent than was actually found in the envelope. This can happen quite innocently with elderly patients who may have a poor memory.

If you are employed by a surgeon, the mail will contain copies of hospital summaries and operative notes. These can be filed directly in the patient chart. Often copies are sent to the referring physician. Other hospital, laboratory, or special examination reports received should be seen by the physician and initialed before they are filed. Requests regarding patients or other office matters should be placed in a designated area for the physician to see and respond to each day.

The medical assistant can perform a valuable, timesaving service for the physician by **annotating** the incoming mail, or identifying important points to be noticed. If any correspondence or a patient chart will be needed to answer mail, it should be pulled and placed with the mail to be answered.

Notifications of meetings, miscellaneous correspondence, and professional journals are placed under the stack of mail. Some physicians want to see all supply catalogs and pharmaceutical company descriptions of products. In other offices, many of these items are disposed of immediately, especially if they concern areas of practice the office does not provide. Items that may be needed for future reference should be placed in a designated file.

Drug samples that may be used should be placed in a designated area for future use. Samples that will not be used should never be placed in the trash where they could cause harm to individuals taking them without medical evaluation and advice. Often, community clinics and service organizations can make good, safe use of unwanted samples. The office should have a box to collect samples for this purpose.

VACATION MAIL

When the physician is away from the office for professional meetings or on vacation, the medical assistant may be asked to carefully read all mail and decide how each piece will be handled. You should discuss what to do with urgent mail before the physician leaves. The physician may want you to call to discuss, or in some cases, to copy and forward the mail. Never send the original. If the physician will be away

for a long time, you may need to send urgent mail more than once. If so, be sure to number the envelopes **consecutively** and keep track of what you send so that you can be sure all the urgent mail is received. When responding, you may also wish to send a brief note explaining the reason for the delay in answering. If the office will be closed temporarily or permanently, be sure to go to the post office and complete a form to have mail held or forwarded to another address. Never send this form by mail as it may be delayed. The USPS cannot take verbal orders for this purpose. Allowing mail to accumulate invites theft.

ADDRESSING ENVELOPES

The United States Postal Service (USPS) uses optical character readers (OCRs) and bar code sorters (BCSs) to read the addresses on envelopes you mail. The BCS equipment is capable of sorting over 30,000 pieces of mail per hour but only if envelopes are properly addressed.

The bar code is a series of little lines you often see at the bottom of letters from utility companies, banks, retailers, and other businesses, Figure 6–22.

Each piece of mail passes by the computer's scanner for a quick read of the delivery address. Then, it goes to the OCR's printer, which sprays on a bar code representing the zip code or ZIP + 4 code for the address. Next, the mail piece goes to one of the OCR's sorting channels reserved for the proper delivery area. From there, the bar coded mail is fed to BCSs for the final separations. The BCS processes mail just as quickly and in much the same way as the OCR reads addresses, except its scanner recognizes only one thing—the bar code. As the bar code on your mail piece passes the BCS lens, it is quickly read and sent to the appropriate channel for delivery.

Addresses should be typewritten or machine printed to be processed on automated equipment. Script or Executive type should not be used. The USPS prefers that the entire address be printed in upper case letters and, except for the hyphen in the ZIP + 4 code, all punctuation should be omitted. Lines of the address should be formatted with a uniform left margin.

ADDRESS BLOCK LOCATION

The shaded area in Figure 6–23 illustrates the area on the face of the mail piece where address information should be located to be read by the OCRs. The OCRs and BCSs register mail pieces on the bottom edge; therefore, all vertical measurements are relative to the bottom edge.

Where possible, the entire address (exclusive of the optical lines above the name of recipient line) should be contained in an imaginary rectangle which extends from $5/8''$ to $2\frac{3}{4}''$ from the bottom of the mail piece, with $1''$ margins on each side. At a minimum, all characters of the last line of the

FIGURE 6–22 Example of bar code (Courtesy of United States Postal Service).

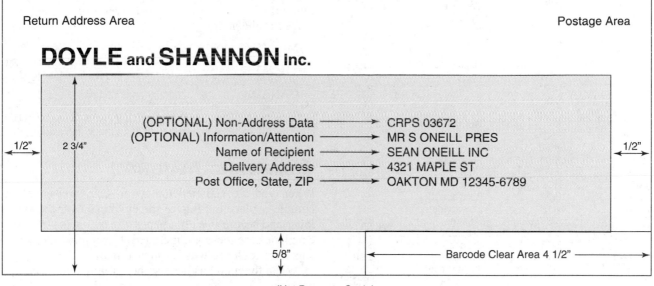

Return Address Area

Postage Area

DOYLE and SHANNON inc.

1/2"   2 3/4"

(OPTIONAL) Non-Address Data ——————→ CRPS 03672
(OPTIONAL) Information/Attention ——————→ MR S ONEILL PRES
Name of Recipient ——————→ SEAN ONEILL INC
Delivery Address ——————→ 4321 MAPLE ST
Post Office, State, ZIP ——————→ OAKTON MD 12345-6789

1/2"

5/8"

Barcode Clear Area 4 1/2"

(Not Drawn to Scale)

FIGURE 6–23   Example of address block location (Courtesy of United States Postal Service).

address block—the post office (city), state and zip code or ZIP + 4—should be located within an imaginary rectangle which extends from ⅝" to 2¼" from the bottom of the mail piece with 1" margins on each side.

Care must be taken to make the lines straight, as slanted lines cannot be read by the OCR process. The only **abbreviations** permitted in the name of the city are those found in the "Abbreviations" section of the *National Zip Code Directory*. The OCR cannot read a non-standard abbreviation.

Special notations for the post office such as *Special Delivery* or *Certified Mail* should be typed in all capitals two lines below the postage. Be sure you are above the address zone. Special notations for the recipient such as *Personal* or *Confidential* should be typed in all capitals aligned with and two lines below the return address.

The zip code is critical to the rapid delivery of mail. The first number of the zip code refers to a region of the United States, from 0 for the East coast to 9 for the West coast and Hawaii. The next two numbers refer to the major post office in the region, and the final two identify the local delivery post offices. The newer ZIP + 4 coding will allow even better use of automated processing in that the first two additional numbers denote a delivery sector, which may be several blocks, a group of streets, several office buildings, or other small geographic area. The last two numbers denote a delivery segment, which might be one floor of an office building, one side of a street, specific departments in a firm, or a group of post office boxes. If your office has a large volume of mail, use of ZIP + 4 offers a discount in postal rate. The USPS will offer assistance in converting to ZIP + 4, but the confidential nature of medical office records means that patient interests would best be served by converting your own records. The customer service representative at the post office can answer your questions on the use of the *ZIP + 4 National/State Directory*.

Now that you know how to address an envelope correctly, it is time to put the pieces together. The name of the intended **recipient** (business or individual) should appear on the first line. The line above the name of recipient line is an optional line for additional address information. When needed, it should be used to direct mail to the attention of a specific person when a business name has been placed on the name of recipient line or to provide other information that will facilitate delivery (i.e., the name of a department within a company).

The line immediately below the recipient line is designated the *delivery address line*. The street address, post-office box number, rural route number and box number, or highway contract number and box number should appear on this line. Mail addressed to multiunit buildings should include the apartment number, suite, room, or other unit designation immediately after the street address of the building, on the same line. When the length of the delivery address is such that it prevents the placement of the unit number or other designation on the same line, the number or designator should be placed on the line immediately above the delivery address line. When use of the building name in the address is necessary, it should also be placed on the line above the delivery address line, Figure 6–24.

For **domestic** mail, the post office (city), state, and zip code or ZIP + 4 should appear in that order on the bottom line of the address. However, if all three elements will not fit on that line, the zip code or ZIP + 4 may be placed on the line immediately below the post office and state, aligned with the left edge of the address block. The standard two-letter state abbreviations should also be used, Figure 6–25. The ZIP + 4 codes should always be printed as five digits, a hyphen, and four digits. The hyphen should be treated as any other character as far as spacing and stroke width are concerned.

Annex	ANX	Park	PK
Apartment	APT	Parkway	PKY
Association	ASSN	Pike	PIKE
Attention	ATTN	Place	PL
Avenue	AVE	Plaza	PLZ
Boulevard	BLVD	Post Office	PO
Canyon	CYN	President	PRES
Causeway	CSWY	Ridge	RDG
Circle	CIR	River	RIV
Court	CT	Road	RD
Department	DEPT	Room	RM
East	E	Route	RT
Expressway	EXPY	Rural	R
Freeway	FWY	Rural Route	RR
Heights	HTS	Secretary	SECY
Highway	HWY	Shore	SHR
Hospital	HOSP	South	S
Institute	INST	Southeast	SE
Junction	JCT	Southwest	SW
Knolls	KNLS	Square	SQ
Lake	LK	Station	STA
Lakes	LKS	Street	ST
Lane	LN	Terrace	TER
Manager	MGR	Treasurer	TREAS
Meadows	MDWS	Turnpike	TPKE
North	N	Union	UN
Northeast	NE	Vice President	VP
Northwest	NW	View	VW
Palms	PLMS		

FIGURE 6–24 Examples of USPS approved address abbreviations (Courtesy of United States Postal Service).

Mail addressed to **foreign** countries should include the country name printed in capital letters (no abbreviations) as the only information on the bottom line. For example:

MR THOMAS CLARK
117 RUSSELL DRIVE
LONDON WIP6HQ
ENGLAND

Alabama	AL	Montana	MT
Alaska	AK	Nebraska	NE
Arizona	AZ	Nevada	NV
Arkansas	AR	New Hampshire	NH
California	CA	New Jersey	NJ
Canal Zone	CZ	New Mexico	NM
Colorado	CO	New York	NY
Connecticut	CT	North Carolina	NC
Delaware	DE	North Dakota	ND
District of Columbia	DC	Ohio	OH
Florida	FL	Oklahoma	OK
Georgia	GA	Oregon	OR
Guam	GU	Pennsylvania	PA
Hawaii	HI	Puerto Rico	PR
Idaho	ID	Rhode Island	RI
Illinois	IL	South Carolina	SC
Indiana	IN	South Dakota	SD
Iowa	IA	Tennessee	TN
Kansas	KS	Texas	TX
Kentucky	KY	Utah	UT
Louisiana	LA	Vermont	VT
Maine	ME	Virginia	VA
Maryland	MD	Virgin Islands	VI
Massachusetts	MA	Washington	WA
Michigan	MI	West Virginia	WV
Minnesota	MN	Wisconsin	WI
Mississippi	MS	Wyoming	WY
Missouri	MO		

FIGURE 6–25 Two-letter state abbreviations.

Mail addressed to Canada may use either of the following formats when the postal delivery zone number is included in the address:

MRS HELEN SAUNDERS
1010 CLEAR STREET
OTTAWA ON K1AOB1
CANADA

MRS HELEN SAUNDERS
1010 CLEAR STREET
OTTAWA ON CANADA
K1AOB1

The post office will furnish additional information on mailing to foreign countries if assistance is needed.

COMPLETING MAILING

When you are satisfied that your letter and envelope are complete, place the flap of the envelope over the top of the letter and secure it with a paper clip. If enclosures are indicated, be sure these are included. It is a good idea to have a signature folder in which finished mail is placed.

When the mail has been signed, fold it and place it in the envelope. A standard-size letter should be folded by bringing the lower third of the letter up and making a crease, then folding the top third of the letter down to about half an inch from the creased edge and making a second crease. The second crease goes into the envelope first. To fold a standard-size letter for a 6¾ envelope, bring the bottom edge to within half an inch of the top edge and crease. Fold from the right side about one third the width of the sheet and crease. Fold from the left edge to within half an inch of the second crease. Insert the left-edge crease into the envelope first.

If you have a large number of envelopes to seal you can speed up the process by placing eight or ten envelopes address side down with flaps open in fan fashion. Use a damp sponge to wet all the flaps at once and then starting with the lower letter turn down each flap and seal. Be sure that the sponge is not too wet as it will wet the envelopes and may spread glue so that letters stick together before you can seal them.

STAMP OR METER MAIL

The cost of sending mail is an expenditure that must be examined to be sure you obtain the most for your money. Your local post office can furnish you with current information. Postage rates, categories, and regulations are changeable, so you need to be current.

Mail may be either stamped or metered. Stamps may be purchased at a post office or obtained through the mail by using a specially printed envelope available through the post office. If you have a large volume of mail, it is preferable to use a postage meter. This machine can be leased from several authorized dealers, but the license to use it must be obtained from the USPS. A medical office can obtain a license by submitting an application to the post office where the metered mail will be deposited.

Postage meters contain a sealed unit that houses the printing die and two recording counters. One counter adds up all postage printed by the meter. The other counter subtracts and shows the balance of postage remaining in the meter. When you purchase an amount of postage, the post office will open the meter with a key, set the counter for the amount of postage purchased, and relock the meter. When the prepaid

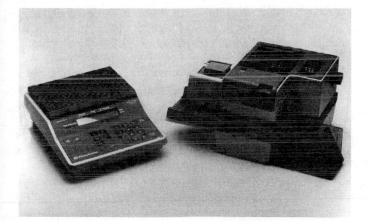

FIGURE 6-26 Postage scale and meter (Courtesy Pitney Bowes).

amount runs out, the meter will lock automatically. The postage meter prints prepaid postage either directly on the mail or on adhesive strips that are then affixed to the mail. The metered mail imprint, or metered stamp, serves as postage payment, **postmark**, and **cancellation** mark. All mail classes, amounts of postage, and quantity of mail may be metered. Metered mail, when bundled, can provide faster service than stamped mail because it is already postmarked and will bypass postal cancellation equipment.

To expedite the processing of metered mail, remember to: (1) change the date on the meter daily, (2) apply the correct amount of postage by weighing the mail before affixing postage, (3) check the imprint to be sure it is clear and readable, and (4) use fluorescent ink in the meter, Figure 6-26.

MAIL CLASSIFICATIONS

Mail is classified according to type, weight, and destination. **First class mail** includes handwritten and typewritten messages, payments from patients or insurance companies, laboratory reports, and any other business mail which weighs up to 11 ounces. (Postage is figured by the ounce.) All first class mail over 11 ounces is considered **priority** mail. The cost of priority mail is determined by the weight and zone of destination. The maximum weight for priority mail is 70 pounds. If you need to send first class mail that is larger than the usual number 10 business envelope, the envelope should have a green diamond border which signals the post office that the letter is to go first class.

The office should have a mail scale so that you can determine the amount of postage necessary for your mail. The second ounce does not cost as much as the first.

Second class mail includes newspapers and other periodicals issued regularly at least four times a year. You are not likely to use this classification unless you work for a medical society that mails its own journal.

Third class mail includes circulars, printed booklets, catalogs, newsletters, and merchandise weighing up to but not including 16 ounces, which is not required to be mailed at first class rates or as priority mail. Anything 16 ounces or more must be mailed fourth class or priority mail.

Fourth class mail is commonly known as parcel post. The classification also includes bound printed matter, books,

16 mm or narrower films, sound recordings, and manuscripts. Fourth class postage is computed by weight and the zone of destination.

In combination mailing, a first class letter is sent with a parcel, either by placing the letter in an envelope and attaching it to the outside of the package or by enclosing it within the parcel, in which case you write *letter enclosed* just below the postage. This method is used frequently in the field of medicine for sending x-rays with an accompanying report. Separate postage is paid for the two items.

Express mail service is a reliable, speedy delivery service available in most major metropolitan areas for anything mailable up to 70 pounds and 108 inches in combined length and girth. You are given a receipt when the letter or package is mailed and the addressee is required to sign a **confirmation** of delivery. Each express shipment is insured against loss or damage at no additional charge. Postage varies according to weight and the type of express mail service chosen. A form with a large *A* or *B* on it will be attached to express mail. *A* designates post office-to-post office service: mail which is deposited by 5:00 P.M at an express post office will be shipped to the destination post office for customer pickup the next day as early as 10:00 A.M. *B* designates post office-to-addressee service: mail which is deposited by 5 P.M at a designated post office will be delivered to the addressee no later than 3:00 P.M. the next day (weekends and holidays included). A full refund of postage will be made if shipments are delivered later than the service standard called for. You apply at the originating post office for the refund. Express mail envelopes and labels are available at the post office as well as a network directory of all destinations that can be accessed.

Special delivery may be purchased for all classes of mail to provide prompt delivery *to the destination post office*. Smaller post offices and rural routes do not offer this service, so it is best to check before mailing a letter to such an address. Do not send special delivery to a box number because it is considered delivered when it is put in the box.

A *certificate of mailing* provides evidence of mailing. The postal clerk will date and initial the slip you prepare to show that a piece of mail was sent from that post office on a particular date. The service is inexpensive and is often used as evidence that a document was mailed or a deadline was met. For an additional fee **certified** mail provides an opportunity to restrict delivery to addressee only and to request a signed return receipt. This method of mailing should always be used when you need to be certain a patient, and only the patient, receives specific communication. It could be a sensitive lab report, a copy of a consult, an important physical examination report, or anything that is highly personal or contains important information. It is also appropriate to use certified mail to notify a patient that because instructions and treatments are not being followed as ordered, medical services will no longer be provided and that another physician should be contacted. A certified letter ensures you have verification that the patient received notice. The signed return receipt needs to be filed in the patient's chart as your proof that the patient received the letter.

Registered mail is the best method to use if sending valuable articles. Paying the extra fee for this service **guarantees** extra security in the form of locked mail bags and signed releases for each step through which the mail passes. The full value of the mailing must be declared, and it can be insured up to $10,000. Only first class and priority mail can be registered.

You can insure any class of mail against loss or damage. You can also request a return receipt and restrict the delivery.

If you have deposited mail and find you want it back, you will need to file a written application at the local post office, with an envelope addressed exactly as the one you wish returned. If the post office finds that the letter has left the local post office, the postmaster will telephone or telegraph the destination post office, at your expense, to have the letter returned to you.

If you have mail returned because the patient has moved and left no forwarding address, you can try contacting the employer for a new address or talking with the individual who referred the patient. When a letter is returned, after an attempt has been made to deliver it, you must prepare a new envelope and put on new postage before remailing. This sometimes happens if you have made an error such as transposing numbers in an address.

Alternative Ways to Communicate

There are many ways to receive and send information in today's technological society. Some common methods are FAX, pager, cellular phone, voice mail, conference call, teleconferencing, E-Mail, and the Internet.

FAX Machines

Facsimile (FAX) machines, Figure 6–27, can be used by hospitals, physicians' offices, and clinics to send and receive information over telephone lines, regarding patients. The machine makes it possible to send and receive letters, medical reports, laboratory reports, and insurance claims. Physicians may use the FAX machine to send prescription orders to pharmacies. The office may also use it for ordering office or medical supplies.

A FAX machine is connected to a telephone line. The machine scans a document and converts the image to electronic impulses that are **transmitted** over the telephone lines. The

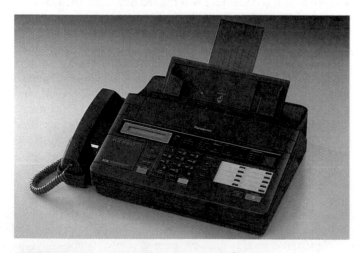

FIGURE 6–27 FAX machine (Courtesy of Panasonic Communications & Systems Co.).

receiving FAX machine converts the impulse to make an identical copy of the original. FAX machines may print on **thermally** treated paper or plain paper. The thermally treated paper fades when exposed to sunlight; therefore, you would usually photocopy an important document onto bond paper.

The FAX machine is available with many special features. Certainly a concern in the medical office is the transmission of confidential material. It is possible to have a secret code that will lock out unauthorized **polling**. The FAX machine may also be able to store multiple documents in memory and have automatic dialing with redialing when a busy signal is detected. The paper is automatically cut to the length of each page of the received message. If the recording paper runs out, the message is stored in memory and will be automatically printed out when new paper is loaded. A battery safeguards the document memory in case of power failure. The machine may be equipped with a white line skip function that automatically skips over horizontal blank spaces on a document. This feature allows a standard document to be transmitted in as little as twelve seconds.

You will need to learn the specific procedure for operating the FAX machine you will be using. However, there are general rules which are important to the use of any FAX machine.

1. Always remove paper clips and staples from material to be scanned so you will not damage the FAX machine.
2. Make a test copy if the document has color. Dark colors may block copy and can slow transmission.
3. Do not use correction tape or fluid on documents to be transmitted.
4. Do consider typing words for numbers to avoid problems with interpretation.
5. If the material you are faxing is confidential, before sending, call the recipient to alert them to be watching for the material.
6. The first sheet of any transmission is called the FAX page. It includes the date, name of recipient, recipient's address and FAX number, and the number of pages being sent (includes FAX page). The name and FAX number of the sender will also be included. Any other special information required for routing instructions should be added.
7. Be familiar with the error messages the FAX machine may display and learn how to correct these problems. The machine may be equipped with built-in service diagnostic codes that can be automatically transmitted over the telephone lines to a service provider. Most service calls can be resolved by telephone and therefore reduce costly equipment downtime and labor costs.
8. You may need to resend a message if noise or interference on the telephone line resulted in an unclear transmission.
9. Check to be sure the transmission is completed before you leave. It will indicate the message was sent, identifying the date and time of transmission. Remove the original from the machine.

Pagers

Physician's commonly wear pagers so they can be contacted regardless of where they are or what they are involved in. A pager is a small electronic device that is activated by a telephone signal. When you wish to contact the physician, you simply dial the number. After it rings, a series of beeps will be heard and you then enter the phone number from which you are calling. Meanwhile, the beeper being worn by the physician will be activated and will produce a beeping sound or, if sound is turned off, will vibrate to alert the wearer of a call. The phone number of the caller will be displayed in the small viewing area and the physician can go to a phone and make the call. Some newer models have the viewing capacity and ability to receive small messages which print out on the pager viewing area. An additional feature provided by some paging services allows voice messages to be left which can be retrieved by the receiver from any phone. Pagers are very beneficial and allow people to stay in contact even when they are not near a phone.

Voice Mail

Voice mail is another way to communicate. It is similar to a telephone answering machine except it can receive messages into your "mailbox" even if your phone is busy. Basically, if you call and the individual is either not there to answer or is talking on the line, a recording comes on. The message is usually spoken by the individual and typically changes daily. It may tell you the date and explain where the person may be. It may also give you the individual's schedule for the next couple of days. It will then typically request that you leave a message. When the individual checks their phone, an audible cue such as an intermittent dial tone alerts them to a message in their box or the phone may be equipped with a message light. Another advantage of voice mail is that a sender, with the proper software, can record a message and then direct it to several mailboxes. This is especially helpful within a company or association to notify several people of an event or a meeting. These messages can also be retrieved from any phone by accessing the "mailbox" using a personal identification number.

Cellular Phones

The ease and portability of cellular phones make them another option for communication. As the phone technology makes them smaller and lighter, they become a more easily carried device. Slim pocket-size phones are now available with some slightly larger than a credit card. Of course their greatest advantage is the familiarity of use and the ability to give and receive information instantly. Perhaps their only disadvantage may be the difficulty of reception within certain environments and within certain locations. The inconvenience of inappropriate times for ringing to occur can be solved for the most part by the adjustment of the ringer.

Conference Calls

The telephone can be used to simultaneously conduct conversations with several people in various locations, at the same time. This allows business to be conducted, meetings to occur, and professional or personal communication to be carried out. Conference calling saves time, travel, and money—all important in managing practice expenses. If your phone system is not equipped to allow multiple connections, conference calls may be arranged with the local phone provider.

Teleconferencing

This means of exchanging information is like a conference call but everyone can see and hear each other at the same time. They are linked together by way of telecommunications equipment. There are cameras, speaker phones, connection devices, and television monitors in each of the locations. The phone company for the meeting originator will contact all other sites and network the phones together. With the aid of the phone, camera, and television, participants can see and talk to each other. A **teleconference** can involve several people in many different locations. Ideas can be presented, concerns expressed, new techniques shown; it is the next best thing to actually being together in a meeting, yet it conserves travel time and expense.

Telemedicine

In January 1997, The Harvard Health Letter reported an exciting long distance medical care that is happening and may become more routine. It enables physicians to "see" patients at other sites miles away from their home base or office. It involves the use of electronic stethoscopes, digitized x-ray transmissions, and interactive video to examine, diagnose, and treat patients. In Kansas, nurses who make home visits to chronically ill patients, began using interactive video to enable them to "see" more people. The home care agency set up a camera and a 13-inch TV in a participant's home. The nurse sends a "buzzer" sound to alert the patient that the call will occur in two minutes. The patient sits in front of the camera and talks with the nurse as they perform a series of tasks using digital equipment attached to the TV. The electronic stethoscope is placed on the chest to check the heart; a blood pressure cuff gets a reading; a finger stick and the glucometer tests the blood sugar level; and the finger oximeter measures the amount of oxygen in the blood. Patients seem to like the approach and it has greatly boosted efficiency. When driving from patient to patient, only five people could be seen in a day, now they are able to see three times as many.

Telemedicine enables primary care physicians to consult with a faraway specialist immediately while the patient is still in their office. As an example, the cardiologist can listen to a patient's heart with the electronic stethoscope and assist the primary physician to diagnose a murmur or irregularity. It has been adapted to permit "house calls" to people who find it physically difficult to visit care facilities or for those who live or are stranded by weather in remote areas. Health care reform may encourage this form of practice as a more efficient use of resources (e.g.: skilled specialists). A California pilot program links physicians at Stanford University with patients at a nursing home, an urban clinic, and a multispecialty medical practice. This allows experts from the university to participate in the examination of high risk or problem cases. Through the use of high-resolution, computerized images, it is possible for the specialist to see a skin rash, fetal ultrasound, or the retina of the eye. The capabilities are endless. In 1996, doctors at the New England Medical Center in Boston conducted about 1,500 consultations with regional and overseas patients—one as far away as South America.

There are some issues to be settled regarding this form of medical practice. Items such as costs to initiate, legal, ethical, and professional concerns need to be addressed. Some physicians see it as threatening since they would have to compete with many more physicians than just those in their local area. And of course, there is the issue of malpractice liability. If the consult is out of state, whose state laws apply? Another factor is privacy when sending personal medical records through telecommunication systems. Congress recently passed legislation requiring federal health officials to develop specifications for a national computer network that will enable doctors, hospitals, insurers, and others to transfer patient records electronically. Now, a way to keep them confidential must be found. Another big question is medical licensure since physicians are licensed only in the state they practice. Currently, ten states are requiring that doctors who practice within their boundaries hold a state license, even if their presence is purely electronic. The AMA went on record recommending full licensure for each state except in emergencies and physician-to-physician consultation. Some states, however, feel a lim-

ited telemedicine credential would be sufficient. Some telemedicine physicians feel it is time for a national licensure to be established for physicians and solve the problem completely. This new form of medical practice will be interesting to watch develop.

E-Mail

This form of communication, "electronic mail," is carried out by a computer and appropriate software. Before you can send or receive messages you need to have an E-mail "address." E-mail can be exchanged within a company or clinic, or outside to anyone with a phone and an address which is obtained through electronic service providers. You are charged a fee for the amount of time you are using the network; it can be by the word or a flat rate time. In order to communicate by E-mail, you will need some form of communication software on your computer. To use it, you need to access the networking system and the connection with a provider of the service. When you wish to send a message, you contact the provider, through your computer and modem; the provider's modem then receives the request and routes it to the electronic address you indicated within your message. Electronic addresses will contain the

Medical-Legal Ethical Highlights

Throughout this chapter you should be mindful of all medical-legal/ethical implications. Listed below are a few important reminders.

1. Use only blue or black ink for documenting messages.
2. Draw a single line through an error then initial, date, and state error.
3. Keep office policy handbook updated on a routine basis.
4. Cover telephones adequately at all times.
5. Chart reasons for all missed appointments.
6. Establish and maintain good rapport with patients.
7. Never give information over the telephone to anyone concerning a patient unless written authorization from that patient is on file.

Mr. Right uses black ink when documenting information about patients. If an error is made, he draws a single line through it, initials and dates it, and then briefly states the error. He is polite in speaking to patients over the telephone and never leaves telephones unattended. When a patient misses an appointment, he records the reason on the chart. He never gives information to anyone on the telephone (or otherwise) unless written permission is obtained

from the patient. When it comes time to revise the office policy handbook, he offers helpful suggestions. He is efficient in office correspondence and in scheduling appointments.

Advancement potential: Excellent.

Miss Wrong never worries about what color she uses in recording patient information. She frequently uses "white out," or erases errors on the patients' records, schedule book, and other documents. She is short and rude with patients over the telephone when she does answer it. She has been known to put callers on hold for long periods or even hang up on them. She is careless about taking messages and forgets to write them down. When a caller requests information about a patient she tells the caller she'll get it if she can find it. She pays no attention to the office policy handbook because she thinks it is silly. She makes appointments when she remembers and is negligent in correspondence.

Advancement potential: None.

person's name or initials, perhaps a location, an employer or association, and the provider, but not necessarily in that order. An address will look something like this: John.Smith@Chicago.AMA.Magnus.ACS.Com. When you receive communication, you can "open" your E-mail and read the information. If you wish to save it, it can be printed or sent to your hard disk and stored.

The Internet/World Wide Web

This communication link allows you access to information from all over the world. It can be a great source of data from health organizations such as the American Cancer Society and the Center for Disease Control. Another capability through the Internet, which your physician may wish you to use, is the ability to schedule airline, hotel, and other services directly without going through various agents. Again, in order to access the "information super highway," as it is called, you will need a computer, the appropriate software, and a modem. A service provider is required in order to allow you access to the various suppliers of information. If you learn how to identify what you are looking for, you probably can find it. All you have to do is give the provider's computer your subject matter. You enter the appropriate key words into a "search engine" such as YaHoo or Alta Vista. In return, you receive a listing from which you can select a more specific entry. When this is viewed, it may be even fur-

ther definable until you are able to pinpoint the topic you want. You can access a source's "home page" to obtain their general information. By identifying your topic more specifically, you can bring the appropriate information to your screen to view. You can read it there, produce a hard copy with your printer, or store it on your disk.

It is possible to enter, obtain, and exchange information as well as conduct business transactions such as banking, all electronically. The amount of material available is mind boggling. It is possible to look at books, museums, association's publications, the world's encyclopedias, and on and on. However, there is some concern about the lack of security. With all the providers and information routing involved, interception of information is possible. Because of this, and the nature of medical records and the need to provide for privacy of information, electronic communication may not be advisable in a medical office.

This new technology will make for great change in the way we access and exchange information in the future. At present, the storehouse of historical data is unbelievable; the ability to have instant connection with virtually every business, university, organization, and even governments is apparently reasonable. It is important that you learn to use new technologies. When things change and go on, you must go with it or be left behind, unable to compete in the new workplace.

Complete Chapter 6, Unit 4 in the workbook to help you meet the objectives at the beginning of this unit and therefore achieve competency of this subject matter.

REFERENCES

Fordney, Marilyn, and Diehl, Marcy. *Medical Transcription Guide: Do's and Don'ts.* Philadelphia: W. B. Saunders, 1990.

Frew, Mary, and Frew, David. *Comprehensive Medical Assistant: Administrative and Clinical Procedures,* 3rd ed. Philadelphia: F. A. Davis, 1995.

Harvard Health Letter (Jan. 1997). *Telemedicine healers in cyberspace.* Boston, MA: Harvard Medical School.

Kinn, Mary, and Derge, Eleanor. *The Medical Assistant: Administrative and Clinical,* 6th ed. Philadelphia: W. B. Saunders, 1993.

U.S. Postal Service. *Creative Solutions for Your Business Needs,* 1992.

Records Management

Medical records consist of a health history, physical examination, diagnostic reports, and treatment notes that allow the physician to provide necessary care for patients. The records must be accurate, complete, and filed so that they may be quickly found when needed.

The confidentiality of the records must be maintained by careful management as they are used. Efficiency is essential to a well-run medical facility. Filing needs to be current at all times.

UNIT 1

The Patient's Medical Record

▮ OBJECTIVES

Upon completion of the unit, meet the following terminal performance objectives by verifying knowledge of the facts and principles presented through oral and written communication at a level deemed competent, and demonstrate the specific behaviors as identified in the terminal performance objectives of the procedures, observing safety precautions in accordance with health care standards.

1. Describe the importance of the medical record as a legal document.
2. List examples of subjective information.
3. List examples of objective information.
4. Describe methods of recording progress notes.
5. Describe the correct procedure for making corrections of progress notes.
6. List the differences between a conventional record and the Problem Oriented Medical Record.
7. Explain the HPIP method of recording patients' medical information.
8. Spell and define, using the glossary at the back of the text, all the words to know in this unit.

▮ WORDS TO KNOW

charting	progress notes
objective	subjective
procrastinator	

The patient history is the most important record kept in the medical office. The dates of any injuries, dates of treatment, and all notes regarding the condition of the patient must be accurate in every detail. In a lawsuit resulting from an injury, the patient chart information could win or lose the case.

Each office has its own method of charting patient information during visits. Some physicians ask the medical assistant to record the findings of a physical examination as it is being completed. Some physicians take the time to write all physical findings and progress notes for each visit. Many physicians prefer to dictate progress notes; then it becomes the duty of the medical assistant to type them, or process data using a word processor or computer. If dictating and transcribing the information is the preferred method, the printed document must be dated and placed in the patient's chart with the notation: e.g., *as dictated by Dr. H.G. Brown.* Keep in mind that confidentiality is vitally important, especially where many staff members have access to patient files and when the patients and their families may have a clear view of the monitor screen at times. Safeguarding personal and private patient information is always necessary.

Computer generated patient records begin with entering the patient's general information for billing and scheduling, which was discussed in Chapter 4. Computerized patient records also include the medical history appropriate for each particular type of medical practice. The extent of computer use in patient records is a decision made by the employer and the office manager. The issue of protection of patient confidentiality still remains a legitimate concern for both physician and patient. Extensive medical histories of patients who have conditions or diseases that may affect their insurance coverage, career, relationships, and so on are an important consideration. Some patients are reluctant to have their personal information accessible to so many people. Patients must be informed that there is a risk of a possible invasion of privacy of their medical information even though every effort is made to protect this confidence. A password should be made known only to a select few employees to access files. This helps to keep information confidential.

Software packages are available to fit the needs of the practice according to the types of functions desired. Computerized medical records, examination formats, as well as billing and insurance with CPT and ICD-9 codes and other helpful and time-saving programs are designed to make processing and retrieving information easy and efficient in the daily practice of managed care of patients.

The complete medical record has several important purposes:

1. It serves as a basis for planning patient care and for continuity in evaluating the patient's condition and treatment. The combination of the personal and family history with the findings of the physician must be combined with the results of laboratory studies, x-rays, and any indicated special tests. The review of all of these facts together help the physician determine the diagnosis and course of treatment. This would not be possible without a well-documented, accurate record. The patient history or family history may alert the physician to certain conditions such as a family history of diabetes or exposure to hazardous substances.

2. The medical record furnishes documentary evidence of the course of the patient's medical evaluation, treatment, and change in condition. The charting of progress notes is extremely important and should give an indication of the patient comments, physician's evaluation, prescribed treatment, and need for further follow-up.

3. The record furnishes evidence of communication between the physician and any other health professional contributing to the patient's care. The chart should include a record of reports from other physicians asked to evaluate the patient with special laboratory, x-ray, or diagnostic procedures.

4. It affords protection of the legal interests of the patient and the physician. The complete accurate record would be necessary if the patient wishes the physician to testify in an injury case. The complete accurate record is also necessary if the patient sues the physician for malpractice. The patient must always sign an authorization form before any information may be released. An authorization must indicate who is to be allowed to receive the information.

5. The medical record helps to establish a data base for use in continuing education and research. The accurate record of patients is a useful resource for research concerning response to medications or procedures in every phase of medical treatment.

The information in the medical record is classified as subjective or objective. The **subjective** information is supplied by the patient. The **objective** information is supplied by the physician. The subjective information includes the routine information about the patient, past personal and medical history, family history, and chief complaint. The objective information supplied by the physician should include examination, results of any laboratory studies, special procedures, x-rays, the diagnosis, treatment prescribed, and progress notes.

The progress notes should be arranged in chronological order with the most recent date on top. If several notes are recorded on a page, the last on the page should be the most recent. The chart should be carefully dated for each visit. As discussed in the chapter on medical-legal considerations (see Chapter 3), each no-show, cancellation, telephone call, or prescription needs to be recorded as a progress note in the record of the patient, along with the date each took place, and initialed by the individual making the entry.

Some examples of progress notes might be:

12/14/__ Patient returns 10 days postop left 2d metatarsal osteotomy, some symptoms of pain on walking, area well healed, sutures removed. Continue boot, limited activity and return in 3 weeks. (Initials)

1/6/__ Patient returns, some slight complaint of pain with increased activity. Able to wear flat leather walking shoe. AP and lateral x-rays reveal healing, advised activity to tolerance. Return necessary only if symptoms remain after 2 weeks. (Initials)

2/8/__ Patient called and reported feeling fine. (Initials)

2/9/__ Patient canceled appointment. (Initials)

2/15/__ Prescription for Aldomet renewed at ABC Pharmacy. (Initials)

2/15/__ Patient did not keep appointment. Notified physician of this. (Initials)

DATING, CORRECTING, AND MAINTAINING THE CHART

It is extremely important that the date and time be recorded on the page for progress notes each time the patient is seen. The date may be written in ink or stamped. Every time a patient is given a prescription over the phone or is given a report or advice should also be recorded with the date and time. Failure of a patient to keep an appointment should always be recorded by the date stamp on the chart. When it is necessary to start a new page, the patient's name and the date should always be written at the top of the new page. If office staff other than the physician are making notes on the chart, these should be initialed by the person making the notation.

In making a correction on progress notes, a handwritten entry should have a single line drawn through it and the correction written above or following it. An indication of correction should be made in the margin and should bear the initials of the person making the correction. Using correction fluid or erasing the error is not recommended because it looks as if one were trying to cover up or completely eliminate what was written. This could raise suspicion if there is ever a legal question regarding a patient and treatment. Write or print in a neat and legible manner. Be very careful to spell the patient's name correctly and learn how to pronounce them accurately. (If necessary, you should ask the person to give you a way to record an easy way of remembering.) Charting becomes a part of the permanent record and one should respect this fact. Using black ink will make much better photo copies of the record. When you finish with a patient's chart, always try to straighten up the forms and make the chart neat before filing it. Forms and other documents tend to shift with handling and they sometimes become folded or tattered, which eventually makes them difficult to read. After you have completed recording or filing additional information in a patient's chart, you should return it to the files as soon as possible. Having stacks of files pulled too far in advance of the patients' appointments is not necessary and is not practical. Making many outguides is time consuming and not necessary for patients being seen on the present day. Patient charts should be filed when not in use for a specific purpose.

Typing should be corrected at the time of error by use of correcting ribbon or correction fluid. An error found at a later time is corrected in the same manner as in a handwritten record, but there should be no need to do this if typed material is carefully proofread in the typewriter.

Each medical field has its own specialized terms. You should make a correctly spelled list of these terms so you won't have to continually refer to a dictionary. These may be anatomical terms, surgical terms, appliances, medications, or simply English vocabulary the physician uses frequently. You will also find that the physician frequently uses abbreviations in handwritten notes or even in dictation, and a knowledge of these is also useful. See Figure 7–1 for steps to follow.

The medical assistant should check the charts each day to see whether notes have been dictated or written. Some physicians find it useful to keep a chart each day that reflects patients seen and has a check-off block for progress notes, referring physician if any, report dictated, and charges for service rendered. The physician can then see at a glance if all necessary work is completed on each patient.

Example:

DATE	PATIENT NAME		
10/1/93	Jane Doe		

Progress Notes	Referring M.D.	Letter Dictated	Charges
X	John Smith	X	25.00

Many fine physicians are **procrastinators** when it comes to completing paper work in the office. It is the duty of the medical assistant to see that it gets done even if this requires daily reminders.

THE PROBLEM ORIENTED MEDICAL RECORD

In the early 1970s Lawrence L. Weed, M.D., a professor of medicine at the University of Vermont's College of Medicine, originated a system of record keeping for patients

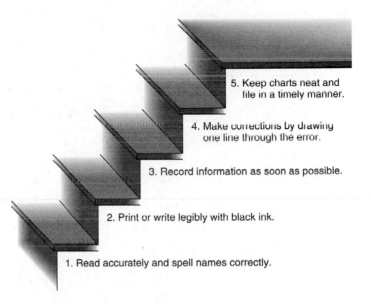

FIGURE 7–1   Follow these steps for proper records management.

5. Keep charts neat and file in a timely manner.

4. Make corrections by drawing one line through the error.

3. Record information as soon as possible.

2. Print or write legibly with black ink.

1. Read accurately and spell names correctly.

that he named the Problem Oriented Medical Record (POMR). In the traditional medical record, the progress notes are recorded according to the source they come from—the physician, laboratory, or physician's assistant—with no special attempt to record a relationship between them. The POMR record begins with the standard data base, which includes patient profile, chief complaint, review of systems, physical examination, and laboratory reports. The patient chart is then further built up by adding a numbered and titled page for each problem the patient has that requires management. Each problem is then followed with the SOAP approach for all progress notes:

S —Subjective impressions
O—Objective clinical evidence
A—Assessment or diagnosis
P —Plans for further studies, treatment, or management

This process makes the chart easier to review and helps in follow-up of all problems the patient may have, Figure 7–2.

Another similar system of recording medical information about patients is the HPIP method. This format provides the same information as the SOAP method in different terms, as you can see outlined as follows:

H— history (objective findings)
P —physical exam (subjective findings)
I —impression (assessment/diagnosis)
P —plan (treatment)

Complete Chapter 7, Unit 1 in the workbook to help you meet the objectives at the beginning of this unit and therefore achieve competency of this subject matter.

FIGURE 7–2 Example of POMR progress note page (Courtesy of Bibbero Systems, Inc., Petaluma, CA).

UNIT 2

Filing

OBJECTIVES

Upon completion of the unit, meet the following terminal performance objectives by verifying knowledge of the facts and principles presented through oral and written communication at a level deemed competent, and demonstrate the specific behaviors as identified in the terminal performance objectives of the procedures, observing safety precautions in accordance with health care standards.

1. Explain basic filing methods.
2. List the steps used in filing.
3. Describe methods of removing and replacing patient files.
4. List the storage media used for "paperless" filing systems.
5. Spell and define, using the glossary at the back of the text, all the words to know in this unit.

WORDS TO KNOW

accumulated	chronologically
caption	data
expedite	supplemented
illuminating	systematically
purge	unproductive
sequence	warranty
subsequent	

IMPORTANCE OF FILING

Assembling and filing the patient's medical record are necessary to good patient care. Records must be filed accurately and **systematically**. Accuracy in assembling and filing the patient's medical record is necessary in providing quality managed care. Carelessly filed records produce chaos in the office. Reports that are lost or filed in the wrong chart or hidden in stacks of unfiled material will result in many hours of **unproductive** time spent searching for them. An efficient office requires accurate filing daily. Not only does this maintain efficiency, it also reduces the chance of accidental loss of correspondence and reports.

FILING STEPS

Folders or cards are easily filed alphabetically or numerically, but the procedure for filing reports and letters requires several steps, Figure 7–3.

The first step is to inspect each report or piece of correspondence to see if it is released for filing. After the physician looks at a report, a call or dictation of a letter may be required to give results to the patient or to the referring physician. The physician will place a check mark or initials on the form (usually in the upper righthand corner) indicating that the report has been seen, Figure 7–4.

The second step is indexing. This requires that you make a decision as to the name, subject, or other **caption** under which you will file the material. Materials for patients should be filed under the patient name. Research papers can be filed

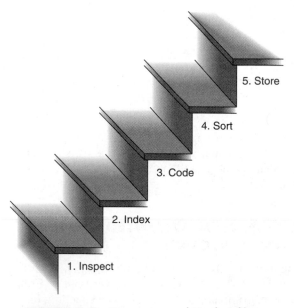

FIGURE 7–3 Steps to remember when filing.

Patient: Carol Sue Lamp ✓

City Hospital
Troy, Ohio

ROENTGEN FINDINGS

Examination of the pelvis. AP supine including the upper thirds of the femora bilaterally visualizes advanced degenerative arthritis of the right hip with narrowing almost to obliteration of the hip joint space and with degenerative changes and cystic formation affecting the articulating surfaces of the head of the femur as well as the acetabulum. The remaining pelvis and left hip appears essentially normal.

Impression: Advanced degenerative arthritis right hip, otherwise normal pelvis and left hip.

FIGURE 7–4 The check mark in the upper right-hand corner of this report is an example of a report released by the physician for filing.

Patient: <u>Marsha Leonard</u>

Tri-County Hospital
Miami, Ohio

ROENTGEN FINDINGS

Films of 8/31 _____. Review of the PA and lateral chest film of 8/31 _____ shows the traches to be shifted slightly to the left by a soft tissue mass in the right thoracic inlet in the superior mediastinal area. This probably represents tumor and is again seen on the lateral view lying in the anterior portion of the thoracic inlet on the right. Heart is otherwise normal. Lungs are otherwise clear.

FIGURE 7–6 Underlining the patient's name is one way of coding in preparation to file the report.

under illness, procedure, treatment, medication, or author. A cross-reference may be helpful in finding things later, Figure 7–5. For example, a research paper might be filed under the title, *Diabetes,* and a cross-reference to the article placed under the author's name, *Allen, John.*

Coding is the third step, and is done by marking the index caption on the papers to be filed. If the name, subject, or a number appears on the paper, you can underline or circle it, preferably with a colored pencil or a color highlighter. (Your employer may have a preference as to the color to be used for the coding process.) If the name, subject, or other caption does not appear on the material to be filed, write the caption in the upper right-hand corner, Figure 7–6.

The fourth step is to sort the material. A desk sorter may be used to put papers in alphabetical order after they have been coded. This speeds up the process of filing, Figure 7–7. Using this sorter or an expanding alphabetical file to sort re-

ports, mail, and other items can provide a temporary file of these records until they can be placed in the patient's permanent chart. On days when it is especially hectic and all the filing has not yet been completed, this means of sorting can help you locate a particular report quickly. This can be a practical answer to more efficient filing because when all items are arranged alphabetically, it saves steps because each letter of the alphabet is in groups and filing goes much more quickly. Also, there are times when the patient's chart is in another department and mail, for example, can be placed in this temporary file for ease in obtaining information to answer a phone call without having to take time out to go and get the entire chart.

PATIENT   <u>JANKOWSKI, EMILY LOUISE</u>
CROSS REFERENCE

<u>PENDEN-JANKOWSKI, EMILY LOUISE</u>

PATIENT   <u>PENDEN-JANKOWSKI, EMILY LOUISE</u>
CROSS REFERENCE

<u>JANKOWSKI, EMILY LOUISE</u>

FIGURE 7–5 Example of a cross-reference card for efficient filing.

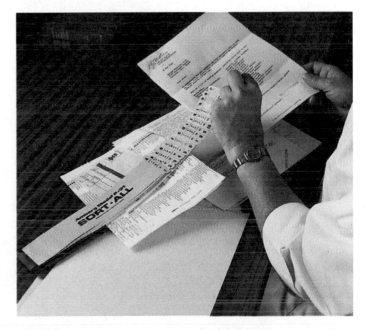

FIGURE 7–7 This photo shows a medical assistant using a desk sorter to alphabetize reports to make filing easier.

The final step is storing. You must first locate the file drawer or shelf with the appropriate caption. Then find the folder in which the reports will be stored. Lift the folder and place it on a flat surface before adding any material. This procedure makes it easier for you to make sure the caption on the folder agrees with the caption on the paper to be filed. Place the papers with the heading to the left and the most recent material on top. Some offices attach laboratory reports to the folder in a "shingle" fashion, Figure 7–8. The first is attached at the bottom of the page and each **subsequent** report partially overlaps the previous ones.

FILING UNITS

Every office that requires you to file paper records will have storage units for this purpose. Files come in many different styles, shapes, and sizes. There are vertical or lateral file cabinets, card index files, open shelf files, tub files, various types of movable or automated files, and special-purpose file units, such as those used to store computer printouts. It is reasonable for employers to expect you to understand how to use these storage units, Figures 7–9 and 7–10.

Safety is an important consideration when you work with file cabinets. When you leave a file drawer open at floor level where someone can fall over it, you are setting up an accident scene. If you pull out more than one file drawer at a time in a vertical file cabinet, it can tip over and injure you.

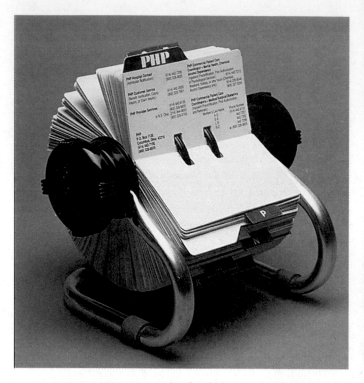

FIGURE 7–9 Example of a desk top rolodex file.

Be careful when pulling a file drawer out to reach material in the back because some drawers do not have a stop to prevent the entire drawer from falling out. **CAUTION:** There can also be the danger of a file cabinet tipping over and falling on you if you pull the entire top drawer out as far as it can open and do not have enough weight in the bottom drawer(s). This can be a problem especially with new file drawers as they are being filled with charts. It is best to start placing files in the bottom drawers first to avoid the possibility of injury as well as the avoidance of a potential mess of papers and forms if a drawer were to fall. You always should be mindful to keep all drawers, cabinet doors, step

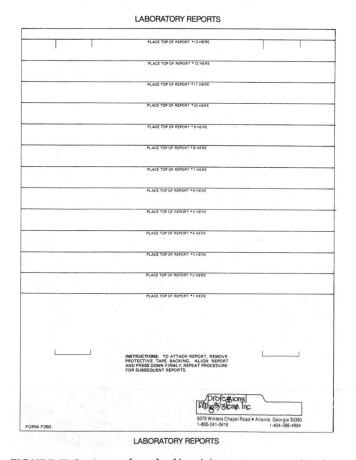

FIGURE 7–8 Report form for filing laboratory reports shingle fashion (Courtesy Professional Filing Systems, Inc.).

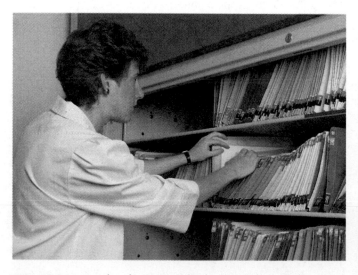

FIGURE 7–10 This shows a medical assistant looking for a chart in these shelving storage files.

stools or any other source of a possible accident closed or out of the path of others.

FILING SUPPLIES

Filing supplies include guides, OUTguides or OUTfolders, folders, vertical pockets, index tabs, various colored self-stick number and letter labels, as well as the standard office equipment such as stapler, staple remover, tape, and so on, Figures 7–11 and 7–12. A properly organized filing system will have many dividers or guides that identify sections within the file. The guides should be constructed of heavy material to stand up under continual wear. They reduce the area to be searched and allow you to locate a folder more quickly. Some authorities recommend a guide for every eight or ten folders, but this would occupy a great deal of space. The number of guides used is a matter of personal preference and will be determined by each office.

An OUTguide or folder is used to temporarily replace a folder that has been removed. It is thick and may be of a distinctive size and color for easier detection. The use of OUTguides makes refiling much easier and also alerts the medical assistant to missing files. The OUTguide may also have lines for recording information, such as where the missing folder may be located, or it may have a plastic pocket for inserting an information card. In a large office, with several physicians and employees, it is essential to know who has the folder when it is out of the file. Occasionally, a record may be sent to another physician or treatment facility and it is extremely important that this information be recorded. The OUTfolder is also useful in providing a place to file material until the original folder is returned. Make sure you check with the physician before allowing a patient to take an entire chart. This is not an accepted practice and requires written permission and signatures with an expected date of return. It is only allowed in exceptional cases. A copy of, or a written summary of, a patient's health records is the usual procedure in sending information regarding a patient to another physician or health care facility.

A color coding system may be used to **expedite** both filing and finding of folders. Ordinary manila folders may be coded with colored strips or dots along the edge of the folder. The coding may be used to identify portions of the alphabet or patients of different physicians within an office. Color coding is also useful in identifying different types of insured patients. Everyone should have a key to the color coding through use of a procedure manual or posted chart.

PAPERLESS FILES

With computers outputting volumes of information at unbelievable speeds and the cost of office space steadily increasing, many offices have installed "paperless" filing systems. These systems record information for storage on such media as magnetic tape reels, cartridges, or cassettes; magnetic disks; and/or microforms. The use of such media has dramatically reduced the need for storage space. It is estimated that microforms (microfilm and microfiche) use less than 2% of the storage space required for traditional paper files. (Microfiche is a rectangular sheet of clear film containing rows of tiny negatives. Each negative represents a separate page of a document or report. See Chapter 4).

Storage units used to house such paperless media are either card files, drawers, open shelves, or racks. Shelves or drawers are used to store boxed rolls of microfilm. Card files are used for microfiche and aperture cards. (Aperture cards are one tiny negative mounted on a data processing card.) These types of records require an **illuminating** and magnifying viewing device to read the stored information.

If you are hired to work with a paperless filing system, you will be taught how to use the special filing equipment on the job. You will learn about the camera used to produce reduced images on film and the viewers used to read the blown-up film images. You will be using word processors and duplicating equipment to handle **data** and printers to produce hard copy from film images. There will be automatic storage and retrieval units to master. Paperless files have become common with the use of the computer. Storage of a vast array of information regarding patient records, employee information and payroll, scheduling, statistics regarding medical conditions, office management,

FIGURE 7–11   Example of OUTguide cards (Courtesy of Professional Innovations).

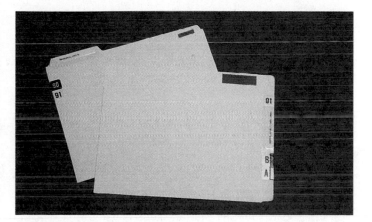

FIGURE 7–12   Examples of top cut and end cut file folders (Courtesy of Professional Innovations).

taxes, inventory, and a host of other records can be filed and stored on a computer system with easy retrieval whenever necessary. This eliminates clutter and the need for filing space. Software companies provide advice for practical use to fit particular needs of the practice.

FILING SYSTEMS

Most filing systems are based directly or indirectly on an alphabetic arrangement. In alphabetic filing, the names of persons, firms, or organizations are arranged as in the telephone directory. This is the simplest and most commonly used method of filing. In numeric filing, the material is arranged in numerical order in the main file. The main file is **supplemented** by an alphabetically arranged card index. The number under which a given item is to be filed can be determined by referring to the alphabetical card index file.

A subject file is based on an outline or classification of the subject matter to which the material refers. In a physician's office, it is customary to maintain files or reference materials **accumulated** by subject matter.

In geographic filing, material is arranged alphabetically by political or geographic subdivisions such as country, state, city, and even street, and each subdivision is alphabetized.

Chronological filing refers to filing according to date. Arranging documents with the most current date on top, is recommended.

HOW TO FILE ALPHABETICALLY

The most common method of filing is alphabetical, Procedure 7–1. The rules for filing material alphabetically must be learned. They are as follows.

Rule 1. In filing the names of persons, the surname or last name is considered first, the first name or initial second, and the middle name or initial third.

Example: John E. Brown is filed as Brown, John E.

Rule 2. Names are filed alphabetically in an A to Z **sequence** from the first to the last letter, considering each letter in the name separately and each unit separately. The following names are listed in correct filing order:

> Allard, Wm.
> Allen, E. S.
> Allen, Edna
> Allen, Wm. A.
> Allen, William C.
> Allens, M. R.

- When the surnames of two persons are spelled differently, the first and middle names or initials need not be considered. See the first two names in the preceding list. The order of these two names is determined by the fourth letter in the surname.
- When a shorter surname is identical with the first part of a longer surname, the shorter name is listed first. The rule is sometimes stated as "nothing before something." See the fifth and sixth names in the preceding list.

- When the surnames are alike, the order in filing is determined by the first names or initials. When the surname and first names or initials are alike, the filing order is determined by the middle names or initials. See the fourth and fifth names in the preceding list.
- An initial is listed before a name beginning with the same letter. See the second and third names in the preceding list. This again is the example of "nothing before something."
- An abbreviated first or middle name is treated as if it were spelled out in full. See the fourth and fifth names in the preceding list.

Rule 3. A prefix (also called a surname particle), such as Mc, Mac, De, Le, and von, is considered as part of the surname.

Examples:

> MacAdams, Bruce
> McAdams, Helen
> VonBergen, T. R.

Rule 4. In filing the name of a married woman, her legal name is used. The title Mrs. is disregarded in filing, but is placed in parentheses after the name.

Example: Mrs. R. A. (Betty A.) Smith is filed as Smith, Betty A. (Mrs. R. A.).

Rule 5. Most firm names are filed as they are written. The apostrophe is disregarded in filing.

Examples:

> Herb's Auto Service
> Walters Printing Company

Rule 6. Firm names that include the full name of an individual are filed with the name of the individual transposed.

Example: Edward Wenger Company is filed as Wenger, Edward Company.

Rule 7. When the article *the* is part of a title, it is placed in parentheses and disregarded in filing.

Examples: Sam the Barber is filed as Sam (the) Barber; The Family Steak House is filed as Family Steak House (The).

Rule 8. *And, for, of,* etc. are disregarded in filing but are not omitted.

Example: Adams & Smith Pharmacy is filed as Adams (&) Smith Pharmacy.

Rule 9. Abbreviations such as *Co., Inc.,* or *Ltd.,* in a firm name are indexed as though spelled out.

Example: Frank Smith Co. is filed as Smith, Frank Company.

Rule 10. Hyphenated surnames and hyphenated firm names are indexed as one unit.

Examples: Dunning-Lathrop & Assoc. Inc. is filed as Dunning-Lathrop (&) Associates, Incorporated; Lester Smith-Mayes is filed as Smith-Mayes, Lester.

Rule 11. Numbers are usually filed as though spelled out.

P R O C E D U R E

7-1 File Item(s) Alphabetically

PURPOSE: To file and store patient file(s) or other items accurately in alphabetical order.

EQUIPMENT AND SUPPLIES: Items to be filed, cabinet for files.

TERMINAL PERFORMANCE OBJECTIVE: In a simulated situation, given the patient's file or other items, accurately file and store the file(s) and/or other items within an acceptable time limit according to accepted medical standards.

1. Use the rules for filing items alphabetically. **NOTE: Double check the spelling of the name for accuracy when using the cross-reference file.**

2. Determine the appropriate storage file.

3. If you are filing new material, scan the guides for the area nearest to the letters of the name(s) on the items that you have to file.

4. Place the folder in the correct alphabetical order between two files. **NOTE: Be sure to insert the new file *between* two other folders and NOT within another folder where it could be lost.**

5. If you are filing material previously in the file, scan for the OUTguide. Remove the OUTguide after you have removed the file. **NOTE: Check to be sure it was marking the space for the file you just returned and not another.** (Procedure 7–3 discusses pulling a file folder from alphabetical files.)

Example: 5th Avenue Store is filed as Fifth Avenue Store.

Rule 12. Professional or honorary titles are not considered in filing but should be written in parentheses at the end of the name for identification purposes.

Examples: Dr. Anne Lewis is filed as Lewis, Anne (Dr.); President John Kennedy is filed as Kennedy, John (President); Prof. William S. Smith is filed as Smith, William S. (Prof.).

■ Titles are filed as written when they are part of a firm name. Foreign or religious titles followed by one name are also filed as they are written.

Examples:

Dr. Scholl's Foot Powder
Prince Phillip

Rule 13. Terms of seniority, such as *Junior, Senior, Second,* or *Third,* are not considered in filing. If two names are otherwise identical, the address is used to make the filing decision in the order: state, city, street.

Examples:

Willard Keir, Sr.
Willard Keir, Jr.
Filed as:
Keir, Willard, Sr. (Cleveland, Ohio)
Keir, Willard, Jr. (Columbus, Ohio)

Rule 14. File the names of federal, state, or local government departments first by political division and then by name of department.

Example: Drug Enforcement Administration, Cincinnati, Ohio is filed as Cincinnati, City, Drug Enforcement Administration, Cincinnati, Ohio.

HOW TO FILE NUMERICALLY

The second filing method used, especially in very large clinics, is the numerical system, Procedure 7–2. This system provides the most patient privacy, as all that is visible on the folder is the patient number. As mentioned before, a cross-index or cross-reference is required in the form of an alphabetical card file, and a number is assigned to each patient. You first locate the alphabetical card to determine the patient's number and then locate the numbered file.

Most offices use the same number of digits for each number assigned, and the numbers are always filed in order from smallest to largest. If the zero (0) falls before another number, it is disregarded when filing. A system using six digits would begin 000001, 000002, 000003, and so on.

Some systems use the same terminal digit or digits to designate shelves or drawers. The patients are assigned numbers, which are separated into twos or threes. The numbers are then read from the right hand group of numbers to the left hand group. After the last two or three digits are sorted together in numerical order, you next consider the middle digits and sort them in order. Finally, you consider the first group of digits and sort them in order.

For example, the numbers of charts in one series might end in 25 and another series might end in 35. Charts labeled 10-07-25 and 02-17-25 would then be filed separately from charts labeled 08-17-35 and 12-25-35. The order of the charts numbered above would be:

02-17-25
10-07-25
08-17-35
12-25-35

PROCEDURE

7-2 File Item(s) Numerically

PURPOSE: To file and store patient file(s) or other items accurately in numerical order.

EQUIPMENT AND SUPPLIES: Items to be filed, cabinet for files.

TERMINAL PERFORMANCE OBJECTIVE: In a simulated situation, given the patient's file or other items, accurately file and store the file(s) and/or other items within an acceptable time limit according to accepted medical standards.

1. Use the rules for numerical filing. **Note: Double check the spelling of the name for accuracy when using the cross-reference file.**

2. Determine the appropriate storage file.

3. Match the first two or three numbers with those already in the file. If using terminal digits, match the last two numbers.

4. Match the remaining numbers with those in the file. **Note: If you have assigned a number to a new patient, it should probably be at the very end of the file.**
   (Procedure 7–4 discusses pulling a file folder from numerical files.)

How to File by Subject

In the medical office it is necessary to have files for business information. You must file financial records, copies of inventory, copies of orders, and records of supplies and equipment received. You should have a file for tax records, insurance policies, and canceled checks. The subject headings of the above would be relatively easy to determine, but it is more difficult to determine where to file some general correspondence or reprints of medical research publications.

Very often reprints are filed with a cross-index, one file for the subject and one for the author with a listing of reprint subjects available. The miscellaneous folder is an important subject file. When you have one letter on a subject it should go into the miscellaneous file indexed by subject or names. The material in each subject file is filed in chronological order with the most recent entry on top. When five papers are assembled in the miscellaneous file on one subject or person, a separate folder should be prepared and the material removed from the miscellaneous file.

How to Use a Chronological File

This file is commonly called a "tickler file" and is used as a follow-up method for a particular date. The file may be an expanding file, a card file, or even a portion of a file drawer. It consists of dividers with the names of all the months and dividers numbered from one to thirty-one for the days of the month. Some offices have patients fill out a card to be sent as a reminder to return for examination, testing, or injections. The patient addresses the card and the office retains it in the tickler file to be mailed by you at the appropriate time. You place the month card in the front of the file each month and check each day to see if anything needs to be done. The patients who would benefit are those who need regular or long-range follow-up for Pap tests, tests for follow-up of cancer therapy, or any long-range follow-up care. This file can be used to remind you to order supplies or to renew subscriptions, send tax information, or any task you need to be reminded about.

PROCEDURE

7-3 Pull File Folder from Alphabetical Files

PURPOSE: To obtain the correct patient file(s) from the file cabinet.

EQUIPMENT AND SUPPLIES: Name of patient file to be pulled, OUTguide (card), pen, cabinet of patient files.

TERMINAL PERFORMANCE OBJECTIVE: In a simulated situation, given the patient's name, accurately prepare the OUTguide and pull the file, replacing the file with the OUTguide within an acceptable time limit according to accepted medical standards.

1. Find the name of the patient in the alphabetical file. Double check the spelling of the name for accuracy.

2. Complete the OUTguide with the date and your name. **NOTE: If you are pulling files for the day, OUTguides may not be necessary. When pulling files for another person, write that person's name and your initials.**

3. Pull the file(s) needed and replace with the OUTguide.

Periodically you will find it necessary to **purge** inactive files to storage to make room for the current files. File boxes may be used for this purpose, but they do need to be easily available in the event the patient returns. Transferring records of deceased patients should be delayed until you are sure there will be no more requests for forms to be completed. At that time, the files are closed.

You are far too busy in an office to spend time trying to locate a misplaced file or misplaced material regarding a patient. You need to be extremely careful when filing to be sure you are placing material in the correct folder. You should remove the folder and place the material to be filed in the folder with the top of the material toward the top of the folder when it is opened. The material is placed in chrono-logical order with the most current date on top. File laboratory reports according to your office policy, usually in shingle fashion from bottom to top of the page with the latest on top.

All office records should be in closed files when not in use. Professional liability insurance policies, life insurance policies, canceled checks, wills, licenses, deeds, stocks, and bonds should be kept in a safe or at least in a fireproof file. Receipts for business equipment and any **warranties** should also be kept in fireproof storage until you no longer have the equipment.

Complete Chapter 7, Unit 2, in the workbook to help you meet the objectives at the beginning of this unit and therefore achieve competency of this subject matter.

P R O C E D U R E

7-4   Pull File Folder from Numerical Files

PURPOSE: To obtain the correct patient file(s) from the file cabinet.

EQUIPMENT AND SUPPLIES: Name of patient file to be pulled, OUTguide (card), pen, cabinet of patient files.

TERMINAL PERFORMANCE OBJECTIVE: In a simulated situation, given the patient's name or account number, accurately prepare the OUTguide and pull the file, replacing the file with the OUTguide within an acceptable time limit according to accepted medical standards.

1. Find the name of the patient in the card file to obtain the account number. Double check the spelling of the name for accuracy.

2. Complete the OUTguide with the date and your name. **NOTE: If you are pulling files for the day, OUTguides may not be necessary. When pulling files for another person, write that person's name and your initials.**

3. Locate the corresponding section of the numerical file.

4. Scan the files for the number.

5. Pull the requested file and replace with the prepared OUTguide.

Medical-Legal Ethical Highlights

Throughout this chapter you should be mindful of all medical-legal/ethical implications. Listed below are a few important reminders.

1. Keep patient records according to your state statute of limitations.
2. File timely, accurately, and systematically to prevent loss of records.
3. Secure important documents in a safe or fireproof storage.
4. Obtain and file patient authorization for release of information.

Miss Right . . .

keeps the filing caught up by organizing her work so that she can file a few items between other duties. She purges files and stores them safely according to the state statute to prevent loss of important records. All important documents are placed in a fireproof storage box as they are received. She always obtains and files the proper authorization to release information about a patient. She checks the patient's chart for this signed form before giving information to anyone whether in person or by phone request.

Employment outlook: Continuous.

Ms. Wrong . . .

doesn't like to file, so she lets it pile up and does it only after several reminders by her supervisor. She leaves important documents wherever she puts them and isn't concerned about their safe-keeping. She sometimes obtains the signature of patients for release of information when she remembers it. If she can't find the proper authorization form in a patient's chart, she gives out information without prior consent so the party won't call back about it.

Employment outlook: Termination.

REFERENCES

Kinn, Mary and Derge, Eleanor. *The Medical Assistant: Administrative and Clinical,* 7th Ed. Philadelphia: W. B. Saunders, 1993.

Simmers, Louise. *Diversified Health Occupations.* 4th Ed. Albany: Delmar, 1997.

8

Collecting Fees

The medical assistant must be concerned with the collection of fees from patients, as there are many expenses to be covered in the practice of medicine. The medical assistant needs to know the local clinics where limited income patients can be referred for care at a reduced fee. The medical assistant can help patients plan a payment schedule for a costly surgical procedure, therapy, or for the birth of a baby. It is important to determine who is responsible for the payment for the services of the physician. If it is not the patient, it may be an employer, an insurance company, or a school.

UNIT 1

Medical Care Expenses

■ OBJECTIVES

Upon completion of the unit, meet the following terminal performance objectives by verifying knowledge of the facts and principles presented through oral and written communication at a level deemed competent, and demonstrate the specific behaviors as identified in the terminal performance objectives.

1. Name the factors in determining fees for patient care.
2. List the types of patients who pay no fees or reduced fees.
3. Discuss the pitfalls of reducing fees.
4. List the information that should be obtained about every new patient.
5. Spell and define, using the glossary at the back of the text, all the words to know in this unit.

■ WORDS TO KNOW

complexity	pitfalls
indigent	subsequent
nominal	verify

Physicians traditionally are reluctant to discuss fees with patients. It is fairly common for the medical assistant to be the one who must answer these questions. When a patient is unhappy about medical costs, it is important to listen and try to explain why the charges are as stated. The physician should always be told when a patient is un-happy with the cost of treatment. It may be necessary for the physician to talk with the patient about the concern regarding cost of care.

Physicians must set their fees based on their professional financial profile and the fees appropriate for similar specialists in the community.

In considering the fee for services to the patient the physician must consider the time spent with the patient, the **complexity** of the diagnosis, and the treatment. In addition, the cost of maintaining an office and staff must be considered. The physician can obtain usual and customary fee schedules from the local medical society or a medical practice management firm.

In some instances now, you will find that insurance companies and government agencies will establish a fee profile for the physician based on the charges averaged over a period of time. This is one of the reasons it is so critical to learn to code patient visits accurately. When such a profile is established, it represents the highest payment the insurance company or government agency will make for the services listed in the profile.

NO CHARGE OR REDUCED FEE

Although most physicians accept patients of all socioeconomic levels, the medical assistant should be aware of various **pitfalls** of reducing fees. **Indigent** patients receive the same care as paying patients and the same records are kept. The charge will be recorded as *n/c* (no charge) on the financial records for the day. Most physicians find it necessary to limit the number of indigent patients they accept, for obvious reasons. Therefore, you may be faced with the task of telling a patient who wishes to be seen, and who indicates indigent status, that your office cannot accept new patients. You should know the names, addresses, and eligibility requirements of local clinics operated by social service agencies for such referrals. These clinics provide services from qualified physicians as well as other health care at no cost or a **nominal** cost.

When your employer has treated a patient and the patient encounters difficulty in paying the bill, it is important to check for possible insurance coverage and the possibility of local or state public assistance. Physicians may simply write off an account they feel cannot be collected. They may also decide to reduce the fee. In that case, it should be done in writing with a date setting the time limit within which the account is to be paid. The words *without prejudice* should be part of the written agreement. This precaution will allow the physician to collect the total bill if the reduced amount is not paid. Two copies of the written statement should be made, and should be witnessed as they are signed. The original should be kept in the office and the copy given to the patient. You should continue to bill for the total amount with the understanding that when the reduced amount is paid the remainder will be written off. A fee should not generally be reduced for a patient who has died, because the family may see this as an indication that the physician was at fault. It is also not considered good practice to reduce a fee because of a poor result or to avoid sending the bill to a collection agency.

Physicians traditionally treat one another and the immediate family of close physician friends without charge or accept any insurance payment as payment in full, writing off any difference. This is considered a professional courtesy. Physicians may also treat members of the clergy and allied health professionals employed in their own offices or offices of close associates without charge or at a discount. If any of these individuals insist on paying or offer insurance to cover the charges, payment should be accepted.

Personal Data Sheet

A personal data sheet should be completed the first time patients are seen in the office, Figure 8–1. On **subsequent** visits you should routinely **verify** the address, place of employment, and insurance information. You may type the form while interviewing the patient in private, or the patient may complete the form. The following information should always be obtained.

- Patient's full name correctly spelled.
- Date of birth. This is useful if you have two people with the same or similar names.
- Social Security number. This is used as the identification number with insurance carriers in many cases.
- Marital status.
- Current address and length of time at that address. A person who moves frequently may lack stability in payment of bills.

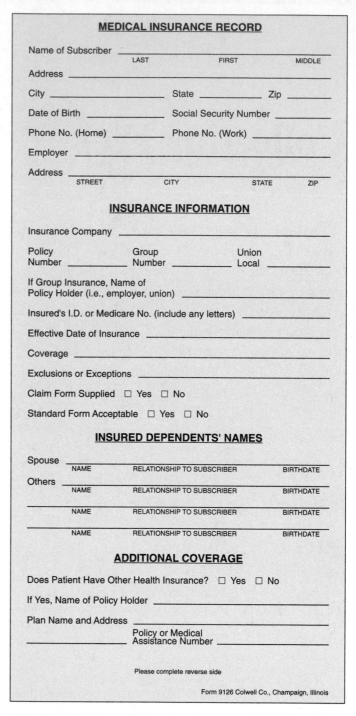

FIGURE 8–1 Personal data sheet (Courtesy of Colwell Systems).

- Telephone number at home and at work or availability of pager number.
- Name and relationship of person legally responsible for charges. Under normal circumstances parents are considered responsible for the charges of their children. However, if a third party is involved, an oral agreement is not binding and the individual who will pay the bill needs to sign a simple statement before care is given. This statement may be a form you have prepared or it may be a handwritten statement, Figure 8–2.

Samuel E. Matthews, M.D.
Suite 120
100 East Main Street
Yourtown, US 98765-4321

Date _____

Name of patient _____

I _____ agree to pay for the
　　　(name of responsible party)

examination and treatment of _____
　　　　　　　　　　　　　　　　　　　(name of patient)

on _____
　　　　　　(dates of treatment)

Witness _____

Date _____

FIGURE 8-2　Third party liability statement.

BEST CLINIC ASSOCIATION
PHILLIP H. BEST, M.D.
DEAN E. MCLAUGHLIN, M.D.
P.O. Box 136
LOVINGTON, ILLINOIS 61937

RECORDS RELEASE　　　Date

To _____

_____

I hereby authorize you to release to

_____

_____

any information including the diagnosis and records of any
treatment or examination rendered to me during the period from
_____ to _____

　　　　　　　　　　　　_____
　　　　　　　　　　　　　　　　SIGNATURE

_____　_____
　　　WITNESS　　　　　　　　　　　ADDRESS

FIGURE 8-3　Records release form (Courtesy of Colwell Systems).

- Patient's occupation, with name and address of employer. If a patient has a spouse, you should also obtain spouse's occupation and name and address of employer.
- Name of person referring patient. This information can be valuable if the patient later moves without leaving a forwarding address.
- Health insurance information. Ask to see the patient's identification card or cards, if they are covered by more than one plan. You need to make a copy of both sides of the card(s) on your copy machine to be sure you have all the information. Some states require a consent for release of information separate from the printed one on insurance forms. If this is the case in your state, be sure that this form also is completed at the time of the first visit, Figure 8–3. Be sure you have complete information on all insurance carried.

Complete Chapter 8, Unit 1 in the workbook to help you meet the objectives at the beginning of this unit and therefore achieve competency of this subject matter.

UNIT 2
Credit Arrangements

OBJECTIVES

Upon completion of the unit, meet the following terminal performance objectives by verifying knowledge of the facts and principles presented through oral and written communication at a level deemed competent.

1. List circumstances when you may need to discuss payment planning with a patient.
2. Describe credit arrangements used to finance medical care.
3. Describe the reason for accepting credit cards as payment for services rendered.
4. Spell and define, using the glossary at the back of the text, all the words to know in this unit.

WORDS TO KNOW

solicit　　　　　　　　　　　　substantial

PAYMENT PLANNING

The medical assistant can be a great help to patients who are going to have a baby, elective surgery, or extensive therapy by helping plan for payment. When the patient knows in advance that there will be costly medical expenses, the medical assistant should review the patient's health insurance coverage. Some physicians use a cost estimate sheet to give the patient an idea of the cost for surgery or long-term treatment, Figure 8–4. The estimate may include the approximate cost of the anesthetist, any consultants, and hospital charges.

SURGICAL COST ESTIMATE

NAME OF PATIENT   DATE

Procedure _____

_____

Your surgery is scheduled at _____

Hospital on _____. You should report to the Admitting Office

between the hours of _____ (a.m.)(p.m.) and (a.m.)(p.m.).

Although medical and hospital expenses are often covered by
insurance, knowing in advance what expenses to expect and how to plan
for them is beneficial to the patient. This estimate is prepared to assist
you in budgeting, if necessary, to cover your surgical costs.

PROFESSIONAL FEES

When you have major surgery, the surgical team includes the
operating surgeon, the assistant surgeon and the anesthetist. Each has an
important part in your care, and each will render a separate statement
for services. While each physician will set his/her own fee, it is usually
possible to make an estimate in advance of the approximate range of
fees. Assuming an uncomplicated course for your surgery, the charges
are estimated as follows:

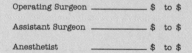

Operating Surgeon _____ $ to $

Assistant Surgeon _____ $ to $

Anesthetist _____ $ to $

The assistant surgeon and anesthetist usually base their fees on the
length of the operating time; consequently, if a surgical procedure
requires more time, the charges may be correspondingly increased.

The estimated duration of your hospital stay is _____ days at
$ _____ a day for a (semi-private) (private) room. During your
hospital stay there will be charges for laboratory tests, medications as
required, and other services. It is impossible to estimate in advance what
these charges will be, they will be itemized on your hospital bill. If you
have health insurance, please take the appropriate forms and I.D.
information with you on the day you are admitted to the hospital.

PLEASE KEEP IN MIND THIS IS ONLY AN ESTIMATE

FIGURE 8–4 Estimate sheet.

LEONARD S. TAYLOR, D.D.S.
2100 WEST PARK AVENUE
CHAMPAIGN, ILLINOIS 61820
____
TELEPHONE 381-5400

FEDERAL TRUTH IN LENDING STATEMENT
For professional services rendered

Patient _____

Address _____

_____

Parent _____

1. Cash Price (fee for service)	$	_____
2. Cash Down Payment	$	_____
3. Unpaid Balance of Cash Price	$	_____
4. Amount Financed	$	_____
5. FINANCE CHARGE	$	_____
6. Finance Charge Expressed As Annual Percentage Rate	$	_____
7. Total of Payments (4 plus 5)	$	_____
8. Deferred Payment Price (1 plus 5)	$	_____

"Total payment due" (7 above) is payable to _____
_____ at above office address in
_____ monthly installments of $ _____. The first
installment is payable on _____ 19 _____,
and each subsequent payment is due on the same day
of each consecutive month until paid in full.

_____   _____
Date   Signature of Patient, Parent if Patient is a Minor

FORM 9402 COLWELL SYSTEMS INC. CHAMPAIGN, ILLINOIS

FIGURE 8–5 Federal truth in lending form (Courtesy of Colwell Systems).

If it appears that the patient will need to pay a **substantial** sum out-of-pocket, the medical assistant should discuss the manner in which payments will be made. If the patient does not have current resources to pay the full amount in one payment, the medical assistant should offer the option of a fixed sum as a down payment and regular payments of a fixed amount on specified dates. The Truth in Lending Act, which is enforced by the Federal Trade Commission, specifies that when there is an agreement between the physician and a patient to accept payment in more than four installments, the physician is required to provide disclosure of finance charges. Most medical offices do not charge for financing but this makes no difference; the form still must be completed, Figure 8–5. The patient must sign this form in your presence and the disclosure statement must be kept on file for two years. If the physician makes no specific arrangement for more than four payments and bills each month for the full amount, rather than installment amounts, there is no need for the signed statement.

CREDIT CARD USAGE

Patients are currently using many methods of financing medical care. The AMA Code of Ethics includes several guidelines for physician participation in credit card programs. Physicians may not increase their charges for services to patients who wish to use credit cards; they may not encourage patients to use credit cards or use the credit card as a way to **solicit** patients; physicians may offer credit card payment as a convenience for patients but cannot advertise this fact outside the office.

The advantage of credit card use for paying for medical services is the monies are generally available to the physician within twenty-four hours of depositing. Also, it removes the responsibility from the physician for collection. This service does not come without cost to the physician. Generally, a fee of 1% to 3% is assessed, based on the volume of credit cards used. Many physicians feel this is to their advantage because the office time is not used for collection of any delinquent accounts.

Some banks have set up financing programs in which the bank sends the money directly to the physician after deducting a handling charge. It is important for the physician to be sure that any outside financing arranged for patients is managed in a professional manner and that no unreasonable pressure tactics are used. In larger cities the physician may want to check credit references before extending credit for a large surgical fee. Some large medical societies have Bureaus of Medical Economics that perform a collection service and also provide credit information.

If you should receive a request from a credit bureau, you can say when a patient's account was opened, the current balance, and the largest amount of the account at any time. You will be in violation of the law if you make any statements regarding paying habits of the patient or the character of the patient.

Complete Chapter 8, Unit 2 in the workbook to help you meet the objectives at the beginning of this unit and therefore achieve competency of this subject matter.

UNIT 3
Bookkeeping Procedures

■ OBJECTIVES

Upon completion of the unit, meet the following terminal performance objectives by verifying knowledge of the facts and principles presented through oral and written communication at a level deemed competent, and demonstrate the specific behaviors as identified in the terminal performance objectives of the procedures.

1. Transfer charges from charge slip to daily log.
2. Post charges from daily log to patient ledger card.
3. Type itemized statement.
4. Describe exceptions to usual billing procedures.
5. Describe the advantages of one-write bookkeeping system.
6. Spell and define, using the glossary at the back of the text, all the words to know in this unit.

■ WORDS TO KNOW

assets	ledgers
bankruptcy	petition
bookkeeper	posted
chemotherapy	trial balance
journalizing	

BOOKKEEPING TERMS

Some of the basic terminology used in recording office business transactions includes:

- *Daily journal* or day sheet. All patient charges and receipts are recorded here each day.

- *Account.* Record for each patient, which will show charges, payments, and balance due.
- *Accounts receivable.* All of the outstanding accounts (amounts due).
- *Posting.* Transfer of information from one record to another.
- *Debit.* A charge, added to existing balance.
- *Credit.* A payment, subtracted from existing balance.
- *Balance.* Difference between debit and credit.
- *Adjustment.* Professional courtesy discounts, write-offs, or amounts not paid by insurance. If no adjustment column is included, discounts are listed in red in the debit column.
- *Debit balance.* Shows that the patient paid an amount less than the total due.
- *Credit balance.* Shows that the patient paid more than was due or is paying in advance. A credit balance is written in red ink, circled, or noted in parentheses.

Daily Log

The medical assistant should record the charges for each patient on the daily log sheet, Figure 8–6. They should be itemized and a total only put in the charge column. Payments should be placed in the credit (paid) column. The daily log sheet will reflect the names of all patients treated in the office each day as well as any payments received in the mail or from patients who come to the office just to pay the bill.

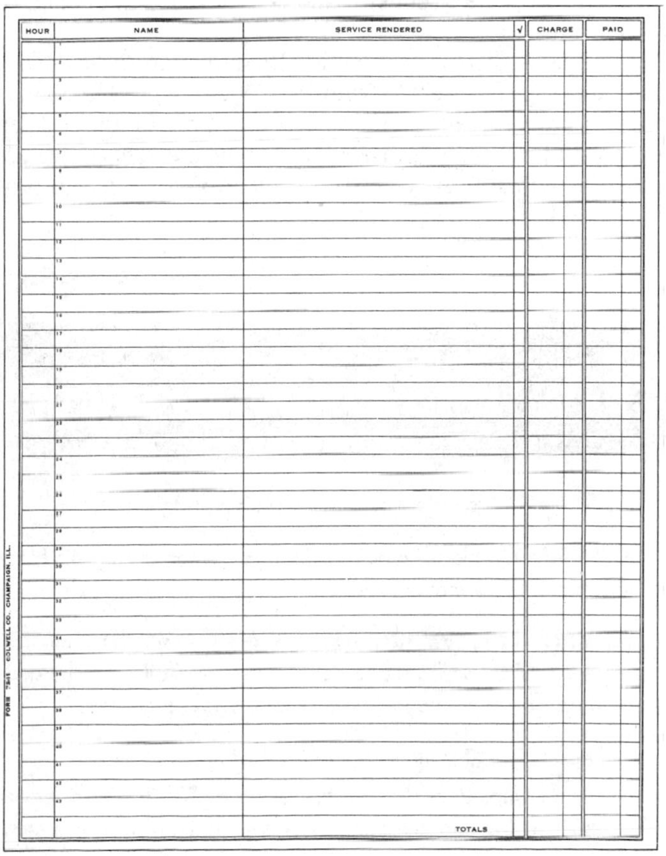

FIGURE 8–6 Daily log sheet (Courtesy of Colwell Systems).

Unassigned columns on the daily log may be used to distribute charges or receipts among partners or to distribute charges by departments, such as laboratory, x-ray, physical therapy, or medication in such cases as **chemotherapy**.

Ledger Cards

The medical assistant who must transfer the charges from the day sheet to the patient account card should do this when there will be a minimum of interruptions, Procedures 8–1 and 8–2. The variety of ledger cards available makes it possible to increase efficiency by using the one which best suits your needs. It is a good policy to place a small check mark on the day sheet after each entry has been **posted** to the account card. Then if you are interrupted you will know where to begin again in your posting job.

Statements

Statements (Procedure 8–3) must be accurate in every detail, from the name of the patient to the figures for charges and payments, Figure 8–7. If your office uses monthly billing, send the bills on the last day of the month. Your patients are more likely to pay if statements are received on a regular basis. If you have a large number of statements to send, cycle billing should be used. With this system, you divide your account cards into groups to correspond to the number of times you will be billing. You then maintain the same cycle each month so that patients learn when to expect your statement. You might send A through F on the tenth of each month, G through M on the twentieth, and N through Z at the end of the month.

Medical assistants are generally more concerned with bookkeeping as an entry level employee. A **bookkeeper** is one who records information. You may be required to keep a record of accounts receivable and payable. The office accountant will inform you of any records you need to provide to prepare summary reports of financial information, which are as important in the practice of medicine as in any well-run business. The accountant will analyze the figures and prepare reports that not only tell the present status of accounts receivable and payable, but compare current reports with other years or periods of time. A breakdown of the most cost-efficient pro-cedures and least cost-efficient procedures may be revealed in such a summary. The accountant may be the person designated to prepare payroll checks and pay the quarterly amounts due to government agencies for taxes withheld.

The medical assistant who is going to do bookkeeping must be accurate in every detail. There is no "almost right" in bookkeeping. The work is 100% correct or it is incorrect and must be corrected. The bookkeeper must enjoy detail work and must make clear, legible figures using a fine point black ink pen. Care must be taken to record figures in correct columns as debit or credit and always in straight columns. Care must also be taken to place the decimal point correctly and always double-check figures on a calculator or adding machine. An adding machine tape is helpful in that you can double-check figures easily. Employees have been fired from their jobs because of carelessness with figures in simple math. You should practice adding and subtracting numbers without the use of paper or pen or computer. The bookkeeper who can independently compute answers quickly and accurately is considered an asset to any office.

BOOKKEEPING

As a bookkeeper, the medical assistant prepares the daily log or journal and posts charges and payments on the patient **ledger** card. The patient ledger card is a record of all charges or services rendered, any payments made by the patient or the insurance carrier, and any adjustments, such as courtesy discounts or discounts determined by contracts with insurance carriers. The entries on the daily log are

P R O C E D U R E

8-1 Prepare Patient Ledger Card

PURPOSE: Accurately prepare a patient ledger card.

EQUIPMENT: Blank ledger card(s), typewriter or pen with black ink, patient information sheet.

TERMINAL PERFORMANCE OBJECTIVE: In a simulated medical office situation, prepare a patient ledger card following the steps in the procedure. The instructor will observe each step.

1. Type name of patient, last name first.

2. Type complete address with zip code. **NOTE: On a ledger card to be photocopied the name and address are com-** pleted in the same manner as an address on an envelope since the copy of the card is folded and mailed in a window envelope.

3. Type name and address of person responsible for charges if different from patient.

4. Type telephone number of patient.

5. Type the name of the insurance company.

6. Type the referring individual.

7. If this is a continuation of a previous card, carry forward any balance due.

PROCEDURE

8-2 Record Charges and Credits

PURPOSE: Accurately record charges and payments on patients' ledger cards.

EQUIPMENT: Ledger cards, typewriter or pen with black ink, daily log.

TERMINAL PERFORMANCE OBJECTIVE: In a simulated medical office situation, record charges and credits following the steps of the procedure. The instructor will observe each step.

1. Pull ledger card for the patient.
   NOTE:
   - If you can record charges near your ledger file it will be efficient to do one at a time. Tilt up the card behind as a marker.
   - If you must post away from your ledger file pull all the cards you need at one time; then return all to file.

2. Post all charges and credits for a patient and check them off on the day sheet before you go on to the next patient.

NOTE:
- Use small, neat figures.
- Note the dividing line between dollars and cents. In some cases this is a darker line.
- Never use dollar signs on account cards.

3. Charges are posted in the debit column.
   Key Point: If a balance is shown on the card add the new debit to get a new balance.

4. Payments are posted in the credit column and are subtracted from the balance due. **NOTE: If the credit is greater than the balance due, the difference is a credit balance and is shown in red.**

5. The balance column should always reflect the current status of the account.

PROCEDURE

8-3 Type Itemized Statement

PURPOSE: Accurately prepare an itemized statement.

EQUIPMENT: Ledger cards, typewriter (or computer and printer), appropriate stationery for statement.

TERMINAL PERFORMANCE OBJECTIVE: In a simulated medical office situation, type itemized statements with 100% accuracy following the steps in the procedure. The instructor will observe each step.

1. Stack ledger cards beside the typewriter.
2. Assemble statement forms and window envelopes.
3. Stamp the ledger card on the line below the last entry with a date stamp.
4. Type the name and complete address in an area that will show in window envelope.
5. If there is a balance from the previous month, list that first under services.
6. Type each service charge and payment for the current month.
7. The last line should show the current balance due.
8. Fold and place in envelope with the address showing through window in envelope.
   NOTE:
   - You may want to stuff all the envelopes after you have typed all the statements.
   - Be careful to place only one statement in each envelope.
9. Fan out several envelopes with flaps exposed.
10. Dampen a sponge and wipe over all flaps at once.
    NOTE: Be careful not to overwet.
11. Fold down flaps and seal.

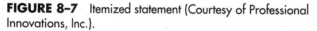

KERRY PEOPLES, M.D.
101 Fitness Lane
Anywhere, U.S.A. 00000

Marsha Leonard
777 Pine Tree Lane
Troy, Ohio 47100

| DATE | | DESCRIPTION | CHARGE | CREDITS | | CURRENT BALANCE |
				PAYMENTS	ADJ.	
			BALANCE FORWARD →			
8/31/XX	Marsha	Office visit	35.00			35.00
8/31/XX	Marsha	SMAC w/CBC & diff	30.00			65.00
9/15/XX		ROA - cash		15.00		50.00

276L
PLEASE PAY LAST AMOUNT IN THIS COLUMN ▲

THIS IS A COPY OF YOUR ACCOUNT AS IT APPEARS ON YOUR LEDGER CARD

FIGURE 8–7 Itemized statement (Courtesy of Professional Innovations, Inc.).

called **journalizing**. The entries should be kept in chronological order. The total amount of cash and checks should be recorded on a cash control sheet. This may be a daily record sheet or a monthly record showing an entire month with a line used each day to show income in cash and checks, any deposits made, and any amounts not deposited and therefore carried over to the next day.

When the balance is carried forward it is important to record it under "previous balance" for the next day, where it will be added to the total received to calculate "total on hand."

This kind of record is also helpful in double checking your bank deposit slips. The cash and checks should equal the amount shown on the cash control sheet, Figure 8–8.

An accounts receivable record should be kept daily. This record represents the total amount owed to the physician for services rendered. The total should be the same as the total of balances on all the active patient ledger records. The process of running such a total is called a **trial balance**. The accounts receivable balance is carried forward from month to month and added to the daily charges. The payments made by the patient and any adjustments are subtracted to determine the true account receivable each day.

This single entry method of bookkeeping records all increases and decreases in the **assets** of the practice. Assets are anything that have value which are owned by a business. Examples of assets are office furniture, equipment, the building itself, and the land on which the building stands.

EXCEPTIONS TO USUAL PROCEDURES

There are a number of exceptions to the usual billing procedures. Many companies make arrangements for annual physical examinations to be completed by community physicians. In these cases, the statements are sent to the employer rather than the patient. Some physicians complete physical examinations for individuals applying for insurance coverage. In this case the bill is sent to the insurance company. Physicians who specialize in sports medicine and examine athletes may be paid by the school or team referring the patient.

When it is necessary to collect a bill owed by a deceased patient, the statement is sent to the estate of the deceased in care of any known next of kin at the patient's last known address. You do not address the statement to a relative unless you have a signed agreement that that person will be responsible for the bills. You may need to contact the Probate Court to obtain the name of the administrator of the estate if the patient died in a nursing home and had no known next of kin.

When your office receives an official notice that a patient has filed for **bankruptcy**, you send no more statements and can make no attempt to collect the account. The patient who has filed a wage earner's bankruptcy will pay a fixed amount to the court to be divided among the creditors. Your office may receive only a dollar at a time. Accept this and credit the account. You will be notified of a creditors' meeting in a

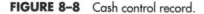

CASH CONTROL
January 19___

Day	Total Received	Total Cash	Total Checks	Previous Balance	Total on Hand	Deposit	Balance Carried Forward
5	7,650.00	250.00	7,400.00	——	7,650.00	7,650.00	
6	500.00	——	500.00	——	500.00	——	500.00
7	5,950.00	550.00	5,400.00	500.00	6,450.00	6,450.00	

FIGURE 8–8 Cash control record.

straight **petition** for bankruptcy, but it is usually best just to be sure they have a copy of the statement and wait to see if you will receive any money. Sometimes the patient wishes to continue seeing the physician and will make payments on the account independently on a cash basis.

The physician may examine a patient in consultation in a legal claim, and in this case the person or agency requesting the consultation is responsible for the charges. The statement is sent with the consultation report. Other examples of third party billing are auto accidents, Workers' compensation, and Medicaid.

Some offices send copies of charge slips to an outside billing service. In this case you need to be sure all charges and payments are sent so that the statements will be accurate and complete. The disadvantage of this system is that you do not have records in your office of current balances for your patients.

PEGBOARD SYSTEM

Many offices use the one-write pegboard system mentioned earlier for their accounting records. The base or board has pegs, which you should place up and to the left. This log holds all of your daily entries; it becomes a listing of patients seen, as well as a complete financial record of charges made and payments received. You position a shingle of receipt/charge slips on top of the daily log, with the notches fitted over the pegs. Working downward from the top of the daily log, the shingle must be placed so that the charge/receipt slip nearest the top of the pegboard has its posting line directly over the first available line on the daily log. At the beginning of each day this will be at the top of the daily log. These forms are prenumbered in the lower right corner; be sure to use them in numeric sequence to preserve the strong audit trail designed into the system. The receipt/charge slip serves several functions. It is the charge slip for current fees; a receipt for any payment received either by check or cash; a statement of account showing previous balance, today's charges, today's payments, and the new balance; it also shows the next appointment if there is one. When this is completed you are ready for your first patient of the day, Figure 8-9(a) and (b).

When you check in a patient, pull the appropriate ledger card from your file tray. If the patient is new to your practice, prepare a ledger card. Post to the first available charge/receipt slip the existing balance (if zero, write —0—), and the patient's name. What you are writing on the charge/receipt slip is being written simultaneously on the daily log sheet. You then detach the charge slip portion at the perforation and forward it to the doctor with the patient's clinical record. The doctor will check the services received by the patient and give the slip to the patient to return to the receptionist. This gives the patient an opportunity to review the services and to ask any questions about the charge. The medical assistant will then position the ledger card so that the posting line of the receipt slip is directly over the first available line on the ledger card and post the receipt number, date, and professional services rendered, using the codes preprinted on the form. The total charges are figured from the charge slip and entered in the charge space on the receipt slip. This is the time to ask for payment. If there is no charge the entry is written *n/c*.

Post any payment received in the paid space on the receipt slip. If no payment, record as —0—. Post the new balance in the appropriate space and again, if zero, write —0—. In one writing you have created for the patient a combination receipt and statement. With the same one-write system, you have recorded the financial data you need on both the patient's ledger card and the daily log sheet. You

FIGURE 8–9(A) Pegboard charge, receipt and appointment slip (Courtesy of Colwell Systems).

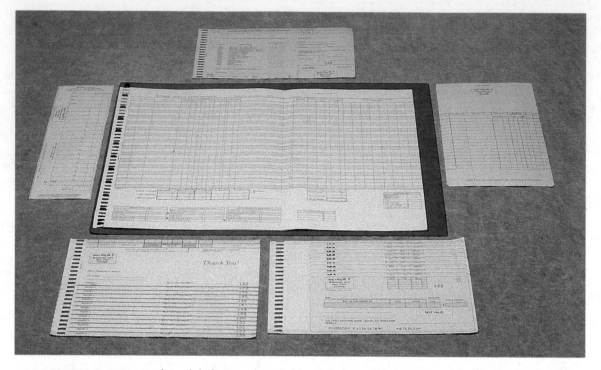

FIGURE 8–9(B)   Pegboard, ledger card, and charge slip assembled (Courtesy of Colwell Systems).

are now ready to detach the receipt slip from the shingle at the perforation and remove it from the pegboard.

Arrange a new appointment, if necessary, and record the date and time in the appropriate spot on the receipt slip. Also be sure to record the appointment in the appointment book before handing the receipt to the patient. Never write in the appointment space while the receipt is still attached to the shingle.

The last step is to return the patient ledger card to its proper position in the file tray.

If payment is made other than when service is rendered, the receipt slip is used if the payment is made in person. If the payment is received in the mail, it is written directly on the ledger card and through it to the daily log sheet. The new balance is then posted on the ledger card after it is removed from the daily log sheet.

At the close of the day, remove remaining charge/receipt slips from the pegboard and verify that all receipt numbers are listed on the daily log. You will usually have several blank lines at the bottom of the sheet; on the last line write "End of (date)." Use a new log sheet each day. Add each column and post totals in spaces provided. Save your tapes and double-check the figures. It is a simple matter to have an up-to-date account of accounts receivable at all times with this system. The total owed to the physician by all patients is increased by the day's charges and reduced by the day's receipts. The total of the receipts should be the amount of the bank deposit each day.

To protect the employees of the office against a possible bank error, the daily cash summary and the bank deposit slip should be initialed by at least two persons.

Complete Chapter 8, Unit 3 in the workbook to help you meet the objectives at the beginning of this unit and therefore achieve competency of this subject matter.

UNIT 4
Computer Billing

■ OBJECTIVES

Upon completion of the unit, meet the following terminal performance objectives by verifying knowledge of the facts and principles presented through oral and written communication at a level deemed competent, and demonstrate the specific behaviors as identified in the terminal performance objectives, observing all aseptic and safety precautions in accordance with health care standards.

1. Describe the advantages of computerized billing.
2. Describe different ways to locate an account in a computer system.
3. Describe an account history.
4. List reasons why billing statements would/should be withheld.

■ WORDS TO KNOW

account history   alpha search

Billing is the most common use for a microcomputer in the medical office. Many different computer systems and software packages are available. It is important to determine the needs of the office prior to purchasing. You may also:

■ visit medical offices in similar practice to discuss advantages and disadvantages of their system and software packages

- ask personnel in other medical practices about their equipment, software and service
- attend trade shows and demonstrations of medical practice software
- have representatives from various companies present hands-on inservice presentations of their medical practice systems and software

Practice management software offers a variety of services such as posting electronic claims, providing statistics on the number of patients seen per day (week, year), the diagnoses, month and year-to-date billing information, and so on. Software should also provide CPT and ICD-9 codes for processing insurance claims efficiently. Careful and thoughtful consideration must be given before a new system is purchased. Cost is the primary concern. Often the existing hardware may need to be upgraded, thereby eliminating the additional expense of a complete new system. If the billing system software is self-contained for the practice, patients' questions may be answered by the administrative assistant who handles the billing. Making a back-up file disc of all transactions daily is necessary in order to keep billing records secure. Patients can have a more personalized service if all transactions are done on site. If the billing is sent out to a billing service, patients must deal with yet another person for any billing questions or problems. With planning, each method can be equally efficient.

The computer terminology for a patient ledger is **account history**. This is simply a record of the information that should be obtained for every new patient. You need to know the name and address of the person responsible for payment of the account, all data regarding insurance, and all necessary information regarding family members under the same insurance. Generally, account histories follow the same organized plan you used for ledger records of patients. You may have a choice in determining how you will find an account entered in the computer system. When the system will accept a number only, you must maintain a cross-reference file of an alphabetical listing of patients along with their account numbers. The easiest and fastest method is called an **alpha search**. You type in the first few letters of the name and the screen will automatically list all names of patients starting with those letters. You select the name you wish to make an entry for and type in the appropriate entry. The account history automatically shows the balance of the account and the number of days the account has been due. The entire account activity is available to see on the screen or to make a printout for the patient. Your system should allow you to remove inactive accounts from the computer just as you remove inactive ledger cards. When a physician's office converts to a computerized system, it is important to choose the Current Procedural Terminology (CPT) codes commonly used in the practice. They are then programmed into the computer along with the descriptions of the codes and the fees to be charged for each. The International Classification of Diseases (ICD) diagnostic codes must be programmed into the computer for insurance claims use. The computer can be coded to indicate the source of the payment: insurance, cash, or check. Adjustment codes can be used for returned checks, courtesy discounts, and any cancelled account balances.

Some computers can be programmed to create charge slips. When the patient hands a computer-generated or handwritten charge slip to the receptionist, the charge and payments may be entered on the patient account history. A courtesy discount can also be recorded as an adjustment. In some offices, the receptionist would check to be sure the services rendered were indicated on the charge slips and then send them to the business office for processing in the computer. All charge slips must be accounted for each day. The computer can create a statement or receipt to be handed to the patient before leaving the office.

Computers can be programmed to lead you through the entry of every transaction by means of questions flashed on the screen or statements telling you what to do next. A medical assistant should be an accurate typist to operate a computer efficiently. If an error is posted on a transaction, there are ways to delete the transaction and start over again with a correct entry.

The computer insurance claims can greatly improve cash flow as a claim can be completed in a matter of seconds for every patient visit. This is a great advantage for patients who pay cash and need to be reimbursed as soon as possible. When the physician accepts the insurance payment, the computer can be programmed to print "patient signature on file" in the signature portion of the claim, so that there is no need to have the patient sign the form. Where there is no such system, the form must be signed by the patient or sent to the patient for signature in the hope that it will be forwarded to the insurance company.

The computer can speed up monthly billing and can be programmed to withhold statements on accounts for which you do not need or wish to send statements. Some examples are welfare patients, Workers' Compensation, or families of patients who have recently died. The computer statement is considered to be an efficient collection method for the office because it not only shows an itemized account of all transactions, but the age of the account can also be listed. The statement should show the portion of the amount due that is current, over thirty days, over sixty days, and over ninety days.

The computer can furnish you with a daily journal report. This report can be a record of cash control also, as a listing of checks and cash can be shown separately. All computer systems should be set up to record deleted transactions as a printed safeguard against anyone being tempted to steal money by entering a transaction and then deleting it.

The computer can be used to print out monthly summaries of charges, payments, and accounts receivable. Year-to-date reports can be easily produced. You may print out a record of all outstanding accounts with an analysis of account age.

The computer can provide a detailed list of patients seen by each physician in a large clinic and the services rendered. It can be used to determine the number of patients seen with a specific diagnosis or for a particular procedure for research summaries.

The medical assistant may be able to program the computer to print out a list of hospital and nursing home patients to be seen. Such a list improves the accuracy in recording all out-of-office patient charges.

When you have a computer system with many of the printout possibilities detailed here, you will find the business management of the office much more efficient. You will find you can complete all of these procedures in a fraction of the time required to do them by more conventional methods. For additional computer information and sample medical management computer screens, see the computer section in Chapter 4, Unit 3.

Complete Chapter 8, Unit 4 in the workbook to help you meet the objectives at the beginning of this unit and therefore achieve competency of this subject matter.

UNIT 5

Collecting Overdue Payments

■ OBJECTIVES

Upon completion of the unit, meet the terminal performance objectives by verifying knowledge of the facts presented through oral and written communication at a level deemed competent, and demonstrate the specific behaviors as identified in the pupil performance objectives of the procedure.

1. Define "aging of accounts."
2. Demonstrate use of the telephone for collection of accounts.
3. Compose collection letters suitable for a variety of situations.
4. Define the statute of limitations.
5. Spell and define, using the glossary at the back of the text, all the words to know in this unit.

■ WORDS TO KNOW

antagonize	reputable
convey	specified
expended	termination
harassment	

Computers can help in analyzing accounts receivable for accounts past due. This process is known as *aging of accounts.* It is basically a means of dividing accounts into categories according to the amount of time since the first billing date. Accounts are considered current if within thirty days of the billing date. Some medical assistants place a colored metal tag on accounts sixty days past due to indicate that a reminder was placed on the statement. At ninety days the tag color is changed and a letter is sent requesting prompt attention. Some offices use the numbers 1, 2, and 3 after the stamped date on the ledger card to indicate that past due notices were attached to the statement. The notices can be in the form of pressure-sensitive colored stickers that are progressively more severe in wording and in colors which are sure to attract attention, Figure 8–10. The first one might be a mild yellow, the second an orange, and the third and final one a red. No account should be referred to a collection agency unless the physician has given approval for this to be done. However, federal law requires that when you have

M_____19____

_____

Did you overlook the payment that you were going to mail us last month? Please consider this a gentle reminder of your obligation to this office in the amount of $ _____, due since _____.

Your prompt remittance will be appreciated.

3621

FIGURE 8–10 Sample collection cards (Courtesy of Colwell Systems).

stated you will turn the account over for collection you must follow through and do so if the bill is not paid. You cannot make idle threats.

A personal telephone call will often result in payment of overdue accounts. If you make collection calls, never do so without the consent of your employer, and confine your calling to your normal office hours. If you make calls early in the morning or late at night you can be held liable for **harassment.** Confine your calls to a place in the office where you will not be overheard by other patients. It is generally not a good policy to call a patient at work. If the patient has no home phone it may be necessary to call at work but you should simply ask the patient to return your call at a time when he or she can discuss the problem with you. Remember that you will violate the confidentiality of patient-physician relationships if you talk to anyone other than the patient or the individual responsible for the charges. When the telephone is answered, use the full name of the patient in asking, "May I speak to Jane Ann Jones, please?" Always ask if it is convenient to talk at this time; if it is not try to set a definite time when you may call, or ask the patient to call you at a **specified** time. If the phone is answered by someone other than the patient, identify yourself by name only. When the patient is on the phone, come directly to the point by saying that you are calling regarding the past due account. Approach the task with a positive attitude. Say that you are sure nonpayment of the bill is an oversight and, if not, that you want to help them make arrangements for payment. Make every attempt to establish a date when the bill will be paid, and make a notation on the ledger card indicating when that will be. Be sure you have a reminder file to help you follow up on promises to pay. If the patient indicates dissatisfaction with the results of medical care be sure that you **convey** this information to the physician.

Some physicians feel that collection cards or stickers are a sufficient reminder, but others prefer the use of collection letters, Procedure 8–4. Consult the office procedure manual or your employer regarding preferences for followup on the collection of accounts. You may want to compose a series of standardized letters that you can personalize as needed, Figure 8–11. When composing collection letters, avoid words that tend to **antagonize**, such as *forgot,*

Since your last office visit in May we haven't received any word of how you are feeling or any payments on your account.

If arrangements can't be made to pay the full amount of $_____ by June 12, please let us know so that the office can help you make arrangements for your payments.

You have always paid promptly on your account in the past, so you must have accidentally overlooked the statements we've sent. If that is the case, please accept this as a friendly note to remind you of your account due in the amount of $_____.

We can no longer carry your account on our books. The balance of $_____ must be paid within 10 days.

Our collection agency receives all delinquent accounts on the 25th of each month.

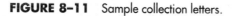

FIGURE 8-11 Sample collection letters.

neglected, overlooked, and *failure.* Decide whether you are going to use a series of three, four, or five letters. The last letter in the series will usually inform the patient that you must resort to a collection agency if you do not receive payment by a *specified* date. Use your knowledge of the patient to decide what type of letter to use. You would use a stronger sounding first letter for someone with a poor payment record. For a patient who has an excellent payment record your first letter would be a gentle reminder. Every effort must be **expended** to collect as many accounts as possible without resorting to a collection agency, which charges a percentage of everything collected. Most offices avoid collection agencies if at all possible.

An example of a form letter that can be used to obtain an answer in writing of reasons for nonpayment of an account is shown in Figure 8–12. If you can get this kind of letter signed by the patients, you not only know the reasons for nonpayment, but you have a signed paper acknowledging the amounts they owe the physician. If you know the reason for nonpayment, it is easier to help work out a solution for payment. If the payment is not made within the prescribed period used by your office, the fact that you have a signed statement from the patient acknowledging the amount owed is helpful in a collection situation. The patient cannot deny the debt.

Each state has laws (called *statutes of limitations*) which establish the number of years during which legal collection procedures may be filed against a patient. If a patient is being treated for a chronic illness, there is no **termination** of the illness or treatment unless the patient dies or changes physicians. The last date of debit or credit on the patient account card is the starting date for that particular debt. If the last date was June 1990, a 2-year statute could be collected through June 1992. In written contracts the statute of limitations starts from the date due. Some states have a shorter time limit on the statute of limitations on single entry (single charge) accounts.

When statements you have mailed are returned marked *moved, no forwarding address,* you have to consider the possibility that the patient is a *skip* (collection agency slang), or has moved to avoid payment of bills. The first step is to check your records to make sure you mailed to the correct name, address, and zip code. If these are all correct, place a telephone call to see if perhaps the old phone number was transferred to a new address. You may call referring individuals to try to obtain a new address for the patient, although you must not indicate your reason for needing the new address other than that you need to verify it. You may call the patient's employer for information regarding address change, identifying yourself by name only and asking that the patient return your call. You may find the patient simply forgot to inform the post office of an address change. You may also find the patient has left his or her place of employment, in which case you should check with your employer about referring the account for collection. The longer you wait, the less chance you have to collect.

Your employer should have arrangements with a **reputable** collection agency. The office reputation can be severely damaged if the agency you work with uses unethical collection methods. When your employer has made the decision to refer an account for collection, send the collection agency the full name of the patient, name of spouse or person responsible for the bill, last known address, full amount of debt, date of last entry on ledger card, occupation of debtor, and business address. Send no further statements, and refer any calls regarding the account to the collection agency. If you should receive any information regarding the account or any payments, you should forward it to the collection agency.

Complete Chapter 8, Unit 5 in the workbook to help you meet the objectives at the beginning of this unit and therefore achieve competency of this subject matter.

Samuel E. Matthews, MD
100 East Main Street, Suite 120
Yourtown, US 98765-4321
(654) 789-0123

(Date)

(Patient name)
(Patient address)

Dear

    Normally, at this time, because your account in the amount of
_____ is long past due, this account would be placed with our
collection agency. However, we prefer to hear from you regarding
your preference in this matter.

   ( ) I would prefer to settle this account. Payment in full
       is enclosed.

   ( ) I would like to make regular weekly/monthly payments of
       $_____ until this account is paid in full. My first
       payment is enclosed.

   ( ) I would prefer that you assign this account to a
       collection agency for enforcement of collection.
       (Failure to return this letter will result in this
       action.)

   ( ) I don't believe I owe this amount for the following
       reason(s):

               signed _____

Please indicate your preference above and return this letter.

              Sincerely,

              Samuel E. Matthews, M.D.

FIGURE 8-12 Collection letter requesting statement from patient of reason(s) for nonpayment of account.

P R O C E D U R E

8-4 Compose Collection Letter

PURPOSE: Compose collection letters appropriate for the aged accounts.

EQUIPMENT: Typewriter, stationery, patient ledgers, envelopes.

TERMINAL PERFORMANCE OBJECTIVE: Compose and type appropriate mailable collection letters for assigned accounts to be collected according to the procedure that follows.

1. Identify patients to whom an initial collection letter should be sent. **NOTE:** If you categorize your collection accounts you will be more efficient. Complete all #1 letters before proceeding to all #2 letters, etc.

2. Compose a rough draft with the first paragraph indicating *why* you are writing.

3. The second paragraph should indicate what response or reaction you expect.

4. Reread the rough draft to be sure you have written clearly, correctly spelled words, and correctly punctuated sentences.

5. Type the letter.
   NOTE:
   - Follow standard letter form (block or modified block).
   - Proofread the letter.
   - Sign the letter with your name unless the physician wishes to sign. Remember to type your position below your name and your title (Mr., Mrs., Miss, or Ms.) before your name.
   - Do not use identification initials if you sign the letter

6. Type the envelope.

7. Fold the letter, seal, and mail.

Medical-Legal Ethical Highlights

Throughout this chapter you should be mindful of all medical-legal/ethical implications. Listed below are a few important reminders.

1. Keep financial records accurate and complete.
2. Respect the privacy and confidentiality of patients' records.
3. Obtain and file written authorization for release of information.
4. Obtain a written contract if a third party is responsible for payment of medical treatment.

Mrs. Right . . .

organizes her work so that she can devote quality time in posting financial transactions on records. She is mindful in keeping this information confidential, respecting the privacy of patients. She makes sure that a signed authorization is obtained and filed when a third party payment contract is made for payment of services.

Promotion outlook: Excellent.

Mr. Wrong . . .

is careless when posting charges on records because he does this between other duties. He delays posting charges and payments because he doesn't like to do this kind of work. He makes errors and doesn't recheck his work. He is also negligent in obtaining proper authorization forms signed by patients regarding third party contract for payments. He confronts patients in hallways or in the waiting area in front of others concerning their accounts. He is known for discussing payments and other confidential information with other patients.

Promotion outlook: Poor.

REFERENCES

American Medical Association. "The Business Side of Medical Practice."

Frew, Mary Ann, and Frew, David R. *Comprehensive Medical Assisting: Administrative and Clinical Procedures,* 3rd Ed. Philadelphia: F. A. Davis Company, 1995.

Kinn, Mary E., and Derge, Eleanor. *The Medical Assistant: Administrative and Clinical,* 7th Ed. Philadelphia: W. B. Saunders Company, 1993.

Simmers, Louise. *Diversified Health Occupations,* 4th Ed. Albany: Delmar Publishers, 1998.

Health Care Coverage

Insurance has long been the way for most people to have some semblance of security in the event of a loss of one form or another. The insurance industry is vast. It encompasses a wide variety of areas to cover all forms of anticipated losses such as life, health, home and auto.

The health insurance industry is quite another matter. The outrageous cost for health care is what has been, and still remains, the cause of concern and the reason for all the attention throughout the nation. News of national health care insurance has been a primary issue for many years. Since the high cost of medical care is apparent to most everyone, health insurance has become a basic necessity. There have been efforts to research the insurance field and determine if reasonable cuts and changes could bring about a plan for the citizens of this country to provide quality health care at a more reasonable cost. This cost containment was a good idea; however, in trying to cut costs, the physicians were penalized by having fees reduced which, in turn, reduced the income of the physician. This also affects the income of the practice. The rippling effects reach out to how much can be expected in employee benefits, as well as many other factors regarding the whole practice. The reality of where these changes in insurance coverage may take us in this arena is uncertain. Of real concern is the quality of health care. Cutting costs could mean that there may be a decrease in the number of diagnostic testing and procedures that a patient may have according to their health insurance plan. This could affect the health of the patient because it would deter the patient from having what could be critical simply because of the cost. The quality of care of patients may also be affected by the realization that reimbursement is not likely for many medical services that may be considered unnecessary by the insurance company.

What is certain is that the traditional type of insurance that once covered the cost of our medical care is fast becoming extinct. Even though traditional private insurance is fading, there are still individuals who choose to pay high premiums so that they may have the flexibility to seek medical care from health care professionals of their choice. This is referred to as fee-for-service care. The different types of plans are mentioned in Unit 1 with their brief definitions, and will be explained further in Unit 2 of this chapter.

Health care reform has, in many cases, changed the way individuals select a physician. Often, there is not a choice in which physician one may seek health care from under a particular plan of insurance or health maintenance organization. Many times this is due to a group plan offered at the patient's place of employment. It is a fact that certain considerations must be made for the welfare of patients in general so that quality care is not jeopardized. Considering that a major portion of the income in the medical office is paid in the form of medical insurance, there are many areas that require careful study on the part of the medical assistant.

Both administrative and clinical medical assistants will find it necessary to keep abreast of changes in insurance billing and coding procedures and learn to **implement** them in a timely manner in order to guarantee the income of the practice. A discussion of the language of insurance, managed care, various medical care plans, and preparing claims for payment is offered in this chapter.

UNIT 1
Fundamentals of Managed Care

UNIT 2
Health Care Plans

UNIT 3
Preparing Claims

UNIT 1

Fundamentals of Managed Care

▪ OBJECTIVES

Upon completion of the unit, meet the following terminal performance objectives by verifying knowledge of the facts and principles presented through oral and written communication at a level deemed competent.

1. Discuss the changes in health care coverage in the last two decades and the reasons for the change.
2. Explain the purpose of HMOs.
3. Discuss the concept of managed care.
4. Distinguish the two major classes of health insurance.
5. Explain the reason for keeping patient insurance information confidential.
6. Discuss and define the terms listed in this unit.
7. List the different types of health insurance discussed in this unit.
8. Spell and define, using the glossary at the back of this text, all the words to know in this unit.

▪ WORDS TO KNOW

cessation	primary
devastating	reimbursement
encompass	secondary
implement	

HEALTH MAINTENANCE ORGANIZATIONS (HMOS)

Managed care is a phrase that became popular in the late 1980s in the United States regarding health insurance. Initially, it was used in the early 1970s to convey the concept of promoting good health and preventive medicine. The contracts of these plans which were negotiated between the insurance company and the employer grew in popularity. This medical insurance coverage is a great employee benefit and has created much competition over the years. These insurance plans are referred to as health maintenance organizations (HMOs). The contracts they offer people are affordable health care plans because they are offered through their place of employment at a very reasonable cost. The employer pays the balance. The employee's cost is a reasonable group premium rate for health insurance coverage (a part of their employee benefits) that requires only a small co-payment at the time of the medical service. This is a good arrangement for individuals and families. These organizations employ physicians and other providers of medical care in their service and patients visit them for their needs. Today, managed care is an organized system of medical team members and groups who provide quality and cost-effective care that **encompasses** both the delivery of health care and the payment of these services.

The initial purpose of HMOs is the containment of health care costs. Promoting wellness by offering members counseling about nutrition, exercise programs, stress management, weight control, low-fat diet, smoking **cessation**, drug rehabilitation, and the like, are efforts to keep people well, and thereby cut the costs of medical care. Encouragement of annual physicals and PAP tests, breast self-exams, testicular self-exam, mammographys, prenatal programs, well baby check ups and immunizations, and in general, requesting that people see their physician as soon as any problems are noticed, all help to reduce medical care costs.

The two major types of health insurance are individual and group. Any individual may buy individual health insurance by paying the required premium. Group health insurance generally costs less and is more comprehensive. The group may be employees, a union, or any other party. Complete coverage may or may not be paid by the employer. The employee may have to pay an additional premium to include other family members in the coverage. Most people have some form of health and accident insurance coverage because they realize that a serious illness or injury can be **devastating** to family or individual finances. Insurance seldom pays all medical costs.

There are many different types of medical care coverage plans, which are third-party payers. They will be discussed further in this chapter. A brief definition of each type can be found in the list of important words on the following pages that are used in working with patients and their various plans. Those you will be in contact with are Medicare, Medicaid, CHAMPUS CHAMPVA, Workers' Compensation, HMOs, PPOs, and private insurance companies.

One of the many helpful points that the medical assistant can stress with patients is to have them check their insurance policy regarding their coverage. Many times there is a misunderstanding or a lack of comprehension on the patient's part as to the types of coverage their insurance allows. If the patient seems to be unclear of the coverage, it is a good idea to suggest to them to phone the insurance company and speak to someone in the customer service area. Often this is helpful to the patient in having questions answered. Even though it would be a kind gesture on the medical assistant's part to go over the policy with the patient, there is not sufficient time for this activity in a professional setting where other patients need attention. It is fair to let patients know that not all physicians are members of all plans. This could be a source of frustration if the patient is not aware of this fact. Each insurance company does send members a packet of information when the contract is issued. Periodic supplemental information should also be received by the patient in the mail. You can ask the patient to gather this together and look for a *provider of services* booklet. This will help the patient to find the names of the physicians who are participating members of the patient's HMO.

Primary and Secondary Insurance Coverage

Another helpful practice upon greeting the patient in the office at the time of arrival for an appointment is to ask the patient for his/her current insurance card(s). Making a copy of both sides of the card(s) is of great help in completing any forms or in requesting information regarding that patient and their coverage, Figure 9–1. Patients may have more than one insurance plan. Often families have coverage which is from each parents' place of work. Many insurance companies include a "non duplication of benefits" or "coordination of benefits" clause in the policy. If both husband and wife carry insurance coverage that overlaps, the insured's coverage is considered **primary** and the spouse's is **secondary**. The charges are filed first with the primary carrier; after payment is received the explanation of benefits and a completed form is then submitted to the secondary carrier for consideration. When the couple has children covered by both policies, the Birthday Rule applies: the parent whose birthday falls first in the calendar year is considered the primary carrier. More information regarding primary and secondary insurance coverage will follow later in this chapter. Also, those who have Medicare may have additional insurance coverage to supplement their insurance costs. Remember to ask for the current information and insurance card(s) each time the patient comes in for an office visit as changes may occur from one visit to another. Posting a sign that says, "Please give your insurance card to the receptionist when you arrive—thank you," Figure 9–2, will help with obtaining current information from all patients served. There are still insurance companies that request a superbill from the physician which the patient attaches to their insurance form that they send in to be processed.

The Insurance Paper Trail

An example of how the paper trail for services rendered to patients is initiated and progresses is provided in Unit 3. The importance of accuracy and completeness is made evident by this series of forms and billing statements generated by only one patient for a relatively minor procedure. The medical assistant must be careful in documenting all information. Legible writing or printing as well as exactness is critical in successful **reimbursement** for services. Another sign which will help in collecting fees for services is one that states clearly, "Payment for services is appreciated at the time of service," Figure 9–3. Even if this payment is the co-pay amount, it can save time and work in ending the potential future paper trail. Submitting a claim form for the services to the patient's insurance provider will speed up the cash flow of the practice. Patients will comply with requests if they are made in a pleasant manner. It is the usual custom to have insurance payments and reimbursements sent directly (direct payment) to the physician. In those cases where the patient is reimbursed for medical services, the payment may be delayed because the patient may put off sending in the payment for one reason or another. This is referred to as indirect payment.

Included in this unit are many of the terms (with brief definitions) used in dealing with insurance claims. As medical terminology and anatomy are necessary for dealing with patients and procedures, so too is the terminology used in preparing insurance claims. You should familiarize yourself with these important words and their meanings to communicate needs and expectations of both patients and insurance companies. Your knowledge will help to expedite the processing of claims accurately and efficiently, thereby bringing payment for medical services to the practice in a timely manner. For those who prepare claims, it is necessary to keep current with any changes in policy, terminology, and procedures. There are newsletters, periodicals, and workshops offered to help in providing data to keep up with the latest information. It is to your advantage and that of the practice where you are employed to participate in these informative offerings. Knowledge in this extremely important task will lessen the frustration that is often associated with the complications of preparing and processing claims for patient services.

> Please present your insurance card to the receptionist when you arrive for your appointment.
> Thank you!

FIGURE 9–2 Posting a sign such as this at the receptionist's window in the office will help with keeping records current.

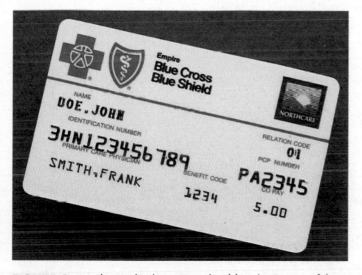

FIGURE 9–1 The medical assistant should make a copy of the patient's insurance card to secure accurate information regarding the type of coverage offered.

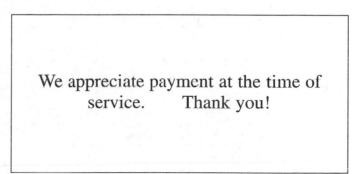

> We appreciate payment at the time of service.   Thank you!

FIGURE 9–3 Receiving payment at the time of medical services saves time and work for the practice.

TERMS USED IN HEALTH INSURANCE

Accounts payable/receivable—The total amount of the charges for services rendered to patients which have not been paid to the physician.

Admitting physician—The physician who admits a patient to the hospital (not necessarily the patient's attending physician).

Advance directives—A printed and signed statement to direct those who will take care of medical decisions for a patient when the patient becomes unable to make decisions. (Also known as a living will)

Assignment of benefits—The authorized signature of the patient for payment to be paid directly to the physician for services.

Attending physician—The physician who cares for a patient in the hospital (not necessarily the physician who admitted the patient).

Authorization to release medical information (Release of medical information form)—A form that must be signed by the patient before any information may be given to an insurance company.

Balance billing—The amount of the charges to the patient that the insurance company did not pay for medical services.

Capitation—The health care provider is automatically paid a fixed amount per month regardless of provided services for each patient who is a member of a particular insurance organization.

Civilian Health and Medical Program of the Uniformed Services (CHAMPUS)—Established to aid dependents of active service personnel, retired service personnel and their dependents, and dependents of service personnel who died on active duty, with a supplement for medical care in military or Public Health Service facilities.

Civilian Health and Medical Program of the Veterans' Administration (CHAMPVA)—Established in 1973 for the spouses and dependent children of veterans who have total, permanent, service-connected disabilities.

Claim—A request for payment under an insurance organization made by either the physician (medical assistant) or the patient.

Coding—Transference of words into numbers to facilitate the use of computers in claim processing.

Coordination of benefits (COB)—Procedures used by insurers to avoid duplication of payment on claims when the patient has more than one policy. One insurance becomes the primary payer and no more than 100% of the costs are covered.

Co-payment or Coinsurance—A specified amount which the insured must pay toward the charge for professional services rendered.

Current Procedural Terminology (Code CPT)—Coding system published by the American Medical Association.

Deductible—A predetermined amount that the insured must pay each year before the insurance company will pay for an accident or illness.

Diagnostic related group—A system developed by Yale University to group together major diagnostic categories, organized by body systems, from which the 470 DRGs are drawn.

Effective date—The date when the insurance policy goes into effect.

Electronic claims—Also referred to as electronic media claims, electronic data interchange, and electronic claims processing.

Encounter form—See "Superbill."

Endorser—The one who writes his/her signature on the back of a check that is made out to another person.

Early and periodic screening, diagnosis, and treatment (EPSDT)—This program requires screening and diagnostic services to determine any diseases or disorders, as well as complete health care, in children ages birth through twenty-one years. (Also called healthcheck)

Explanation of benefits (EOB)—A printed description of the benefits provided by the insurer to the beneficiary.

Fee disclosure—Health care givers informing patients of charges before the services are performed.

Fee schedule—A list of approved professional services for which the insurance company will pay with the maximum fee paid for each service.

Fee slip—A printed (computer) form with the patient's information and listing the services and code numbers with the charges.

Gatekeeper—A term given to a primary care physician for coordinating the patient's care to specialists, hospital admissions, and so on.

Group insurance—Insurance offered to all employees by the employer.

Health Care Procedural Coding System (HCPCS Code)—An alphanumeric coding system devised by the federal Health Care Financing Administration (HCFA) as a supplement to the CPT code and distributed by the regional fiscal agents of Medicare, CHAMPUS, and Medicaid.

Health Maintenance Organization (HMO)—A prepaid group practice serving a specific geographic area with a wide range of comprehensive health care at a fixed fee schedule; HMOs are interested in promoting wellness and good health, thus containing the cost of health care. These can be sponsored and operated by the government, medical schools, clinics, foundations, hospitals, employers, labor unions, hospital medical plans, or the Veteran's Administration.

HCFA 1500—The standard claim form of the Health Care Finance Administration to submit physician services for third party (insurance companies) payment.

Indemnity plan—a commercial plan in which the company (insurance) or group reimburses physician or beneficiaries for services.

Independent Practice Association (IPA)—A group of individuals who prepay a fee for treatment by a group of physicians who continue to practice independently in their own offices.

Individual insurance—Insurance purchased by an individual for self and any eligible dependents.

International Classification of Diseases, Ninth Revision, Clinical Modification (ICD-9-CM)—The coding system used to document diseases, injuries, illnesses, and mortalities.

Loss-of-income benefits—Payments made by an insured person to help replace income lost through inability to work because of an insured disability.

Managed care—An organized system of medical team members into groups to provide quality and cost-effective care that encompasses both the delivery of health care and payment of the services.

Medicaid—A joint funding program by federal and state governments (excluding Arizona) for low income patients on public assistance for their medical care.

Medicare fee schedule—A list of approved professional services that Medicare will pay for with the maximum fee that it pays for each service.

Medigap (Medifill)—Private insurance to supplement Medicare benefits for non-covered services.

Member physician—A physician who has contracted to participate with an insurance company to be reimbursed for services according to the company's plan.

National Committee for Quality Assurance (NCQA)—A non-profit organization created to improve patient care quality and health plan performance in partnership with managed care plans, purchasers, consumers, and the public sector.

Out-of-area—An HMO member is generally covered for emergency services out of his or her geographic area, but other coverages may not always be provided.

Preadmission testing (PAT)—Routine tests required for all patients before hospital admission to screen for abnormal findings that could interfere with the patients' hospital stay or scheduled procedure.

Patient status—Insurance companies frequently have stipulations that services be provided on an inpatient or outpatient basis; there are also requirements for prior authorization from the insurance company for certain services or procedures to be performed.

Point of service (POS) plan—An open-ended HMO, POS encourages their members to choose a primary care physician.

Pre-certification—Prior authorization must be obtained before the patient is admitted to the hospital or some specified outpatient or in-office procedures.

Preexisting condition—A condition that existed before the insured's policy was issued.

Preferred provider organizations (PPO)—This plan offers different insurance coverage depending on whether the patient receives services from a contracting network or non-network physician. The benefits are higher if the physician provider is a member of the PPO (or is a network physician).

Premium—Monies paid for an insurance contract.

Resource-based relative value scale (RBRVS)—Fee schedule based on relative value of resources that physicians spend to provide services for Medicare patients.

Release of medical information form (authorization to release medical information)—A form that must be signed by the patient before any information may be given to an insurance company.

Service area—The geographic area served by an HMO.

Skilled nursing facility—A medical facility which is licensed (defined by Medicare) to primarily provide skilled nursing care to patients.

Subscriber—The person who has been insured; an insurance policy holder.

Superbill—A printed form containing a list of the services with corresponding codes (encounter form).

Third party check—A check from one person which is made out to a second person for payment of a third person.

Third party payer—An insurance carrier who is not the doctor or patient who intervenes to pay the hospital or medical bills per contract with one of the first two parties.

Usual and customary fee—The usual fee is the charge physicians make to their private patients; the customary fee is one within the range of usual fees charged by physicians in a given geographical and socioeconomic area who have similar training and experience.

Utilization management—A panel who keep track of what their members receive and check if their medical care meets the standards of the organization.

Utilization review—A review carried out by allied health professionals at predetermined times to assess the necessity of the particular patient to remain in an acute care facility.

Walkout statement—A printed form with the patient's charges and the amount paid for the services rendered which the patient takes with them.

Workers' compensation—Government program that provides insurance coverage for those who are injured on the job or who have developed work-related disorders, disabilities, or illnesses.

As with any patient information obtained concerning patients, the strictest confidence must be kept to safeguard their privacy. Under no circumstances should any information about a patient be given to anyone without specific instructions from the patient. This permission is granted only by patient authorization by the signature of the patient. The release of medical information form must be kept in the patient's chart for this purpose. Updating this periodically and as insurance carriers change is necessary for legal concerns. If information is given to a third party without the signed authorization of the patient, the one who gave the information may be charged with breach of confidentiality. A contract is legally binding. Those who enter into a contract have certain expectations. A contract is an agreement between two (or more) parties for certain services or obligations to be fulfilled. Where there is a concern as to the competence of the patient or if the patient is a minor, a guardian must sign for any information to be released as well as for any service to be completed. Refer to Chapter 3 regarding legal terms.

Complete Chapter 9, Unit 1 in the workbook to help you meet the objectives at the beginning of this unit and therefore achieve competency of this subject matter.

UNIT 2
Health Care Plans

■ OBJECTIVES

Upon completion of the unit, meet the following terminal performance objectives by verifying knowledge of the facts and principles presented through oral and written communication at a level deemed competent.

1. Describe important health care plans.
2. Describe the important government health insurance plans.
3. Spell and define, using the glossary at the back of the text, all the words to know in this unit.

■ WORDS TO KNOW

annuity	periodic
connotations	statutory
illegible	supplement

COMMERCIAL HEALTH INSURANCE

A large segment of the population is covered by commercial insurance policies. These private, commercial insurance companies control the price of premiums paid and specify the benefits they will provide.

Blue Cross and Blue Shield health insurance plans are generally well known. Physicians helped originate them. Blue Cross was originally set up to pay for hospital expenses but now covers outpatient services as well. Blue Shield was originally used to pay for physician's services. In the early years, Blue Cross and Blue Shield was an indemnity type plan with an annual deductible and co-payment. They have changed with today's health care demands and now also offer a variety of HMO, PPO, POS, and indemnity type plans.

Indemnity type insurance gives the patient the option of the provider of their choice and the patient can see specialists without referrals. The patient assumes a greater financial responsibility for their health care. Indemnity plans require that the insured pay an annual deductible, usually between $100–$250, before the carrier begins to pay any benefits, and then usually 80%. Physicians will often ask the patient to pay at the time of service and provide the patient with a superbill or itemized statement to submit to their carrier for the patient's reimbursement.

HMOs are plans set up to provide comprehensive health care with an emphasis on wellness and preventative medicine. The patient is encouraged to have annual physicals to identify health problems early. Some HMOs have the subscribers choose a primary care physician (PCP) to oversee their medical care. The primary care physician is responsible for referring the patient to a specialist if needed. Another cost containment measure with HMOs is precertification for all inpatient hospital stays, some outpatient surgeries, and referrals to physicians outside the panel of providers. Most HMOs require the patient to pay a co-payment at the time service is rendered, usually $5 to $20. The physician's office staff then files the claim with the insurance carrier for the balance due. Along with the physicians, the HMO also contracts with hospitals, laboratories, and other ancillary services such as pharmacies. There are four types of HMOs.

Types of HMOs

- **Staff model HMO** is where all services (physical therapy, radiology, and so on) are provided at the same location. The primary care physician is responsible for routine care and referrals. True emergency (life threatening) care does not require preauthorization. If the patient is traveling outside the HMO geographic area, they must call and preauthorize any non-emergency care. Failure to do so will result in the HMO refusing payment of the services.
- **Group model HMOs** are multispecialty practices contracted to provide health care services to members. The physicians are reimbursed on a capitated basis. Capitation means that the physician is paid a set fee per patient on their patient listing each month, whether the patient is seen one or more times or not at all.
- **Open-ended HMOs** allow members greater freedom in their choice of care. They do not have a primary care physician and can self refer to specialists. If they choose to use a non-panel provider the benefit would be more like an indemnity plan with a deductible and coinsurance. If they choose a panel provider they would receive the HMO benefit.
- **Independent Practice Associations** (IPAs) are individual health care providers who join together to provide prepaid health care to groups and individuals who purchase coverage. This is a restricted health plan as only panel providers, hospitals, laboratories, and other ancillary services can be utilized for benefits to be paid. IPA physicians can hire their own staff and maintain private

offices. Primary care physicians are usually paid on a capitated basis while the specialists are paid on a fee-for-service basis.

HMO Accredidation

To qualify as an HMO, an organization must present proof of its ability to provide comprehensive health care. To retain eligibility, the HMO must submit **periodic** performance reports to the Department of Human Services. The National Committee for Quality Assurance (NCQA) is responsible for assessing, measuring, and reporting outcomes of HMOs. They also provide the accreditation for HMOs after reviewing the HMOs' performance and procedures. It is important for the physician's office to keep complete and accurate records for their patients, maintenance records on all equipment, and records of medications dispensed from their offices; office safety procedures, office cleanliness/appearance and accessibility are all components to the NCQA standards. There are four levels of accreditation:

1. Full accreditation is given for three years indicating excellent performance
2. HMOs that are well equipped to make recommended improvements are given a one year accreditation
3. Provisional accreditation for one year is given if it is felt the potential for improving the HMO is there
4. Accreditation is denied because the HMO does not meet the NCQA standards.

Preferred Provider Organization (PPO)

PPO is not an HMO. The PPO affords the patient the option of using network or non-network physicians and hospitals. Benefits are greater if a network physician/hospital is utilized. The patient assumes a greater financial responsibility if non-network physicians and/or hospitals are used. PPOs do not have a PCP, but do have more patient care management than an indemnity type plan due to the limitations of the provider panel. PPOs usually have deductibles and co-payment requirements and the physician's office generally files the claim for services rendered.

Many physicians belong to multiple HMO, PPO, and IPAs, unless restricted by specific terms of an insurance carrier contract or because of certain regulations in their area.

MANAGED CARE DELIVERY SYSTEMS

With the advent of health care reform, managed care delivery systems are gaining prominence in the types of plans employers are offering employees. Managed care plans integrate the financing and appropriate delivery of services to covered persons by contracting with selected providers for comprehensive health care services, with specific standards for the specialty of the provider and programs for quality assurance and utilization review. The primary care physician (PCP) or gatekeeper is responsible for coordinating all care for the patient. The patient must first consult with their PCP for a referral before seeking the services of a specialist. The PCP is encouraged to use the specialists listed with the HMO/IPA panel of physicians. There may be circumstances when a referral is necessary outside the panel as the specialty may not be part of the panel. Some managed care plans will allow a woman only one visit a year to her gynecologist for her annual well-woman exam and Pap smear, but if there are any gynecological problems prior to the next well-woman exam she will need a referral from the PCP to see the gynecologist again. Managed care also encourages mammograms for the female patient based on the American Cancer Society guidelines: a baseline mammogram between the ages of 35 to 40, every two years between 40 and 49, and annually after age 50 to 70 and at the physician's discretion after age 70.

Well child care is also promoted by the HMOs. This includes periodic visits for screenings of height, weight, vision, and hearing, neurological exams, immunizations at appropriate intervals, and TB tine tests. Most managed care plans require that the patient pay a co-payment, usually between $5 to $20, at the time of service. The administrative medical assistant in the physician's office files the claim for reimbursement of the charges for the services rendered for the visit.

Managed care plans employ a large staff of provider/professional relations representatives. These representatives periodically personally call on the physician's offices to provide new information, distribute new policy manuals, and answer questions that the staff or physicians may have regarding their particular company. Also, monthly newsletters are mailed to the provider's office to keep the office apprised of changes between representative's visits. Some managed care plans also offer periodic seminars on their policies and claim filing procedures.

GOVERNMENT HEALTH PLANS

Workers' Compensation

Employees in the United States have the benefit of being covered by Workers' Compensation laws. For many years the name of the coverage was known as Workman's Compensation but it was changed to avoid **connotations** of sex bias. Every state has these laws to cover employees who are injured while working or become ill as a result of their work. In addition to state statutes there are federal statutes covering federal employees injured on the job—United States Longshoremen and Harbor Workers Compensation, Federal Coal Mine Health and Safety Compensation, and special benefits for workers in the District of Columbia. The state compensation laws cover those workers not protected by federal statutes. The employer pays the premium for Workers' Compensation insurance, with the premium based on the risk involved in performance of the job.

Physicians who treat patients under Workers' Compensation plans are usually required to register with the state Workers' Compensation Board on an annual basis. The code assigned to each physician will limit care to a particular medical specialty.

There are four principal types of state benefits: (1) the patient may have medical treatment in or out of a hospital; (2) if there is determined to be a temporary disability, the patient may receive weekly cash benefits in addition to medical care; (3) when a percentage of permanent disability is found, the patient is given weekly or monthly benefits and in some cases a lump sum settlement; (4) payments are made to dependents of employees who are fatally injured. Benefits also include comprehensive vocational rehabilitation for severely disabled employees.

In most states the report of an industrial injury is initiated by the employer and sent to the physician who reports to the insurance company responsible for paying the claims, Figure 9–4. A few states have their own state fund for Workers' Compensation, and in these states the forms must be forwarded to the state office responsible. Time requirements for filing a claim vary. When the physician receives the form, it is considered authorization for treatment.

A patient who has an industrial injury should have a separate file set up for that injury and a separate account card. If the patient record is required in a court case for settlement of the claim, there is no chance of violating the patient's confidentiality if other medical records are a separate file. The patient is never billed in these cases unless treatment was given without authorization or was considered excessive by the Workers' Compensation Commission, in which case the patient may be billed for the portion denied by the commission.

The medical assistant must keep current files of procedures to be followed and forms to be used as these are frequently changed. The public affairs section or office services section of your state Workers' Compensation carrier will furnish any needed information.

Patients who have a continuing partial or permanent disability must usually be reevaluated at intervals and the physician must then promptly furnish a supplemental report. The description of injuries must be exact in the written report, and in case of fracture or amputation the anatomy diagram found on the reverse side of some of the forms must be clearly marked, Figure 9–5.

The medical assistant can help ensure prompt payment by paying close attention to all necessary details in the preparation of forms. An accurate claim number must appear on all forms and bills. The complete name of the patient, date of service, and nature of health care treatments must be on the bill. The payee number and payee name and address must be on the form and the form must be signed by the physician. One common reason for delay in payment of claims is that they are **illegible**. The forms should be typed, and to save time a rubber stamp with the name of the physician, full address, and payee number should be used on each form. The fee totals must be carefully checked for accuracy. If billing includes laboratory work or x-rays, the interpretations must be attached to the bill. Any surgery billing should include a copy of the operative report. A bill may be disallowed if it is not filed within the **statutory** time limit. If your records can prove your original billing was filed within the statutory time limit, that information should be submitted for reconsideration of the claim. You should always retain a copy of your billing and be careful to avoid duplicate billing. If computerized billing is used, a code number should identify each patient.

Medicaid

Title 19 of the Medicare Act of 1965 provides for Medicaid agreements with states for low-income families, the elderly, the blind, families with dependent children, and in some states other specified individuals. The states establish eligibility requirements and these are constantly being reviewed. Eligible citizens are issued monthly cards or coupons to identify their Medicaid status. As a general rule, prior authorization is needed to provide medical treatment except in an emergency. There are usually time limits for submission of claims. Again, the medical assistant must be aware of current rules for submitting claims. You should always check carefully to see if the card is current so that your office can be reimbursed for services. One of the important functions of the medical assistant is to assure the patient that the physician gives the same quality care to all patients regardless of their financial status.

Medicare

Medicare is a program of health insurance under Social Security for people over the age of sixty-five who are eligible and who have filed. The disabled or those insured under the Social Security retirement system are eligible as are kidney dialysis or replacement patients. The patient should show you the red-white-and-blue membership card indicating coverage, Figure 9–6.

Part A Medicare is for hospital coverage, and any person who is receiving monthly Social Security is automatically enrolled. The deductible amount has increased each year. Many patients now feel it is necessary to carry a supplemental insurance plan to pay that deductible amount. One such plan by Blue Cross is called *MediFill*. The term *Medigap* is also used to describe this supplemental insurance program.

Part B of Medicare is for payment of medical expenses outside the hospital, including office visits and the services of a physician in or out of the hospital. The premiums are automatically deducted for those who wish the coverage and are on Social Security, railroad retirement, or civil service **annuity**. Other individuals who are eligible pay premiums directly to the Social Security Administration.

Remember that Medicare B is the coverage that will pay for visits to the physician's office. If you are to assume responsibility for completing the forms, be sure to enter the Medicare identification card number in your records for the patient. The number is the Social Security number followed by a letter. A husband and wife will have separate cards.

The Omnibus Budget Reconciliation Act (OBRA) of 1989 requires that all physicians and suppliers submit Medicare claims for their patients since September 1990. Physicians and suppliers are not responsible for filing the Medicare claim if the service is not covered by Medicare or for other health insurance claims. Claims must be filed within a year of the time the service is received by the patient. In some cases the Medicare insurance carrier will automatically send the amount not covered on to the private insurance carrier, which will pay the deductible and the 20% not covered with no need to fill out additional forms.

INSTRUCTIONS

1. Type answers to All questions and file original with the Workers' Compensation Commission within 72 hours after first treatment.
2. DO NOT FAIL to forward to the Workers' Compensation Commission PROGRESS REPORTS and FINAL REPORT upon discharge of patient.

DO NOT WRITE IN THIS SPACE

WORKERS' COMPENSATION COMMISSION
6 NORTH LIBERTY STREET, BALTIMORE, MD. 21201-3785
SURGEON'S REPORT

This is First Report ☐   Progress Report ☐   Final Report ☐

WCC CLAIM #

EMPLOYER'S REPORT Yes ☐ No ☐

EVERY QUESTION MUST BE ANSWERED AND FORM SIGNED

1. Name of Injured Person: Soc. Sec. No.   D.O.B.   Sex   M ☐   F ☐

2. Address: (No. and Street)   (City or Town)   (State)   (Zip Code)

3. Name and Address of Employer:

4. Date of Accident or Onset of Disease: Hour: A.M. ☐   P.M. ☐   5. Date Disability Began:

6. Patient's Description of Accident or Cause of Disease:

7. Medical description of Injury or Disease:

8. Will Injury result in:

   (a) Permanent defect?   Yes ☐   No ☐   If so, what?   (b) Disfigurement   Yes ☐   No ☐

9. Causes, other than injury, contributing to patients condition:

10. Is patient suffering from any disease of the heart, lungs, brain, kidneys, blood, vascular system or any other disabling condition not due to this accident?
    Give particulars:

11. Is there any history or evidence present of previous accident or disease? Give particulars:

12. Has normal recovery been delayed for any reason? Give particulars:

13. Date of first treatment: Who engaged your services?

14. Describe treatment given by you:

15. Were X-Rays taken: By whom? — (Name and Address)   Date
    Yes ☐   No ☐

16. X-Ray Diagnosis:

17. Was patient treated by anyone else?   By whom? — (Name and Address)   Date
    Yes ☐   No ☐

18. Was patient hospitalized?   Name and Address of Hospital   Date of Admission:
    Yes ☐   No ☐   Date of Discharge:

19. Is further treatment needed?   For how long?   20. Patient was ☐ will be ☐ able to resume regular work on:
    Yes ☐   No ☐   Patient was ☐ will be ☐ able to resume light work on:

21. If death ensued give date: 22. Remarks: (Give any information of value not included above)

23. I am a qualified specialist in: I am a duly licensed Physician in the State of: I was graduated from Medical School (Name)   Year

Date of this report: (Signed)

(This report must be signed PERSONALLY by Physician)

Address: Phone:

SF 2-(REV. 1/87)

FIGURE 9–4   First report form for Workers' Compensation for payment of medical fee only (Courtesy of Ohio Bureau of Workers' Compensation).

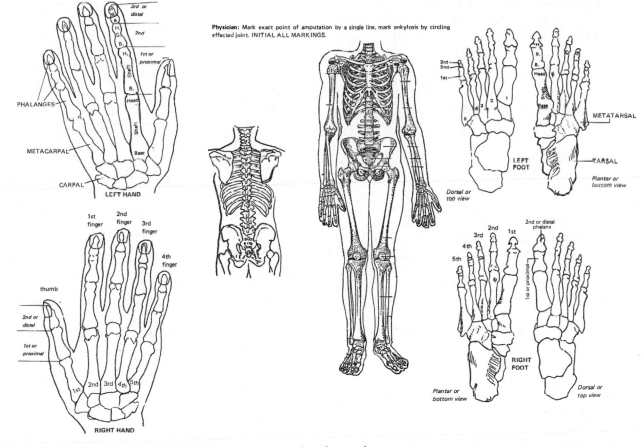

FIGURE 9-5 Anatomy chart for Workers' Compensation.

Physicians who sign a contract with Medicare to be a participating provider will receive payment directly from Medicare for services rendered. Physicians who choose not to be a participating provider must collect only the Medicare approved amount for the service rendered. They cannot balance bill the patient for the difference between what Medicare allows and what the physician charges. Nonparticipating providers are limited to 115% of the Medicare fee schedule for their services.

Patients who have Medicare Part B coverage are responsible for the first $100 of covered services; then, Medicare will reimburse the provider 80% of the allowed charge. The patient or their supplemental insurance would then be responsible for the remaining 20% of the allowed charge.

Most Medicare patients will have some form of supplemental or Medigap insurance to cover the deductible and 20% co-payment. Medigap is health insurance offered by private companies to persons eligible for Medicare benefits and is specifically designed to supplement Medicare benefits. The policy specifically excludes any plan or policy offered by an employer to employees (or retired employees) as well as those offered by unions to members (or former members). Medicare generally forwards the claim information directly to the Medigap carrier, thus saving the office staff time. It is important to ask the patient about any supplemental insurance at the time of service. Make a copy of both sides of the Medicare and supplemental insurance cards for your records. A copy of both sides of *all* insurance cards should be made at each visit. If the patient does not have a commercial supplemental insurance and is unable to pay the co-payment, the patient may be eligible for Medicaid. In this case, Medicare would be the primary insurance and Medicaid would be secondary and balance billed for the co-payment.

Physician payment reform (PPR) is another part of OBRA passed by Congress that made sweeping changes in the payment of physician services by Medicare Part B.

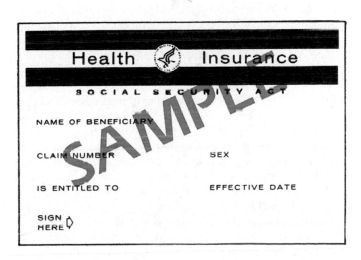

FIGURE 9-6 Medicare identification card (Courtesy of Social Security Administration).

- The PPR payment is based on a fee schedule, which is based on a resource-based relative value system, now referred to as the Medicare fee schedule (MFS).
- Medicare volume performance standards (MVPS) have been established to track annual increases in Medicare Part B payments for physician's services and levels for future years.
- Various financial protections for the beneficiary have been developed.
- Payment and medical policies used by Medicare carriers have been standardized.

Medicare is only permitted to pay for services or supplies that are considered medically reasonable and necessary for the diagnosis given. Medicare will not pay for routine physicals, cosmetic surgery, experimental, unproved or investigational services. If the physician does provide a non-covered service, the patient must be informed in advance and an Advanced Notice statement must be signed by the patient. The notice must state the specific service, the date of service, and the specific reason you believe the service is not covered. The following are some examples of statements which can be used:

- Medicare usually does not pay for this service.
- Medicare usually does not pay for this injection.
- Medicare does not pay for this service as it is considered experimental.

If the patient is not informed in advance of a non-covered service, the patient will not be responsible for payment and any monies collected will have to be refunded to the patient.

Current Medicare requirements specify that nonparticipating physicians must notify all patients, in writing, of the surgeon's estimated charge, the estimated Medicare allowable charge, and the difference between the two in advance of elective operations that involve charges over $500. Preprinted forms will help you comply with this requirement, Figure 9–7.

Claims received after May 1, 1992 must be submitted on the original HCFA–1500 claim form. Copies will not be accepted and will be returned for both assigned and nonassigned claims. You will need to check with the insurance carrier who pays the Medicare claims to find out the approved printers of the HCFA–1500 claim form.

The Health Care Financing Administration (HCFA) has designated the HCFA–1500 as the uniform health claims processing form, Figure 9–8, and requires all Medicare contractors to use it. The special bar code at the top of the form allows the claims processor to assign a unique identification number to the claim during microfilming. Effective March 1, 1996 Medicare adopted a national format for completion of claims. If claims are incomplete they will be rejected and no payment will be made. Additionally, after April 1, 1996, there are no appeal rights for rejected assigned claims. Medicare also encourages all providers to file claims electronically; this speeds up the claim turn-around time for the provider, as data entry errors are eliminated when the infor-

LEONARD S. TAYLOR, M.D.
2100 WEST PARK AVENUE
CHAMPAIGN, ILLINOIS 61820
————
TELEPHONE 351-5400

_____
(date)

Patient Name _____

Address _____

_____
City   State   Zip

My signature below certifies that I have received the following information from my doctor, as required by Medicare regulations.

Surgery proposed: _____

_____

Estimated charge: _____
Estimated charge allowed by Medicare: _____
Estimated difference: _____

It is understood that the planned surgical procedure(s) may need to be changed at the time of the actual surgery, thereby incurring other or additional charges that cannot be estimated at this time.

I also acknowledge receipt of a copy of this form.

_____
Signature

_____
Date

FIGURE 9–7 Form for estimate of surgery charges for Medicare patient (Courtesy of Colwell Systems).

mation does not have to be transferred from a paper claim. Your computer software company should provide regular updates for your system as changes occur with Medicare.

Medical assistants who submit Medicare insurance claims with the stamped statement "patient's signature on file" must be prepared to make these files available in the event the files are audited by the insurance carrier. The only time a signature is not needed is when a patient has services performed without being physically present in the office. An example of this would be the laboratory where a specimen collected in the physician's office was analyzed. In this case, the insurance form should state "Patient not physically present for services." Signatures of welfare patients are not required if the state agency maintains records of the signatures. It was suggested by Nationwide Mutual Insurance Company in a *Medicare Newsletter* that the office have a form prepared for the signature of Medicare patients. This could be signed once and kept on file and it would not be necessary to obtain the signature of the patient on every form. The form should list

PLEASE
DO NOT
STAPLE
IN THIS
AREA

CARRIER

HEALTH INSURANCE CLAIM FORM

PICA ☐☐   PICA ☐☐

1. MEDICARE	MEDICAID	CHAMPUS	CHAMPVA	GROUP HEALTH PLAN	FECA BLK LUNG	OTHER	1a. INSURED'S I.D. NUMBER	(FOR PROGRAM IN ITEM 1)
[X] (Medicare #)	☐ (Medicaid #)	☐ (Sponsor's SSN)	☐ (VA File #)	☐ (SSN or ID)	☐ (DCN)	☐ (ID)	090815621B	

2. PATIENT'S NAME (Last Name, First Name, Middle Initial)
JAMES   MICHAEL   J

3. PATIENT'S BIRTH DATE   MM 08 DD 23 YY 29   SEX M [X] F ☐

4. INSURED'S NAME (Last Name, First Name, Middle Initial)
SAME

5. PATIENT'S ADDRESS (No., Street)
525 N SHORT ST

6. PATIENT RELATIONSHIP TO INSURED
Self [X] Spouse ☐ Child ☐ Other ☐

7. INSURED'S ADDRESS (No., Street)

CITY
YOURTOWN   STATE US

8. PATIENT STATUS
Single ☐ Married [X] Other ☐

Employed ☐ Full-Time Student ☐ Part-Time Student ☐

CITY   STATE

ZIP CODE
12345-6790   TELEPHONE (Include Area Code)
(987) 654-0321

ZIP CODE   TELEPHONE (INCLUDE AREA CODE)
(   )

9. OTHER INSURED'S NAME (Last Name, First Name, Middle Initial)

10. IS PATIENT'S CONDITION RELATED TO:

11. INSURED'S POLICY GROUP OR FECA NUMBER
NONE

a. OTHER INSURED'S POLICY OR GROUP NUMBER

a. EMPLOYMENT? (CURRENT OR PREVIOUS)
☐ YES [X] NO

a. INSURED'S DATE OF BIRTH   MM DD YY   SEX M ☐ F ☐

b. OTHER INSURED'S DATE OF BIRTH   MM DD YY   M ☐ SEX F ☐

b. AUTO ACCIDENT?   PLACE (State)
☐ YES [X] NO

b. EMPLOYER'S NAME OR SCHOOL NAME

c. EMPLOYER'S NAME OR SCHOOL NAME

c. OTHER ACCIDENT?
☐ YES [X] NO

c. INSURANCE PLAN NAME OR PROGRAM NAME

d. INSURANCE PLAN NAME OR PROGRAM NAME

10d. RESERVED FOR LOCAL USE

d. IS THERE ANOTHER HEALTH BENEFIT PLAN?
☐ YES [X] NO   *If yes*, return to and complete item 9 a-d.

READ BACK OF FORM BEFORE COMPLETING & SIGNING THIS FORM.
12. PATIENT'S OR AUTHORIZED PERSON'S SIGNATURE I authorize the release of any medical or other information necessary to process this claim. I also request payment of government benefits either to myself or to the party who accepts assignment below.

SIGNED   SIGNATURE ON FILE   DATE

13. INSURED'S OR AUTHORIZED PERSON'S SIGNATURE I authorize payment of medical benefits to the undersigned physician or supplier for services described below.

SIGNED   SIGNATURE ON FILE

14. DATE OF CURRENT: ILLNESS (First symptom) OR INJURY (Accident) OR PREGNANCY (LMP)   MM DD YY

15. IF PATIENT HAS HAD SAME OR SIMILAR ILLNESS. GIVE FIRST DATE MM DD YY

16. DATES PATIENT UNABLE TO WORK IN CURRENT OCCUPATION   FROM MM DD YY TO MM DD YY

17. NAME OF REFERRING PHYSICIAN OR OTHER SOURCE

17a. I.D. NUMBER OF REFERRING PHYSICIAN

18. HOSPITALIZATION DATES RELATED TO CURRENT SERVICES   FROM MM DD YY TO MM DD YY

19. RESERVED FOR LOCAL USE

20. OUTSIDE LAB?   ☐ YES ☐ NO $ CHARGES

21. DIAGNOSIS OR NATURE OF ILLNESS OR INJURY. (RELATE ITEMS 1,2,3 OR 4 TO ITEM 24E BY LINE)

1. 401.1   3. |___.___|

2. |___.___| 4. |___.___|

22. MEDICAID RESUBMISSION CODE   ORIGINAL REF. NO.

23. PRIOR AUTHORIZATION NUMBER

24. A DATE(S) OF SERVICE						B Place of Service	C Type of Service	D PROCEDURES, SERVICES, OR SUPPLIES (Explain Unusual Circumstances) CPT/HCPCS MODIFIER	E DIAGNOSIS CODE	F $ CHARGES	G DAYS OR UNITS	H EPSDT Family Plan	I EMG	J COB	K RESERVED FOR LOCAL USE
From MM	DD	YY	To MM	DD	YY										
06	18	XX	06	18	XX	11	1	99212	1	35 00	1				4567890123

25. FEDERAL TAX I.D. NUMBER   SSN ☐ EIN [X]
11-0000521

26. PATIENT'S ACCOUNT NO.
1234

27. ACCEPT ASSIGNMENT? (For govt. claims see back)
[X] YES ☐ NO

28. TOTAL CHARGE $ 35 00

29. AMOUNT PAID $ 00

30. BALANCE DUE $ 35 00

31. SIGNATURE OF PHYSICIAN OR SUPPLIER INCLUDING DEGREES OR CREDENTIALS (I certify that the statements on the reverse apply to this bill and are made a part thereof.)

SAMUEL E MATTHEWS MD

SIGNED   DATE 06/20/XX

32. NAME AND ADDRESS OF FACILITY WHERE SERVICES WERE RENDERED (If other than home or office)

33. PHYSICIAN'S, SUPPLIER'S BILLING NAME, ADDRESS, ZIP CODE & PHONE #
SAMUEL E MATTHEWS MD
100 E MAIN ST STE 120
YOURTOWN US 98765-4321
PIN# 4567890123   GRP#

(APPROVED BY AMA COUNCIL ON MEDICAL SERVICE 8/88)

PLEASE PRINT OR TYPE

APPROVED OMB-0938-0008 FORM HCFA-1500 (12-90), FORM RRB 1500,
APPROVED OMB-1215-0055 FORM OWCP-1500, APPROVED OMB-0720-0001 (CHAMPUS)

PATIENT AND INSURED INFORMATION

PHYSICIAN OR SUPPLIER INFORMATION

FIGURE 9-8 Completed HCFA-1500 health insurance claim form.

the name and Medicare claim number of the patient along with the following statement:

> I request that payment of authorized Medicare benefits be made either to me or on my behalf to Dr. _____ for any service furnished me by that physician. I authorize release to the Health Care Financing Administration and its agents any medical information about me needed to determine these benefits or benefits payable for related services.

The form should be signed by the patient and dated.

The HCFA has developed codes for Medicare that allow for uniformity throughout the country. The three levels of codes range as follows:

1. CPT codes established and updated by the American Medical Association. These are five digit numeric codes ranging from 00000 to 99999 for physicians' services, such as examinations, surgeries, radiology, and pathology. Most Medicare B coverage is covered by CPT codes.
2. HCPCS codes are established and updated by HCFA. These alpha-numeric codes range from A0000 to V9999 and are used for physician and nonphysician services not listed in the CPT.
3. W0000 to Z9999 are reserved for local assignment. These codes are not present in CPT and are not common to all carriers.

Another important number necessary for completion of Medicare claims is the physician's National Provider Identification (NPI). In 1997, the NPI replaces the PIN, or physician's identifying number and the UPIN, or unique physician's identifying numbers previously used. The NPI is a ten digit number; the first seven digits are unique to the physician, the eighth digit is a check digit, and the last two have to do with location. If your physician has more than one office, there will be a NPI for each practice location. The NPI will be used in blocks 24k and 33 of the HCFA-1500 form to identify who provided the service. When the physician refers a patient to another practice for services, the referring physician's NPI will appear in block 17a of the HFCA form. If this number is missing from the claim, the claim will be returned.

Medicare provides annual updated policy manuals and monthly newsletters to keep physicians and their staffs current on Medicare policy. Medicare also offers training session to new medical assistants and seminars to keep those who are experienced with Medicare policy up-to-date.

In processing Medicare insurance forms, you must use ICDA codes for diagnosis, CPT codes for treatment, and HCPCS codes for any supplies or appliances used. Coding is discussed in more detail in Unit 3.

CHAMPUS

As part of the United States Department of Defense, the Civilian Health and Medical Program of the Uniformed Services (CHAMPUS) was established to aid dependents of active service personnel, retired service personnel and their dependents, and dependents of service personnel who died on active duty, with a **supplement** for medical care in mili-

tary or Public Health Service facilities. The word *dependents* refers to spouses and dependent children only; this program does not cover active duty military personnel. All members of CHAMPUS over the age of ten are issued an identification card. A patient who lives within forty miles of a uniformed services hospital will need a *nonavailability statement* to be cared for in a civilian or physician's office. This simply means that the necessary services are not available at the service hospital or that for medical reasons it would be better to continue care under the civilian physician who has been treating the patient. Authorization is not necessary if the patient lives more than forty miles from a military medical facility that could furnish the necessary care.

The Civilian Health and Medical Program of the Veterans' Administration (CHAMPVA) was established in 1973 for the spouses and dependent children of veterans who have total, permanent, service-connected disabilities. This service is also available for the surviving spouses and dependent children of veterans who have died as a result of service-connected disabilities. The local VA hospital determines eligibility and then issues identification cards. The insured members can then choose their own private physicians. There are deductibles and cost-sharing requirements your office needs to be aware of.

If your office needs additional information on military benefit programs, you can contact your local health benefits advisor (HBA) at the nearest military hospital or clinic or the office of CHAMPUS, Aurora, CO 80045-6900. The CHAMPUS phone number is (303) 361-3907; the phone number for CHAMPVA is (303) 782-3804.

Easter Seal/Crippled Children

All states operate Crippled Children's Services with federal support under Title V of the Social Security Act. The intent of this service is to locate crippled children under twenty-one or those who have potentially crippling conditions to see that appropriate health care is furnished. Part or all of this treatment may be paid for if the family's resources are not adequate. Some Crippled Children's Services are being changed to Easter Seal rehabilitation centers because of the stigma attached to the words *crippled children*. Some Easter Seal rehabilitation centers are now operated as private nonprofit organizations.

Complete Chapter 9, Unit 2 in the workbook to help you meet the objectives at the beginning of this unit and therefore achieve competency of this subject matter.

UNIT 3

Preparing Claims

■ OBJECTIVES

Upon completion of the unit, meet the following terminal performance objectives by verifying knowledge of the facts and principles presented through oral and written communication at a level deemed competent, and demonstrate the specific behaviors as identified in the pupil performance objectives of the procedures.

1. Tell why claim forms were developed.
2. Discuss the meaning of primary and secondary coverage and how it affects coverage.
3. Name the two main classifications of codes and explain their basic difference.
4. Explain the meanings of both the "reason rule" and sequencing.
5. List four general coding rules.
6. Identify two things to be done <u>before</u> completing a patient's claim form.
7. Demonstrate completion of a claim form.
8. List six common errors made when filing claims.
9. Explain the purpose of an insurance log, listing six of the items to enter.
10. Name four pieces of information to have before calling to follow-up a delinquent insurance claim.
11. Explain the phrase "accept assignment."
12. Describe what action should be taken when a procedure is <u>not</u> covered by insurance.
13. Name five of the seven items necessary for adequate documentation on a patient's record.
14. Identify three ways to stay current with Medicare and other insurance company regulations.
15. Spell and define, using the glossary at the back of the text, all the words to know in this unit.

■ WORDS TO KNOW

bundle	modifier
carrier	nomenclature
contributory	numeric
Current Procedural Terminology	preferred
	primary
encounter	reason rule
fee schedule	reimbursement
Health Care Financing Administration	secondary
	sequenced
International Classification of Diseases	specificity
	third-party reimbursement
Medicare	truncated

THE BEGINNING OF CLAIM FORMS

The preparation of claims for the purpose of receiving payment for medical services is a fairly recent development in the history of health care. For centuries, providers were paid directly with some form of money, "bartered goods," or the exchange of services. With industrialization and the scientific advancement of medicine, this was no longer appropriate. At the same time people began receiving employment benefits such as vacations and pensions. Soon, other benefits such as health care were added and the new industry of health insurance exploded. The phrase "**third-party reimbursement**" was coined to indicate payment of services rendered by someone other than the patient. With this intermediate step came the need for some form of "paper work" to serve as the means of reporting the health care provided to the source of payment: the claim form was developed. Today, the most common third-party reimbursers are federal and state agencies, insurance companies, and Worker's Compensation.

Originally, patients would provide the physician with forms obtained from their employer's benefits office for their insurance coverage. The patient completed their portion of the form and either signed or did not sign the section that authorized payment for services to be made directly to the physician. If it was not signed, the patient paid the charges and then the insurance company sent the payment to the patient. It was customary for physicians to charge a small fee to complete forms after the first one was done. Patients often had multiple coverage and could even "make money" with covered conditions. Medical findings, diagnoses, and treatments were described verbally in medical terminology and fees were paid as requested if they were reasonable. Third-party reimbursement was simple and fairly easy. The contract for services was primarily between the physician and the patient; controls were minimal. As time went by, medicine evolved into a very sophisticated science. Medical care became extremely complicated and technological advances caused a rapid rise in medical costs. Premiums for insurance coverage skyrocketed. Unemployed and retired persons had to resort to community clinics in order to obtain health care.

THE HISTORY OF CODING

While medical care was evolving into highly technical service, another need was surfacing. There needed to be some method of collecting health data so that physicians, scientists, and government agencies could assess the incidences and treatments of diseases. As early as the 1890s, a physician developed a classification of causes of death. From this beginning, The American Public Health Association recommended that this classification system be adopted by those responsible for recording deaths in Canada, Mexico, and the United States. It was decided that the classification should be revised every ten years. In 1938, the fifth revision had evolved into the **International Classification of Diseases** (ICD). A few years later hospitals began trying to classify diseases and their medical records departments used a modified ICD version to code and index records.

By 1978, the World Health Organization published the ninth version of the ICD (ICD-9) and in the United States *The International Classification of Diseases, 9th Revision, Clinical Modification (ICD-9-CM)* was issued. The initial reason for classifying deaths was to provide a means of assessing statistically the prevalence of certain diseases or disorders or the incidences of fatal injuries. Later, codes were used in order to retrieve medical records by diagnosis or surgical procedure to be useful in medical research and education. As other applications became evident, the system provided a method of identifying the incidence of diseases and disorders being treated throughout the world. Reported prevalence provides statistics for assessing the status of people within and among various countries. As the need for greater **specificity** of medical conditions became desirable, the codes were revised, expanded, and refined. The codes now allow for the expression of extensive verbal descriptions into a numerical system. Coding is, in reality, the transferal of verbal and/or written descriptions of disease or injury into numerical designations to achieve uniform data which can be easily entered into electronic processing and storage systems.

CURRENT UTILIZATION OF ICD-9 CODES

The ICD-9 codes became useful for reporting all medical care on claim forms for Medicare, Medicaid, and other third-party payers of medical services. Later, the impact of The Catastrophic Coverage Act of 1988 on the physician's office changed the way physicians manage their practices. Since April 1, 1989, ICD-9-CM coding is no longer an option; it is required on all Medicare and other government health care claims. The act mandates submission of an appropriate diagnostic code or codes for each service provided under Medicare B, or other coverage, for which payment is requested. Specific coding guidelines have been developed for physician's offices. It is very important that coding be done properly. The physician's **reimbursement** is based upon the codes that are submitted. The diagnostic codes (ICD-9) are evidence of the reason for the treatment given, which is another classification of codes (**Current Procedural Terminology** CPT) which will be discussed later. If the two coding systems are not compatible, payment will be rejected. Accurate ICD-9 coding not only helps to optimize reimbursement, it is also essential for **carrier** acceptance. The rules to survive in the new coding climate are very complex and mistakes are common and costly. Not only does the physician pay for coding errors but patients also are affected when services are not covered. NOTE: You communicate with carriers through numbers. You must fully and accurately describe patient services numeri-cally. It is important to code all documented current diagnoses, including underlying diseases and secondary diagnoses.

One of the most important rules to remember has to do with the sequencing of codes. Sequencing is determined by the intensity and acuity of service and the "level of service." Proper sequencing of the diagnosis codes is of utmost importance. Basically, it means listing the primary reason first and others next, in order of importance. Although the coding guidelines are far from perfect, they are the guidelines by which many carriers now pay or reject claims.

PERFORMING CODING FUNCTIONS

To become an accurate and efficient coder, three things are necessary: a working knowledge of medical terminology, an understanding of anatomy and physiology, and the comprehension of ICD-9 characteristics and terminology. This task requires attention to detail. Work experience and a period of learning with the help of an experienced coder would be very beneficial. In this unit, only a brief introduction to the process is presented. This responsibility can best be learned by actual performance using the code materials provided by your employer. Since various companies produce manuals

with the ICD codes and differing methods of organization of the information, specific directions are not practical. Some examples of manuals are *The Educational Annotation of ICD-9-CM, St. Anthony's ICD-9-CM Code Book for Physician Payment,* and *ICD-9-CM Family Practice Easy Coder.*

The standard codes are taken from the Federal Government's official **Health Care Financing Administration** (HCFA) material. Some coding books arrange diseases and injuries in two volumes.

Volume I— is a tabular list, organized into seventeen chapters with conditions listed by body systems in one chapter and by conditions according to their causes in another chapter. Other information in Volume I is in supplementary classifications such as:

- V-codes—Factors influencing health status and contact with health service.
- E-codes—External cause of injury and poisoning.

Volume I also contains appendices of:

- M-codes—Morphology of Neoplasms.
- Glossary of Mental Disorders.
- Classification of Drugs by the American Hospital Formulary.
- Classification of Industrial Accidents According to Agency.

Volume II—is an alphabetical index organized into three main sections:

- Section 1—Alphabetic Index to Diseases and Injuries.
- Section 2—Table of Drugs and Chemicals.
- Section 3—Index to External Causes of Injuries and Poisonings (for assigning E-codes).

Some references have a Section 4—Index to Procedures, while others have a Volume III, which is used by hospital coders to code procedures (physicians' offices use the CPT coding for their procedures so this section or volume is not used for coding in the medical office).

In addition, many code books have enhancement variations. Some are loose-leafed and some have highlighting of codes to avoid or that require additional information. Some carry additional explanations of diseases or disorders while others are color coded to identify cautions, signs, symptoms, external causes, and so on.

The Easy Coder

The Easy Coder is simply an alphabetical system with diagnoses listed in at least one of three ways: by the key word in the diagnosis, the anatomical site, or the first word in the description exactly as written in the patient's record. Every digit and every code necessary for a diagnosis is provided at the listing for the diagnosis. This system uses a series of symbols and formats to provide coding information.

■ If a code is followed by a # sign, you are to choose the appropriate selection from a corresponding menu to take the code to ultimate specificity.

■ If an additional code is given in a bracket, and it corresponds to documentation in the patient's record, the supplemental code must be used and is sequenced secondarily. Sequence multiple codes from left to right.

■ An underlining of a code number and part of a diagnosis description indicates that the code and that part of the description correspond.

■ Parentheses are used to enclose other words that can be used interchangeably in the diagnosis description and for words used to make the meaning of the description clearer.

Since this format is somewhat different, a sample page is shown in Figure 9–9.

Coding Rules

The general coding rules are:

1. Code correctly and completely any diagnosis or procedure that affects the care, influences the health status, or is a reason for treatment on that visit.
2. Code the minimum number of diagnoses that fully describe the patient's care received on that visit. The diagnosis must reflect the patient's need for treatment, x-rays, diagnostic procedures, or medications.
3. Code each problem to the highest level of specificity (3rd, 4th, or 5th digit) available in the classification (see section on page 218).
4. Sequence codes correctly so that it is possible to understand the chronology of events; for example, the reason for the visit and care.

The main rule to remember is the "**reason rule**," which says that the reason for the patient visit (encounter) is coded first.

	ARTHRITIS
716.9#	NOS
716.2#	ALLERGIC
716.3#	CLIMACTERIC
275.4	CRYSTALS [712.9#]
098.50	GONOCOCCAL
274.0	GOUT
711.9#	INFECTIVE
716.3#	MENOPAUSAL
716.6#	MONOARTICULAR
716.1#	TRAUMATIC

5th Digit: 711.9, 712.9, 716.1-3, 6, 9

0. SITE NOS
1. SHOULDER REGION
2. UPPER ARM (ELBOW) (HUMERUS)
3. FOREARM (RADIUS) (WRIST) (ULNA)
4. HAND (CARPAL) (METACARPAL) (FINGERS)
5. PELVIC REGION AND THIGH (HIP) (BUTTOCK) (FEMUR)
6. LOWER LEG (FIBULA) (KNEE) (PATELLA) (TIBIA)
7. ANKLE AND OR FOOT (METATARSALS) (TOES) (TARSALS)
8. OTHER (HEAD) (NECK) (RIB) (SKULL) (TRUNK) (VERTEBRAE)
9. MULTIPLE

	ARTHRITIS (DEGENERATIVE) - OSTEOARTHRITIS
715.9#	NOS
715.9#	DEGENERATIVE JOINT DISEASE
715.3#	LOCALIZED
715.1#	LOCALIZED PRIMARY (BY JOINT)
715.2#	LOCALIZED SECONDARY (BY JOINT)

5th Digit: 715.1-3, 9

0. SITE UNSPECIFIED
1. SHOULDER REGION
2. UPPER ARM (ELBOW) (HUMERUS)
3. FOREARM (RADIUS) (WRIST) (ULNA)
4. HAND (CARPAL) (METACARPAL) (FINGERS)
5. PELVIC REGION AND THIGH (HIP) (BUTTOCK) (FEMUR)

ARTHRITIS-OSTEOARTHRITIS OF SPINE WITH OSTEOPOROSIS [733.0#] (cont.)

721.3	LUMBOSACRAL
721.42	LUMBOSACRAL WITH MYELOPATHY (CORD COMPRESSION)
721.90	SPINE
721.91	SPINE WITH MYELOPATHY (CORD COMPRESSION)
721.2	THORACIC
721.41	THORACIC WITH MYELOPATHY (CORD COMPRESSION)
721.7	TRAUMATIC
	WITH OSTEOPOROSIS [733.0#]

5th Digit: 733.0

0. UNSPECIFIED
1. SENILE
2. IDIOPATHIC
3. DISUSE
9. DRUG INDUCED

ARTHRITIS RHEUMATOID

720.0	SPINE
714.0	ADULT
714.30	JUVENILE CHRONIC OR UNSPECIFIED
714.33	JUVENILE MONOARTICULAR
714.32	JUVENILE PAUCIARTICULAR
714.31	JUVENILE POLYARTICULAR ACUTE
714.2	WITH VISCERAL OR SYSTEMIC INVOLVEMENT

> THE CODE IN THE LEFT MARGIN ALWAYS SEQUENCES FIRST. THE ADDITIONAL CODE IN BRACKETS TO THE RIGHT OF THE DESCRIPTION IS SEQUENCED SECONDARILY. UNDERLINING SHOWS THE CODE NUMBER THAT CORRESPONDS TO THE UNDERLINED VERBAL DESCRIPTION. UNDERLINING NEVER IMPLIES CORRECT SEQUENCING.

> ALL DIAGNOSES THAT MAY CONTRIBUTE TO THE PATIENT'S RISK OF MORBIDITY OR MORTALITY SHOULD BE CODED. THIS HELPS TO GIVE CARRIERS A CLEARER PICTURE OF THE COMPLEXITY OF THE PATIENT ENCOUNTER

ARTHRITIS OTHER SPECIFIED

FIGURE 9–9 Sample page of ICD-9-CM code book (Courtesy of Unicor Medical, Inc.).

This is **primary**; other "side" issues are coded next, in order of importance. The only exception to this rule applies in a situation when, after the physician has "worked-up" the patient, the major effort is directed toward a diagnosis or procedure different from the one for which the patient originally sought treatment. The diagnosis that required the greater amount of effort should be coded first. At first, coding is confusing and difficult, but with experience, it will become easier.

IDENTIFYING THE DIAGNOSIS

Identifying the diagnosis may be a difficult task for the beginning coder. Remember to follow the rules and suggestions above. Physicians usually help by marking indications on the patient's charge slip or a superbill as well as recording diagnoses on the chart. However, it is necessary for the coder to read the chart, or if employed by a surgeon, the operative report, in order to determine any other codes that might apply or to carry those indicated to the next digit. NOTE: Remember, this affects your rate of payment. Some code books provide cues in their listings. Forms with codes that should be carried to the 4th or 5th digit in order to make the diagnosis more specific, but are not, underline{will be rejected and returned}. To complicate matters further, it seems that the rules are always changing. In 1996, Medicare had made five "changes" by July 1 which affected how claims are filed. One referred to rebundling of codes when multiple procedures are performed and said that generally only reimbursement would be given for the underline{major} procedure. To **bundle** refers to the process of considering several parts as a whole. At other times, Medicare will unbundle a multilevel procedure and allow billing on each portion. The new **truncated** (cut off) ICD-9 coding ruling, which became effective July 1, 1996, stated that claims must be coded to the highest level of specificity or they will be rejected and the provider will be required to file a new claim.

HCFA-1500, the standardized underline{required} form will accept up to four diagnostic codes, see Figure 9–8 (p. 179) line 21. Remember: you only receive reimbursement for procedures or services that relate to the identified diagnostic codes. Again, refer to Figure 9–8 line 21. The form asks you to relate the diagnosis code to the procedure and enter that in line 24 D and E. There must be a reason for the procedure to be done. For example, if a patient just wanted to know his or her blood type, but there was no reason (diagnosis) that the information was necessary, the procedure code would probably be rejected.

While the government was busy publishing the ICD code books, the American Medical Association developed and published *The Physicians' Current Procedural Terminology (CPT)* code book. This is a descriptive listing of codes for reporting medical services and procedures performed by physicians. NOTE: These two standard **nomenclature** code books (ICD, CPT) are published annually and are absolutely essential to the function of the medical office. Each year codes are added, deleted, changed or modified for the new editions. Books can be ordered in advance and are released in the Fall for use beginning on the following January 1. Claim forms may use the new codes after January 1 but must

use them after April 1 or forms will be returned to the providers.

CURRENT PROCEDURAL TERMINOLOGY CODES (CPT)

CPT Fourth Edition is a systematic listing and coding of procedures and services performed by physicians. Each procedure or service is identified with a five digit code which is used to report services. The main body of the material is listed in six sections:

1. Evaluation and Management (E/M)
2. Anesthesiology
3. Surgery
4. Radiology (including Nuclear Medicine and Diagnostic Ultrasound)
5. Pathology and Laboratory
6. Medicine (except Anesthesiology)

Within each section are subsections with anatomic, procedure, condition, or descriptor subheadings. The procedures and services with their identifying codes are presented in **numeric** order with one exception: the entire Evaluation and Management section is placed at the beginning of the listed procedures. These items are used by most physicians in reporting a significant portion of their services. At the end of the book are the appendix and the index. Following the index is a page listing instructions for the use of the CPT index. The index has six general categories. Each category has examples to assist the user in understanding the category.

Using the CPT Book

To determine a code, the name of the procedure or service that most accurately identifies the service performed is selected. This could be a diagnostic procedure, radiological examination, or surgery. Other additional procedures performed or pertinent services may be listed including any modifying or extenuating circumstances. Any service or procedure which is coded must be adequately documented in the medical record. As with ICD-9 codes, you can rely on the physician for assistance. Generally, services performed in the office are marked on the patient's charge slip. Care must be taken not to miss items like injections, urinalysis, or blood samples, or the need to use a **modifier** for prolonged E/M services. If you must code from operative reports, it will be necessary to review the description the surgeon dictated to be certain all pertinent codes have been identified.

The introduction in the CPT code book gives excellent instructions on the use of CPT terminology and coding. The book is divided into specialty sections, but codes from any section may be used to give an adequate description of a treatment or procedure rendered by a qualified physician. In reading the introduction, you will find guidelines are presented at the beginning of each section to define items that are necessary to interpret and report the procedure and services to be found in that section. In some instances a specific procedure or service may need to be slightly altered. Instructions and the appendix explains the use of modifiers.

Some examples of when these would be used are if unusual events occurred, if a service was performed by more than one physician, or if a procedure had both professional and technical components. Other examples are listed.

If you cannot find a code listed for a procedure or service your employer has performed, a provision has been made for the use of specific code numbers for reporting unlisted procedures. In these instances a description of the service must also be provided.

It is important to use a current year's code book to check the codes you are using to be sure they have not been changed. A special appendix in the book provides a complete list of the codes deleted, revised, and added to the book. Another detail requiring attention is the superbill or charge slip. Usually they are preprinted with the most frequently used ICD-9 and CPT codes listed in order to facilitate coding by the physician and insurance coder. When new books are issued, these frequent codes especially need to be checked prior to date deadline. If changes have occurred, the slip may need reprinting.

New procedure numbers (codes) added to the CPT are identified throughout the text with a "●" placed before the code number. Where there is a code revision in a substantially altered procedure descriptor, the symbol "▲" is placed before the code number. Figure 9–10 shows codes from CPT 1996. This coding deals with surgery of the nervous system and shows a great deal of new and revised codes. The "*" symbol denotes that the service includes a surgical procedure only. If you look further, you will read of other procedures listed in parentheses and see codes which have been deleted along with one to use for reporting instead.

The AMA also makes available magnetic computer tapes and floppy disk formats of the CPT manual. One tape presentation is the complete procedural text of the manual while the other is a CPT short description tape. The short description tape also contains the complete listing of procedural codes in the manual but each has an abbreviated narrative written in non-technical terms. The floppy disk version is identical in content to the short description tape. The tape formats have some advantages over the floppy disk format: faster and easier coding as well as the elimination of manual coding errors.

E/M SERVICES GUIDELINES

This section is divided into twenty broad categories such as office visits, hospital visits, preventative medicine, and consultations. Most of the categories are further divided into two or more subcategories of services. The subcategories are then classified into levels of E/M services that are identified by specific codes. This classification is important because the nature of the physician's work varies by type and place of service and the patient's status.

The basic format of the levels is the same for most categories. First a unique code number is listed. Then, the place and/or type of service is specified. Third, the content of the service is defined, whether it is problem focused, expanded, detailed, or comprehensive. Fourth, the nature of the presenting problem is described, and fifth, the time typically required to provide the service is specified. Another classi-

▲62274* Injection of diagnostic or therapeutic anesthetic or antispasmodic substance (including narcotics); subarachnoid or subdural, single

62275* epidural, cervical or thoracic, single

62276* subarachnoid

62287 Aspiration procedure, percutaneous, of nucleus pulposus of intervertebral disk, any method, single or multiple levels, lumbar

●62350 Implantation, revision or repositioning of intrathecal or epidural catheter, for implantable reservoir or implantable infusion pump; without laminectomy

●62351 with laminectomy

FIGURE 9–10 Sample CPT-96 codes showing procedures and symbols to denote new, revised, and surgery only changes (CPT codes, descriptions and numeric modifiers only are copyright 1996 American Medical Association. All Rights Reserved.).

fication which affects coding is whether the patient is new or established.

Within each category or subcategory of E/M services, three to five levels are available for reporting purposes. The levels include examinations, evaluations, treatments, conferences with or concerning patients, preventative pediatric and adult health supervision, and similar medical services. The levels encompass wide variations in skill, effort, time, responsibility and medical knowledge required for the prevention or diagnosis and treatment of illness or injury.

In addition to the levels are descriptors which recognize seven components that are used in defining the levels of E/M services:

1. history
2. examination
3. medical decision making
4. counseling
5. coordination of care
6. nature of presenting problem
7. time

The first three are considered key components in selecting a level of E/M services. The next three and the nature of the presenting problem are considered **contributory** factors in the majority of **encounters** (contacts). It is not required that these services be provided at every patient encounter. The actual performance of any diagnostic test or study requires separate specific coding in addition to the appropriate E/M code. Several other items unique to the section are described in the E/M guidelines, which are fairly easy to read and understand. If you refer to the first page of the E/M section of the CPT code book, you will see codes for a new patient that show two levels of history and examination.

COMPLETING THE CLAIM FORM

Before claims are processed, be certain that you have a copy of the patient's insurance coverage card and have secured their signature on a form to permit release of information. This form will also have an "assignment of benefits" clause which authorizes benefits be paid directly to the provider.

Today the patient has little or no responsibility for filing claims. The physician is <u>required</u> to file **Medicare** claims and it is normally an obligation when contracting as a provider with other carriers. Once the physician has billed the primary coverage and they have responded, either the carrier will automatically forward the claim to a secondary carrier, or the physician as a courtesy may choose to file for the secondary coverage. Often this is to the physicians' advantage as the supplemental amount is usually paid directly to them. After primary and secondary carriers have responded, the remaining approved amount must be billed to the patient for payment.

As stated previously, government sponsored health care claims must be filed on the HCFA-1500 approved insurance claim form (refer to Figure 9–8). Regulations also require that the form be an original; copies are not acceptable. Procedure 9–1 "Completing the Claim Form" will give you some practice in preparing a form. Physicians can obtain packages of fifty to as many as 1000 sheets through the AMA. Other suppliers, including the government, are available. The forms come as straight forms or with pinfeed edges for use with computer printers. In addition to government mandatory use, all other insurance companies will accept the form. This is helpful, especially with patients who have **secondary** coverage; it eliminates the need to complete two forms. Even if the secondary carrier has its own claim form, a copy of the HCFA-1500 can be attached and will be acceptable.

It is very important to photocopy all completed forms before mailing in order to have a record of the form. Some offices file claim forms in an insurance folder until payment is received; then, they are filed in the respective patient's chart.

MAINTAINING AN INSURANCE LOG

A method for monitoring the status and payment of insurance claims should be established. It is easy to forget about filed claims and soon a sizeable amount of money is owed to the physician. Some practices use an insurance log. When a claim is filed, it is noted on a log. The log should have columns for recording pertinent information. The following would be helpful in monitoring claim status:

- the date the claim is filed
- the insurance company
- the patient's name
- the amount of the claim
- the amount paid
- secondary company
- date filed
- amount billed
- amount paid
- date the patient was billed
- the follow-up date

By looking at the log, you can quickly see the status of each claim. If claims become delinquent, a carrier can be easily identified and contacted. As a general rule, claims are paid in a timely fashion after billing, usually within thirty to sixty days. At times, a carrier will deny ever receiving a claim. This is when a copy will be helpful because it will be necessary to refile. When claims are <u>not</u> approved or are rejected because of errors, you will be able to refile upon submitting additional information or documenting the charge. When a claim is returned after being denied, it may not be eligible for refiling.

DELINQUENT CLAIMS

If a claim has not been paid and you have not received a denial, it is time to follow up. Most carriers provide a toll-free telephone number on their claim form. Before you make the call, be sure you have the following information available: patient's name, identification number, group name or number, and if the patient <u>is not</u> the insured, the insured's (spouse's) name. Once the account is identified, they will request the date(s) of service and the total amount submitted. The carrier will then give you the status of the claim. If it is still in process, request an anticipated date of payment. If the claim is delayed pending additional information, be sure to follow up quickly and return the material requested. If the company has no record of receiving a claim, ask if you may submit a <u>copy</u> of the claim previously submitted and verify the mailing address. Also ask if you could direct the claim to a specific person to accelerate the process. It is helpful to have a specific contact person in case further discussion is necessary. If the carrier indicates that the claim has been paid, ask when the payment was made and to whom it was sent. If it was sent to the patient, you will need to send the patient a statement.

COMMON CLAIM ERRORS

In a recent survey of insurance companies, the following common errors were listed as causes of claim payment delays:

1. The patient's—not the policyholder's—Social Security number is used as the certificate number. The claim would be rejected for lack of membership.
2. The "Coordination of Benefits" section is not completed, thereby suspending the claim for additional information.
3. Use of incorrect ICD-9 (International Classification of Diseases) codes.
4. Use of an incorrect or deleted CPT code could result in a decreased payment or a rejection.
5. Use of incorrect provider identification number could result in misdirection of payment.
6. Superbills attached to a claim form are sometimes illegible. Always attach additional information to back of claim, upper left-hand corner.
7. Member does not respond to the request for clarification of insurances covering injury or illness when another party might have responsibility.
8. Lack of operative report if procedure is unusual, complicated, or fee is unusual.
9. Incorrect spelling of patient's name.
10. Inconsistent use of patient's name will suspend claim processing; for example, middle name is used as first,

nicknames are used instead of correct first name (Bill instead of William).

11. An incorrect patient birthdate is reported.
12. Use of an incorrect place of service code will suspend a claim.

ELECTRONIC CLAIM FILING

Many offices are now electing to electronically process claim forms to the insurance carrier. The "turn around time" is shortened and there is a reduction in preparation time. The system does require that you purchase a software program that can be accessed by the carrier. A new service has evolved from this technology. Offices can now enter information and codes in a program and then submit it to an intermediary clearing house service. The service screens the forms for coding errors, returns those needing corrections, and forwards claims to the carrier via whichever program the carrier requires. The cost of the service is considered money well spent because the claims are "clean" when submitted and reimbursement is received within a couple of weeks. A hard copy of the claims is kept on file until electronic processing is completed.

ACCEPTING ASSIGNMENT

Medicare and other carriers enlist physicians to "sign up" as approved or **preferred** providers. Usually, the physician agrees to treat people enrolled in the program for an "agreed" rate for services. This rate is referred to as a **fee schedule**. In return for being willing to participate and accept a reduction in charges, the physician is assured a supply of patients enrolled in the health care program of the provider. Physicians often contract with many carriers in order to be able to provide services for a large group of current as well as future patients. (This concept was covered earlier in this chapter when carriers and managed care were discussed.) Particularly with Medicare patients, the contracted provider agrees to accept the "approved amount" as their fee and the agreement is known as "accepting assignment." The difference between the amount charged and the fee received is "written off" by the physician as uncollectible. The physician or any other provider can charge the patient only for the part of the deductible that has not been met and the small "left over" balance from the approved charge. The provider can also charge for any service not covered by Medicare. If your physician is making a charge for a non-covered service, be certain the patient understands that the charges will be their responsibility. It is a good idea to have a statement signed by the patient which states the fee is not covered so that the patient cannot later refuse to pay and claim non-coverage was unknown. NOTE: All physicians, whether they choose to participate or not, must abide by Medicare laws. When the doctor does not accept assignment, they must be paid directly by the patient who is responsible for the entire bill even if it is higher than the Medicare-approved amount. Even though a doctor does not accept assignment, the most that can be charged is 115% of what Medicare approves. Doctors and other providers who exceed limits can be fined.

MEDICARE AUDIT

The importance of complete records and documentation is never as critical as when the office is involved in a Medicare audit. Audits may be conducted if there is any question as to the amount of service rendered in exchange for the claims paid. Records are essential to provide evidence that diagnoses and treatments were appropriate and that the services paid for were actually provided. The level of service must also be documented. Failure to adequately document the level of service could cause a downcoding by Medicare and can result in the charge of "fraud" with a $2000 fine per infraction. Documentation is essential. Remember: when records are reviewed by third-party payers, "If it is not documented, it was never done." Office staffs should monitor physicians' records and inform them if necessary, of what is needed. Not only does it ensure adequate documentation but it also ensures that the physician receives the maximum reimbursement due. Of the following seven items, at least five must be documented in the office medical records:

- Complaints and/or symptoms
- Duration and/or course of illness
- Details of illness
- Examination and findings
- Laboratory and/or x-ray values and findings
- Diagnosis and/or problem
- Treatment, injection, or advice

REIMBURSEMENT

Medicare reimburses the approved fee at the rate of 80% after the year's $100 deductible amount has been paid by the patient. Secondary payment is then sought to cover the 20% not covered. Many secondary carriers likewise will pay 80% of the 20% not covered of the approved amount, after the deductible is met. The remaining small percentage and the initial annual deductible is the responsibility of the patient. Figure 9–11 is a summary of the Medicare and secondary insurance "explanation of benefits" reports, resulting from an actual minor medical situation, in the approximate order they were received. In this example, the patient is a sixty-five-year-old female who had a suspicious mammogram which resulted in an incisional biopsy of two areas of microcalcification within the same breast. The procedure was performed in the "same-day surgery" department of a hospital. The importance of detailed descriptions, procedure codes, and accurate records is very evident. With insurance payment of medical charges, there are several factors to be considered: annual deductibles, approved fee schedules, and percentages of approval rates which all influence the amount paid. Review the summary. Notice how much of the charges are approved and how much is the patient's responsibility. Follow the initial charges through deductibles, Medicare, secondary coverage, sometimes refiling, and finally the patient's responsibility. This excessive amount of "paper work" is a good example of why patients become so confused with insurance coverage and payment, and why medical assistants never get finished filing claims.

9-1　Complete a Claim Form

PURPOSE: To accurately complete a claim form for processing.

EQUIPMENT: Appropriate form, patient record, account ledger/information, typewriter or computer.

TERMINAL PERFORMANCE OBJECTIVE: Given access to all necessary equipment and information, follow the procedure to complete the HCFA-1500 claim form without error within the instructor's prescribed time limit.

1. Check for a photocopy of the patient's insurance card.
2. Check the chart to see if the patient signature is on file for release of information and assignment of benefits.
   NOTE: If not on file, the patient must sign the form. It is best to have it signed before the form is completed. If the completed form is forwarded to the patient to be signed and sent to the insurance company, it is best to send a stamped and addressed envelope so there will not be a delay in forwarding the form to the insurance company.
3. Using Figure 9–8 as a guide, complete the following entries:
   1. Check appropriate box at top of form
   2. Enter name of patient (Be certain the name used on the form is the same as that on the identification card.)
   3. Enter birth date and check box for male or female
      NOTE: Use six digits to write birthdate, i.e., 02/17/21
4. Enter insured's name.
5. Enter patient's full address and telephone number.
6. Enter patient's relationship to insured.
7. Enter insured's full address and telephone number.
8. Enter patient's status.
9. Enter other insured's name.
   - Other insured's policy or group number
   - Other insured's birthdate and box for male or female
   - Employer's name or school name
   - Insurance plan name or program name
     (Fill in "none" or N/A, for not applicable, so there is no doubt you have observed this section.)
10. Check the appropriate box regarding employment and accident. (Do not leave all these boxes blank.)
11. Enter insured's policy number.
    - Insured's birthdate and box for male or female

- Employer or school name
- Insurance plan name or program name
- Is there another health benefit plan?

12. Obtain patients or authorized persons signature.
13. Obtain insured signature or stamp "signature on file" if you have the record to prove it.
14. Record the date current illness began
15. Record the date patient was first treated for same or similar illness.
16. Enter dates unable to work or state N/A.
17. Complete with name of referring physician or state N/A.
17a. Enter ID number of referring physician.
18. Complete with dates of hospitalization or state N/A.
19. Leave blank.
20. Mark appropriate box regarding lab.
21. Enter ICD codes on separate line for each diagnosis.
22. Complete if Medicaid.
23. Complete if applicable with medical authorization code.
24. Complete A through G with appropriate codes for services.
    NOTE: List each service separately with the most important listed first.
25. Add the physician's Social Security number or practice tax identification number and mark the appropriate box.
26. Add patient's account number if applicable.
27. Check one box regarding assignment.
    NOTE: Must be marked "yes" to accept assignment
28. Total charged.
29. Amount paid.
30. Any balance due.
    NOTE: Form will be rejected if not completed.
31. Obtain physician's signature and date.
    NOTE: Medicare will accept stamped signature.
32. Name and address of facility where services were rendered, if other than home or office.
33. Physician's name, address, and telephone number and specific identification numbers for Medicare or other group plan if applicable.

THE FUTURE OF INSURANCE CLAIMS

As long as there are third-party payers, the filing of some sort of claim will continue. Probably the greatest change will come in how the filing is done. It would seem feasible that more providers will take advantage of the electronic process. With the capability of computer programs, it should be possible to develop software that, given a diagnosis, automatically identifies coding, sequences it, and compares it to the treatment codes. An annual update for the program to screen for any changed, added, or deleted codes would also be a benefit. This would eliminate much of the rejection and refiling problems. A built-in fee by the carriers for the physician's filing expenses would also be an excellent update. Currently, additional costs for equipment, personnel, continuing education, and supplies, as well as space, has to be covered from the reimbursement which has been reduced by approval rates.

DATE OF FORM	DATE OF SERVICE	SOURCE OF FORM	PROVIDER OF SERVICE	SERVICE PROVIDED—CODE	CHARGE	MEDICARE APPROVED	MEDICARE PAID	SECONDARY INSURANCE PAID	PATIENT RESPONSIBILITY	COMMENTS
1995										
10/9	9/27	Medicare	Radiologist #1	Mammogram—7609L XA Both Breasts	$135.00	$65.91	-0-	-0-	$65.91	$65.91 applied to '95 deductible
11/2	10/3	Medicare	Surgeon	Office consult—99242	$105.00	$69.16	$28.06	-0-	$41.10	$34.09 applied to '95 deductible
11/10	10/11	Medicare	Primary physician	Office consult—99243 / ECG—93000 / Chest x-ray—71020-XA / Blood draw—60001- / $260.00	$130.00 / 54.00 / 69.00 / 7.00 / $260.00	$85.85 / 26.49 / 32.84 / 3.00 / $148.00	$119.14		$29.04	$3 chg paid at 100%—$145.00 applied to deductible and co-pay
11/30	10/17	Medicare	Radiologist #2	Place needlewire—19290 / X-ray needlewire placement in breast—76096-26 / X-ray specimen—76098-26	$175.00 / 133.50 / 20.50 / $329.00	$69.93 / 29.21 / 8.08 / $107.22	$85.77	-0-	$21.45	1995 deductible met
11/30	10/17	Medicare	Surgeon	Excision breast lesion—19125	$800.00	$348.16	$278.53	-0-	$69.63	—
11/20	10/17	Medicare	Anesthesia-#1	4.3 Anesthesia—00400—Chest skin surgery QKQS	$350.40	-0-	-0-	-0-	-0-	Requested information had not been received.
11/20	10/17	Medicare	Pathologist	1 Tissue exam—88305-26 / 1 Tissue exam—88307-26 / 1 Consult in surgery—88329	$165.00 / 230.00 / 70.00 / $465.00	$50.35 / 86.47 / 38.52 / $175.34	$140.28		$35.06	Deductible met / Other insurance may pay
11/20	10/17	Medicare	Anesthesia-#2	4.3 Anesthesia—00400 QKQS Chest skin surgery	$111.25	-0-	-0-	-0-	$111.25	Charges denied, other insurance may pay
12/2	10/11	Insurance	Primary physician	Medical x-ray, testing	$260.00	$148.00	$119.14	$23.24	$5.80	Deductible met
12/14	10/3	Insurance	Surgeon	Medical	$105.00	$69.16	$28.06	$32.88	$8.22	—
12/15	10/17	Medicare	Hospital	Laboratory / Radiology / Pharmacy / Surgical service	$155.00 / 399.00 / 182.88 / 2317.92 / $3,054.80	$1,527.40	$916.44	-0-	$610.96	Deductible met
1996										
1/5	10/3 and 10/17	Statement	Surgeon	Balance after insurance payments	$110.73	—	—	$32.88	$77.85	Remaining balance due
1/16	10/11	Statement	Primary physician	Balance after insurance payments	$260.00	$148.00	$119.14	$23.24	$5.80	Remaining balance due
1/27	10/17	Insurance	Hospital	Surgical services	$3,054.80	$1,527.40	$916.44	$610.96	-0-	Paid in full by insurance
2/12	10/17	Statement	Radiologist #2	X-ray services balance after insurance payments	$329.00	$107.22	$85.77	-0-	$21.45	Balance due
1/26	10/17	Insurance	Radiologist #2	X-ray services balance after insurance payments	$329.00	$107.22	$85.77	$17.16	$4.29	Remaining balance due

FIGURE 9-11 Summary of insurance explanation of benefits form and medical statements received in connection with one routine breast incisional biopsy procedure.

MAINTAINING CURRENCY

Staying informed and up-to-date with Medicare is a never ending process. Ideally, in each practice, someone is designated as the claims filer and is expected to maintain currency. This can be done in various ways. Medicare updates are discussed in bulletins sent monthly to the practice. Many practice specialty organizations will have newsletters, specific to their needs, to keep members informed. Other insurance carriers will send newsletters to their participating physicians describing any changes in their coverage or processing. Seminars are conducted frequently. The annual major update seminar sponsored by your state medical association is practically a requirement in order for any practice to survive. Other seminars are conducted by private companies and can prove very informative. The con-

tent, of course, depends upon the amount of time and the expertise or focus of the presenting organization. It is very important that you closely review any inservice advertisement. It should identify the content, perhaps include an outline, and if objectives are listed, give you a good idea of expected outcomes. Another assurance of its value is the approval for CEUs by the AAMA or the ARMA. If not preapproved, however, remember that you can submit information and request CEUs for educational seminars you attend, but approval is not ensured. Make certain you understand what is being offered and to what extent it will be presented so that your investment of time and money will be worthwhile.

Complete Chapter 9, Unit 3 in the workbook to help you meet the objectives at the beginning of this unit and therefore achieve competency of this subject matter.

Medical-Legal Ethical Highlights

Throughout this chapter you should be mindful of the medical-legal/ethical implications. Listed below are a few important reminders.

1. Obtain and file written authorization for release of information.
2. Obtain written contract if third party is responsible for payment of medical treatment.
3. Maintain careful records in handling patient claim forms.
4. Respect patients' privacy and confidentiality.

Ms. Right . . .

keeps proper authorization forms and other important documents filed in patients' charts as they are received. She checks for signatures as necessary on claim forms and never releases any information to anyone unless she first checks for the appropriate forms. She keeps abreast of any changes in claims processing or coding procedures to ensure a proper

and efficient payment schedule. She makes sure that a copy of each claim form is made and placed in the patient's chart before sending it to be processed. She respects patients' privacy.

Advancement potential: Excellent.

Miss. Wrong . . .

obtains and files proper authorization forms with signatures when she remembers it. She is careless in her filing of claim forms and other important information. She neglects to read about changes in claims processing or coding procedures and therefore payment is held up until corrections are made. She never makes copies of forms before sending to be processed. She has a habit of discussing patient information with other patients and friends, as well as in public.

Advancement potential: None.

REFERENCES

American Medical Association. *The Physicians' Current Procedural Terminology,* 1996.

Andress, A. A. (1996). *Saunder's Manual of Medical Office Management.* Philadelphia, PA: W. B. Saunders.

Fordney, Marilyn. *Insurance Handbook for the Medical Office.* Philadelphia: W. B. Saunders, 1989.

Harvard Health Letter, special supplement. (April, 1996). Boston MA: Harvard Medical School.

Health Care Management Advisors, Inc. Introduction of CPT- (videos), 1993.

Nationwide Insurance Enterprises. *The Medicare Part B Medical Policy Manual,* Columbus, OH: January, 1996.

Rowell, Jo Ann. *Understanding Medical Insurance: A Step-By-Step Guide, 2E,* (1994). Albany, NY: Delmar Publishers.

Unicor Medical, Inc. *Easy Coder,* Montgomery, 1996.

United States Department of Health & Human Services. *International Classification of Diseases,* 1996.

Webster's New Dictionary, (1994). Springfield, MA: Merriam-Webster.

Medical Office Management

Many different methods are used to affect the overall management of the medical office. A one- or two-physician office that employs only a few people could assign someone to deal with all the office management duties. Most physicians find that a professional accounting firm or professional management company is best suited for the preparation of tax forms and financial statements and maintenance of salary records. Medical assistants with adequate office experience and management abilities are often selected to be the office manager. However, large group practices, clinics, and physician corporations with several physicians and many employees may choose an individual with a business background or degree to be the office manager or elect to use a professional management service, in addition to an accountant.

It would be impossible to include specific management instruction in this text to cover all variables because individual physician preference results in a wide array of possibilities. Therefore, this chapter discusses the general administrative duties and responsibilities of the medical assistant and also includes information regarding the role of an office manager. Regardless of who is serving as manager, you should be aware of the records the accountants will need. You will probably be responsible for maintaining certain financial and tax records.

The physician places great confidence in a manager to handle efficiently and accurately the business affairs of the office. The following units outline the skills and duties related to the fiscal and physical operation of a medical office and include such things as:

- Processing received payments for banking
- Preparing checks for office expenses
- Maintaining office accounting records
- Maintaining employer records

- Maintaining office equipment
- Obtaining essential reference materials
- Attending office management update seminars

UNIT 1
The Language of Banking

UNIT 2
Currency, Checks, and Petty Cash

UNIT 3
Salary, Benefits, and Tax Records

UNIT 4
General Management Duties

UNIT 1

The Language of Banking

■ OBJECTIVES

Upon completion of the unit, meet the following terminal performance objectives by verifying knowledge of the facts and principles presented through oral and written communication at a level deemed competent.

1. Differentiate between savings and checking accounts.
2. Explain the significance of the ABA and MICR codes.
3. Define the banking terms listed in this unit.
4. Differentiate between cashier's, certified, limited, postdated, stale, traveler's, and voucher checks.
5. Explain the difference between overdraft and overdrawn.
6. Discuss the "stop payment" process.

7. Spell and define, using the glossary at the back of the text, all the words to know in this unit.

■ WORDS TO KNOW

agent	issue
certified	negotiable
currency	payee
deposit	power of attorney
endorsement	warrant
insufficient	withdrawal

This unit presents the most common banking terms with their definitions to help you understand financial transactions. The medical assistant must have a good working knowledge of banking and basic accounting procedures. These skills are not only important in the physician's office but also in the management of your own personal finances.

BANKING TERMS

■ *ABA number.* A code number found in the right upper corner of a printed check. It may be above the check number on a business check or below the check number on a personal check. This number was originated by the American Bankers Association. The purpose is to have a method of identifying the area where the bank on which the check is written is located, and to identify the bank within the area. It may be written as a fraction: $\frac{51-44}{119}$ on a business check, or 25-2/440 on a personal check.

■ *Agent.* An agent is a person authorized to act for another person. You are the agent for your employer in the office. Bank officials are agents for the bank.

■ *ATM.* An automated teller machine (ATM) is a banking machine operated with the insertion of a credit or bank card and the entering of a personal identification number (PIN) code. Deposits, transfers, withdrawals, and other banking functions can be performed at the ATM location.

■ *Bankbook.* In the case of a savings account it is called a savings passbook and contains a record of deposits, withdrawals, and interest earned, with the dates of all the transactions. This book must be presented with each deposit or withdrawal. At regular intervals, usually quarterly, interest earnings are credited to an account. These earnings should be entered in the passbook by the bank. Some banks indicate the passbook should be presented for interest entry at least once in a three-year period.

■ *Bank statement.* A record of a checking account sent to the customer, usually on a monthly basis, showing the beginning balance, all deposits made, all checks drawn, all bank charges, and the closing balance. The customer's canceled checks are returned with the statement.

■ *Cashier's check.* The purchaser pays the bank the full amount of the check. The bank then writes a check on its own account payable to the party specified. This type of check "guarantees" to the recipient that the full amount of money indicated on the check will be paid on processing.

■ *Certified check.* The bank stamps the customer's own check *certified* and then holds the certified amount in reserve in the customer's account until the check is cashed. This is a guaranteed check and so is always acceptable when a personal check is not.

■ *Check register.* Also referred to as a check stub. It is a record showing the check number, person to whom check is paid, amount of check, date, and balance, and is kept by the person writing the check, as a record of the transaction.

■ *Checking account.* A bank account against which checks may be written. The bank will **issue** the checks and deposit slips.

■ *Currency.* Paper money issued by the government.

■ *Deposit.* An amount of money (cash and/or checks) placed in a bank account.

■ *Deposit record.* A record of a deposit that is given to the customer at the time of the deposit. It is important to keep the deposit record as proof of the deposit in case the bank fails to list the deposit on the bank statement.

■ *Deposit slip.* An itemized list of cash and checks deposited in a checking account. It is important to keep a copy of all deposit slips.

■ *Electronic fund transfer systems.* Methods of crediting or debiting accounts by computer without checks or deposit slips.

■ *Endorsement.* The payee's signature on the back of a check. It is a transfer of title on the check to the bank in exchange for the amount of money on the face of the check.

■ *Endorser.* The payee on a check. If the name is spelled incorrectly on the face of the check, it should be endorsed in the same way and then endorsed correctly.

■ *Insufficient funds.* A bank term used to indicate that the writer of the check did not have enough money in his or her account to cover the check. An office usually has a policy regarding returned checks, which normally involves contacting the patient immediately, asking the person to pick up the check and bring a cash payment. These checks are sometimes described as *bounced,* and the account is called *overdrawn.*

■ *Limited check.* A check that will be marked void if written over a certain amount. These checks are often used for payroll or for insurance payments. A check may also list a time limit during which it must be cashed. It must be cashed within the time limit or you will find it is not **negotiable**.

■ *Maker.* The individual who signs a check or the corporation that pays it.

■ *MICR.* Magnetic Ink Character Recognition. This technique consists of characters and numbers printed in magnetic ink at the bottom left side of checks and deposit slips, Figures 10–1 and 10–2. This information is specific to each checking account and is imprinted on each check and deposit slip by the company printing the checks. The first series of numbers is the routing information that identifies the bank and area. The second series identifies the account numbers. The last series corresponds to the check number. When the bank processes the check, additional magnetic ink

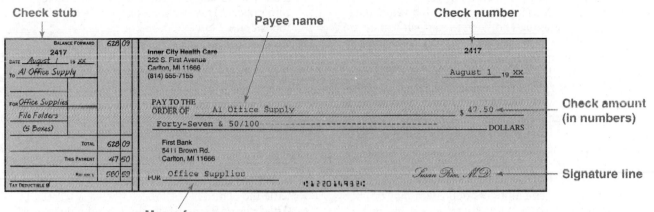

Check stub

Payee name

Check number

Check amount (in numbers)

Signature line

Memo for disbursement

FIGURE 10–1 Check, check stub, and register.

numbers are printed across the bottom identifying the amount of the check. These characters and numbers can be read by high-speed machinery, which greatly enhances the bookkeeping procedures in the bank by simplifying the sorting of checks and the printing of individual monthly statements.

- *Money order.* Negotiable instrument often used by individuals who do not have checking accounts or to meet the requirement for purchasing an item or service. Money orders may be purchased for a fee from banks, credit unions, post offices, and many other money order service locations.
- *Note.* Legal evidence of a debt. A promissory note is a written promise to pay. A collateral note is a written promise to pay with the additional requirement that the maker of the note must list marketable securities that may be sold by the creditor if the maker does not pay the note within the time limit promised.
- *One-write check writing.* System that makes it possible to make a record on a check register as you write a check. This is excellent for payroll because you can record deductions for the employee and office records in one writing.
- *Overdraft checking accounts.* Accounts that allow checks to be written for a larger amount than is currently in the account. The overdraft is covered by the bank in the form of a loan for which interest is charged.
- *Payee.* The person to whom a check is written. The name of the payee is listed on the check after the words *Pay to the order of.*

CHECKS LIST SINGLY	DOLLARS	CENTS
1		
2		
3		
4		
5		
6		
7		
8		
9		
10		
11		
12		
13		
14		
15		
16		
17		
18		
19		
TOTAL		

ENTER TOTAL ON THE FRONT OF THIS TICKET

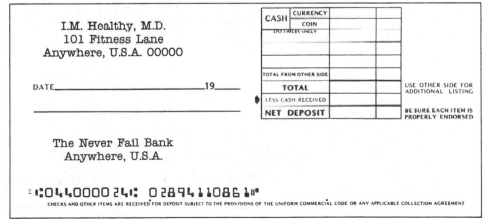

FIGURE 10–2 Deposit slip.

■ *Payer.* The person who signs the check.

■ *Postdated check.* A check made out with a future date. You may have patients who wish to pay while they are in the office but will not have the money in their account until next pay day, which is the date they will put on the check. Never deposit these checks until the date for which they are made out. This practice is illegal in some states; be sure you know the law in your state.

■ *Power of Attorney.* A legal procedure that authorizes one person to act as an agent for another. This is often necessary when patients are not physically or mentally capable of taking care of their own financial affairs.

■ *Savings account.* A bank account upon which the depositor earns interest. The amounts deposited may be recorded in a passbook. (Note that many banks now also give interest on checking accounts if a minimum balance is maintained.)

■ *Service charge.* Fees charged by the bank on a monthly basis for services rendered. If a specified minimum balance is maintained in the account the bank may not charge because they have the use of that money. Some banks charge for every transaction, whether putting money in or writing checks.

■ *Special checking account.* Many different names and definitions apply, depending on the area of the country. It may be an account on which interest is paid if an established minimum balance is maintained in the account; an account for senior citizens for which no handling charges are made; or a fee for checks only. Banks are continually offering new plans to attract depositors.

■ *Stale check.* A check presented too long after it was written to be honored by the bank. Some checks specify that they must be cashed within ninety days and if presented after that date the bank will not honor payment. A period of six months is generally considered enough time for a check to be presented for payment.

■ *Stop payment.* A method by which the maker of a check may stop payment. The bank charges a sizable fee for this service. Some banks will accept a stop order by phone if it is promptly followed by completion of a form, which the bank furnishes. The payer must furnish the number of the check, date issued, name of payee, amount of check, and the reason for stopping payment. The bank will then refuse to honor the check. A stop payment order is used when a check is lost or if there is a disagreement regarding a product or service received.

■ *Teller.* The bank employee who is the main contact between the customer and the bank.

■ *Traveler's check.* A special check used by individuals who are traveling and do not wish to carry a large amount of cash. Personal checks are usually not accepted outside of the area of the bank upon which they are drawn. Therefore, in exchange for cash, banks will issue traveler's checks. These must be signed individually at the time of purchase and again when they are used. They are usually considered the same as cash, but some merchants still require some identification before they accept a traveler's check. Lost traveler's checks can usually be replaced if you can produce a list of their serial numbers. Traveler's checks are listed as checks on a deposit slip.

■ *Voucher check.* A check with a detachable voucher form that is used to show the reason for which the check was drawn. This kind of check is often used by insurance companies. The voucher form is removed before the check is endorsed and deposited.

■ *Warrant.* This evidence of a debt due but is not negotiable. It can be converted into a negotiable instrument or cash. An insurance adjustor may issue a warrant as evidence that a claim should be paid. The warrant authorizes the insurance company to issue a check to settle the claim.

■ *Withdrawal.* Removal of funds from a depositor's account. This may be done by means of a passbook, a withdrawal slip, a check, or electronic fund transfer.

Complete Chapter 10, Unit 1 in the workbook to help you meet the objectives at the beginning of this unit and therefore achieve competency of this subject matter.

UNIT 2

Currency, Checks, and Petty Cash

■ OBJECTIVES

Upon completion of the unit, meet the following terminal performance objectives by verifying knowledge of the facts and principles presented through oral and written communication at a level deemed competent, and demonstrate the specific behaviors as identified in the terminal performance objectives of the procedures.

1. Write a check.
2. Discuss precautions with checks received from patients.
3. Explain blank and restrictive endorsement.
4. Prepare a bank deposit.
5. Discuss special concerns with mail deposits.
6. Reconcile office records with bank statements.
7. Discuss establishing and maintaining a petty cash fund.
8. Spell and define, using the glossary at the back of the text, all the words to know in this unit.

■ WORDS TO KNOW

authorization	third party
depleted	transaction
reconcile	void
register	voucher

WRITING CHECKS

The medical assistant may often be required to write checks to pay for equipment, supplies, or wages. These are then given to the physician for signature before being mailed or otherwise distributed, see Figure 10–1. Some physicians will give check signature power to an office manager to eliminate the need for their personal signature. A signature **authorization** card obtained from the bank must be completed to allow someone other than the recorded owner of the account to execute checks. Some offices, as a means of monitoring expenditures and preventing employee embezzlement, require two signatures on a check or have a policy that the individual writing the check (e.g., bookkeeper) must have another authorized person (often the office manager) sign the check. This also provides an opportunity to question expenditures and maintain a sense of cash flow. Practice preparing checks by following Procedure 10–1 and using the workbook samples.

One area of expenditure that must be carefully monitored is payment of invoices for office equipment and supplies. When a statement is received from a supplier, it is essential to know that everything on the invoice and the amount or number of each item(s) has, in fact, been received. The shipment must be compared to packing slips or invoices at the time they are received and notification of any discrepancy made to the supplier. Frequently, partial shipments are sent and some items are on back order. Payment of the total amount of the invoice would represent payment for goods not received. Some difficulty may also arise in trying to obtain materials not sent once you have paid in full for the shipment. The provider assumes everything was shipped as stated on the invoice because no questions were raised when the shipment was received.

If a mistake is made in writing a check, it is necessary to write "VOID" across the check and stub and rewrite the check.

CHECKS RECEIVED FROM PATIENTS

The medical assistant should take certain precautions when accepting checks from patients:

- Be sure the check has the correct date, amount, and signature, and that no corrections have been made.
- Do not accept a **third party** check unless the check is from an insurance company. A third party check is generally one made out to the patient by someone unknown to you. Since you do not know how creditworthy the check writer is or have any personal information about the individual, it is unwise to accept a check that person has written.
- You might have patients who want to write a check for more than the amount due so they can have some cash in hand. This is generally not a good policy, and it would be advisable to refuse such a check. When you accept the check as payment and give out an additional amount in office cash, you risk the check not being honored by the bank. Your office will lose not only the

PROCEDURE

10-1 Write a Check

PURPOSE: Accurately write a check.

EQUIPMENT: Check book and register, pen with black or blue ink or typewriter.

TERMINAL PERFORMANCE OBJECTIVE: In a simulated medical office situation, prepare a check following the steps of the procedure. The instructor will observe all steps.

1. The check must be dated, identify the payee, the correct numerical and written amount, and must have appropriate signature. Fill out check **register** or stub with the check number, date, name of person or business to receive check, and amount of check. Also enter balance from previous stub.
   NOTE:
   - Always complete register before writing check.
   - Use only black or blue ink.
   - The stub may have the check number preprinted.
   - If a deposit has been made, add to previous balance.
   - Subtract amount of check and enter new balance.

2. Enter the date on check. **NOTE: May be typewritten or entered in black or blue ink.**

3. Enter the name of the payee on check.

4. Enter numerically the amount of the check. **NOTE: Keep numbers close to the dollar sign so other numbers cannot be inserted to change the amount of the check.**

5. Write out the amount of the check in words beginning as far to the left as possible.
   NOTE:
   - After writing the amount, fill in remaining space with a line to prevent insertion of words that would increase the amount.
   - All amounts are written in terms of dollars and fractions of dollars. A check for $10 is written "Ten and no hundredths." A check for $12.65 is written "Twelve and sixty-five hundredths."
   - When writing a check for less than a dollar, write the word Only and then the amount. ("Only ninety-five hundredths.")

6. The check should be signed with the same signature used on the authorization card to open the checking account.

amount owed by the patient, but also will lose the cash given out.

■ Do not accept a check marked "payment in full" unless it does pay the account in full including charges incurred on the day the check is written. If there is still a balance, you will be unable to collect if you accept and deposit such a check. The statement "payment in full" should be written on the back of a check where it is to be endorsed. When you receive a check, you should stamp it with the deposit endorsement (see below) to protect against theft. If you do this, you will be sure to see any statement written on the check and you can be sure the payment is indeed in full before accepting the check.

■ Do not accept a postal money order with more than one endorsement because two are the limit honored.

ENDORSEMENT

An endorsement is a signature or a signature plus other information on the back of a check. The endorsement of a check transfers all rights in the check to another party. Endorsements should always be made in ink and may be made with a pen or rubber stamp. The end of the check to be endorsed can be identified by holding the check on the right end as you look at it, turning it over, and endorsing the opposite or left end. All checks received in the office, whether in person or through the mail, should be protected by endorsement at the time received.

The two kinds of endorsement commonly used are blank endorsement and restrictive endorsement. A *blank endorsement* is a signature only. It should not be used until the check is to be cashed, because if the check is stolen with such an endorsement, someone else could endorse the check below your name and cash the check. A *restrictive endorsement* is used to endorse checks when they are received. It is a stamp or written information that states, "PAY TO THE ORDER OF (name of bank where check is to be deposited)" followed by the name of the physician. If such a check is stolen it could not be used in any way.

If the name of the payee is misspelled, it should be endorsed the same way followed by the correct signature directly below.

Effective September 1, 1988, new federal regulations required all endorsements to be within $1\frac{1}{2}''$ of the "trailing edge" of all checks. Checks on which the endorsement extends beyond the $1\frac{1}{2}''$ area may be refused by the financial institutions for improper endorsement. To avoid processing delays, be sure to endorse all checks as described, Figure 10–3.

MAKING DEPOSITS

The medical assistant is also expected to deposit cash and checks received in the office. This may be a daily task or it may be as infrequent as once a week for a physician with a limited practice. Deposit slips (Procedure 10-2) are imprinted with the account number in magnetic ink character recognition numbers, which match those on the checks. These numbers make it possible for checks and deposit slips to be sorted and recorded by computer. Banks will accept a list of deposited items on something other than the bank-provided deposit slip as long as the bank deposit slip is attached (see Figure 10–2) p. 193.

DEPOSIT BY MAIL

Checks may be deposited by mail. You should avoid sending cash or currency by mail, but if you must, then send it by registered mail. The deposit slip and money are prepared as for any deposit. The checks should be endorsed by restrictive endorsement only. If no stamp is available, the handwritten notation "for deposit only to the account of (name of your employer)" will suffice. You should request a receipt, as this record is necessary to prove a deposit was made. It is extremely important that you have an accurate record of all checks deposited with the check number, whom the check is from, and the amount of check so that you can follow up if the mail is lost. If this should happen, it will be necessary to notify all payees to stop payment and issue you new checks.

```
ENDORSE HERE:

X _____ Your name _____

_____

_____

DO NOT SIGN / WRITE / STAMP BELOW
THIS LINE, FOR FINANCIAL USE ONLY*
- - - - - - - - - - - - - - - - - - - -




*FEDERAL RESERVE BANK REGULATION CC
```

FIGURE 10–3 Proper placement of signature endorsement.

PROCEDURE

10-2 Prepare a Deposit Slip

PURPOSE: Accurately prepare a deposit slip.

EQUIPMENT: Deposit slip, pen with black or blue ink or typewriter, cash and/or checks to be deposited.

TERMINAL PERFORMANCE OBJECTIVE: Prepare a bank deposit slip, following the steps in the procedure.

1. Separate money to be deposited by check or currency.

2. Currency is usually listed first.
   NOTE:
   - All bills should be sorted so that the bills of each denomination are together, facing in the same direction, and with portrait side up.
   - Place highest denomination to lowest (i.e., 20s, 10s, 5s, and 1s).
   - Total currency and record on deposit slip.

3. If a large number of coins are included they should be placed in wrappers. Record the total on the slip.

4. List checks by number, name of maker, and amount.

NOTE:
- List checks from largest amount to least. This makes a search easier if there is a question.
- The check number is sufficient if you have an office copy on which you list the names also.
- Money orders are listed as money order and name or MO and name.
- Be sure checks are endorsed.

5. Total all amounts.

6. Total currency, coin, and checks.

7. Make a copy of deposit slip for your office files.

8. Enter deposit total in checkbook.

9. Deposit at bank. **NOTE: Be sure you receive a record of deposit either personally or by mail if you make a mail or night deposit. This record is necessary to prove a deposit was made if the bank fails to give credit for it on the monthly statement.**

RECONCILING BANK STATEMENTS

An important part of banking is the reconciliation each month of the bank statement with the office records. You need to be sure that you and the bank agree as to the amount of money in the account. You will receive a statement that shows all banking **transactions** concerning the account along with the checks which the bank has received and processed. Most statements contain a section similar to Figure 10–4 that allows you to list outstanding checks and do other calculations to **reconcile** the amounts. Follow Procedure 10–3 and workbook exercises to practice reconciling a bank statement.

PETTY CASH AND OTHER ACCOUNTS

Since it is not reasonable to write checks for small office transactions, most physicians have a petty cash fund. The physician will determine the amount of the fund and for what it will be used. The fund is established by writing a check payable to Cash or Petty Cash. The check is then cashed and the money kept in a locked cash box. (All patient payments should be kept in a separate money box.) The money is often used for postage due letters, inexpensive office supplies, and small charitable donations.

A **voucher** form or expenditure list should be completed each time payment is made from this fund. When the amount

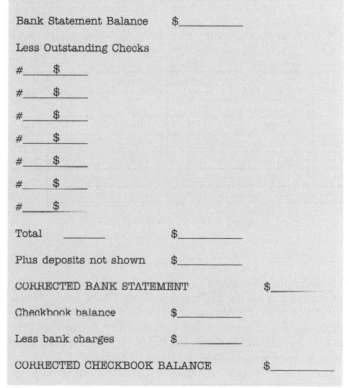

RECONCILING THE BANK STATEMENT

Bank Statement Balance $_____

Less Outstanding Checks

#_____ $_____

#_____ $_____

#_____ $_____

#_____ $_____

#_____ $_____

#_____ $_____

#_____ $_____

Total   _____ $_____

Plus deposits not shown $_____

CORRECTED BANK STATEMENT $_____

Checkbook balance $_____

Less bank charges $_____

CORRECTED CHECKBOOK BALANCE $_____

FIGURE 10–4 Reconciliation form.

P R O C E D U R E

10-3 Reconcile a Bank Statement

PURPOSE: Accurately reconcile a bank statement.

EQUIPMENT: Bank statement and cleared checks, reconciliation worksheet, pen or pencil, calculator or adding machine.

TERMINAL PERFORMANCE OBJECTIVE: Follow the steps in the procedure to reconcile a bank statement.

1. Compare the opening balance on the new statement with the closing balance on the previous statement. **NOTE: If they do not agree, contact the bank.**

2. List the bank balance in the appropriate space on the reconciliation worksheet.

3. Compare the check entries on the statement with the returned checks. **NOTE: The bank may have your checks in numerical order; if not, you should place them in order.**

4. Determine if you have any outstanding checks.
   NOTE:
   - An outstanding check is one you have written that does not appear on your bank statement and has not been returned by the bank.
   - Put a check mark on each check stub or register entry that matches an entry on your statement.

- Any stub or entry not checked indicates an outstanding check, which you list on your worksheet in the column provided.
- Total the outstanding checks.

5. Subtract from your checkbook balance items such as withdrawals, automatic payments or service charges that appear on the statement but not in the checkbook. **NOTE: These items are indicated by a code such as *AP* for automatic payment or *SC* for service charge.**

6. Add to your checkbook balance any interest earned as indicated on your statement. **NOTE: Some banks pay interest if a specified minimum amount is maintained in the account.**

7. Add to the bank statement balance any deposits not shown on the bank statement (*e.g.*, deposited since statement prepared).

8. The balance in your checkbook and the bank statement should agree. **NOTE: If they do not agree, subtract the lesser figure from the greater for a possible clue to the error and recheck all figures.**

DATE	DESCRIPTION	VOUCHER NUMBER	TOTAL AMOUNT	OFFICE EXPENSE	DONA-TIONS	MISC.	BALANCE
10/1	Fund established						25.00
10/5	Postage due	1	.40	.40			24.60
10/8	Parking fee	2	1.60			1.60	23.00
10/10	Coffee	3	2.98				20.02

FIGURE 10–5 Petty cash form.

in the fund is nearly **depleted**, another check is written for the difference between the original fund and the amount remaining. The expense records are kept in a file to verify the use of the petty cash fund. Figure 10–5 shows a petty cash fund ledger form to monitor expenditures.

Complete Chapter 10, Unit 2 in the workbook to help you meet the objectives at the beginning of this unit and therefore achieve competency of this subject matter.

UNIT 3

Salary, Benefits, and Tax Records

■ OBJECTIVES

Upon completion of the unit, meet the following terminal performance objectives by verifying knowledge of the facts and principles presented through oral and written communication at a level deemed competent.

1. Explain the W-4, W-2, and I-9 forms.
2. Differentiate between hourly wage and a salary.
3. Identify the information required for payroll records.
4. List the four factors that affect the amount of federal tax withheld.
5. Differentiate between gross and net salary.
6. Discuss salary benefits, identifying six examples.
7. Spell and define, using the glossary at the back of the text, all the words to know in this unit.

■ WORDS TO KNOW

accountant
benefits
deductions
disability
exemption
gross

longevity
net
profit sharing
unemployment
vested

EMPLOYEE REQUIREMENTS AND RECORDS

All employees in a physician's office must have a Social Security number. This is a nine-digit number which is obtained from the Social Security Administration. Forms to apply for a Social Security number can be obtained from local Social Security office, Internal Revenue office, and post offices. Each employee must also complete an Employee's Withholding Exemption Certificate (W-4 form) indicating the number of **exemptions** claimed, Figure 10–6. Any employee who fails to complete a W-4 form will have withholding figured on the basis of being single with no exemptions. A new W-4 form must be completed if there is a change in marital status or a change in the number of exemptions.

Recent federal legislation requires employees to complete an Employment Eligibility Verification Form I-9. The form is issued by the Department of Justice, Immigration and Naturalization Service. Its purpose is to ensure all persons employed are either United States citizens, lawfully admitted aliens, or aliens authorized to work in the United States. By law, this form must be completed before an individual can be officially hired. **Accountants** will not permit salary to be paid to individuals who do not have a form I-9 on file.

In addition to these federal requirements, forms must also be processed for state and local tax records. Local government tax is paid to the city where employment occurs regardless of where the employee lives.

MEDICAL OFFICE REQUIREMENTS AND RECORDS

The physician's office must have a federal tax reporting number, which is obtained from the Internal Revenue Service. In states that require employer reports, a state employer number must also be obtained.

When payroll checks are prepared, a record must be kept showing Social Security, federal taxes, any state and city taxes, and insurance amounts deducted from earnings. Employees may be paid an hourly wage or a salary (a fixed amount paid on a regular basis for a prescribed period of time). The Federal Fair Labor Standards Act regulates the minimum wage and requires that overtime be paid to wage earners at a minimum rate of one and one- half times the regular rate for hours over and above forty hours per week. It is necessary to keep records of hours worked, total pay, and all **deductions** withheld.

All employees are expected to work the assigned number of hours per day, week and month. Any time off must be reconciled on the payroll records and the salary adjusted according to office policy.

Several office supply houses furnish forms for payroll record keeping. There should be a page for each employee's payroll record. The heading should give the name, address, telephone, Social Security number, and date of employment. In columns there should be a record of date of check, hours worked (regular and overtime), **gross** salary, and individual deductions (including federal income tax, Social Security tax, and any state and local taxes). There might also be deductions for insurances or uniforms. The final column should show the amount of **net** pay, that is, the actual amount of the paycheck after deductions. When an accountant or management firm is employed to prepare payroll, office records must be given to them by a designated date(s) each month in order that payroll can be prepared and records maintained.

The amount of federal tax withheld is based on the amount earned, marital status, numbers of exemptions claimed, and the length of the pay period. The Internal Revenue Service will provide the charts used to figure deductions for federal income tax and Society Security tax. State and local taxes are usually a percentage of gross earnings. The net pay (pay actually given to the employee) is the gross earnings minus taxes and other deductions. The physician must provide the employee with a statement of gross pay and deductions along with the check each pay period. The tax deductions withheld must be sent on a quarterly basis to the federal, state, and local government offices along with the reporting forms provided by the tax offices. The local, state, and federal governments supply the guidelines necessary to complete these reports.

A W-2 form, which is a summary of all earnings for the year and all deductions withheld for federal, state, and local taxes, must be provided to each employee by January 31st of each year. The Social Security Administration must receive a report of W-2 forms each year. The physician who has several employees may also need to submit reports to the state and federal government for **unemployment** taxes. This tax is not deducted from the employee's earnings for federal tax but may be deducted in some cases for state unemployment tax.

BENEFITS

Full-time employed medical assistants and other medical office employees can expect **benefits** in addition to their salary. These are sometimes known as "fringe benefits." Benefits will vary according to the situation of the employee and the generosity of the physician(s). The following are examples of benefits that may be offered.

■ Vacation. Usually a minimum of two weeks with pay after completing a year of full-time employment; will increase with **longevity**.
■ Holidays. A minimum of six paid holidays per year— New Year's, Memorial Day, July 4th, Labor Day, Thanksgiving, and Christmas.

19XX Form W-4

Department of the Treasury
Internal Revenue Service

Purpose. Complete Form W-4 so that your employer can withhold the correct amount of Federal income tax from your pay.

Exemption From Withholding. Read line 7 of the certificate below to see if you can claim exempt status. *If exempt, complete line 7; but do not complete lines 5 and 6.* No Federal income tax will be withheld from your pay. Your exemption is good for one year only. It expires February 15, 1993.

Basic Instructions. Employees who are not exempt should complete the Personal Allowances Worksheet. Additional worksheets are provided on page 2 for employees to adjust their withholding allowances based on itemized deductions, adjustments to income, or two-earner/two-job situations. Complete all worksheets that apply to your situation. The worksheets will help you figure

the number of withholding allowances you are entitled to claim. However, you may claim fewer allowances than this.

Head of Household. Generally, you may claim head of household filing status on your tax return only if you are unmarried and pay more than 50% of the costs of keeping up a home for yourself and your dependent(s) or other qualifying individuals.

Nonwage Income. If you have a large amount of nonwage income, such as interest or dividends, you should consider making estimated tax payments using Form 1040-ES. Otherwise, you may find that you owe additional tax at the end of the year.

Two-Earner/Two-Jobs. If you have a working spouse or more than one job, figure the total number of allowances you are entitled to claim on all jobs using worksheets from only one Form

W-4. This total should be divided among all jobs. Your withholding will usually be most accurate when all allowances are claimed on the W-4 filed for the highest paying job and zero allowances are claimed for the others.

Advance Earned Income Credit. If you are eligible for this credit, you can receive it added to your paycheck throughout the year. For details, get Form W-5 from your employer.

Check Your Withholding. After your W-4 takes effect, you can use Pub. 919, Is My Withholding Correct for 1992?, to see how the dollar amount you are having withheld compares to your estimated total annual tax. Call 1-800-829-3676 to order this publication. Check your local telephone directory for the IRS assistance number if you need further help.

Personal Allowances Worksheet   For 19XX, the value of your personal exemption(s) is reduced if your income is over $105,250 ($157,900 if married filing jointly, $131,550 if head of household, or $78,950 if married filing separately). Get Pub. 919 for details.

A Enter "1" for **yourself** if no one else can claim you as a dependent . . . . **A** _____

B Enter "1" if:
- You are single and have only one job; or
- You are married, have only one job, and your spouse does not work; or
- Your wages from a second job or your spouse's wages (or the total of both) are $1,000 or less. } . . **B** _____

C Enter "1" for your **spouse.** But, you may choose to enter -0- if you are married and have either a working spouse or more than one job (this may help you avoid having too little tax withheld) . . . . **C** _____

D Enter number of **dependents** (other than your spouse or yourself) whom you will claim on your tax return . . . . **D** _____

E Enter "1" if you will file as **head of household** on your tax return (see conditions under "Head of Household," above) . **E** _____

F Enter "1" if you have at least $1,500 of **child or dependent care expenses** for which you plan to claim a credit . **F** _____

G Add lines A through F and enter total here. **Note:** *This amount may be different from the number of exemptions you claim on your return* ▶ **G** _____

For accuracy, do all worksheets that apply.
- If you plan to **itemize or claim adjustments to income** and want to reduce your withholding, see the Deductions and Adjustments Worksheet on page 2.
- If you are **single** and have **more than one job** and your combined earnings from all jobs exceed $29,000 OR if you are **married** and have a **working spouse or more than one job,** and the combined earnings from all jobs exceed $50,000, see the Two-Earner/Two-Job Worksheet on page 2 if you want to avoid having too little tax withheld.
- If **neither** of the above situations applies, **stop here** and enter the number from line G on line 5 of Form W-4 below.

- - - - - - - - - - - - - - - - **Cut here and give the certificate to your employer. Keep the top portion for your records.** - - - - - - - - - - - - - - -

Form **W-4**
Department of the Treasury
Internal Revenue Service

Employee's Withholding Allowance Certificate

▶ **For Privacy Act and Paperwork Reduction Act Notice, see reverse.**

OMB No. 1545-0010

19XX

1 Type or print your first name and middle initial	Last name	2 Your social security number

Home address (number and street or rural route)	3 ☐ Single ☐ Married ☐ Married, but withhold at higher Single rate.
	Note: *If married, but legally separated, or spouse is a nonresident alien, check the Single box.*
City or town, state, and ZIP code	4 If your last name differs from that on your social security card, check here and call 1-800-772-1213 for more information ▶ ☐

5 Total number of allowances you are claiming (from line G above or from the Worksheets on back if they apply) **5** ____

6 Additional amount, if any, you want deducted from each paycheck . . . . **6** $ ____

7 I claim exemption from withholding and I certify that I meet **ALL** of the following conditions for exemption:
- Last year I had a right to a refund of **ALL** Federal income tax withheld because I had **NO** tax liability; **AND**
- This year I expect a refund of **ALL** Federal income tax withheld because I expect to have **NO** tax liability; **AND**
- This year if my income exceeds $600 and includes nonwage income, another person cannot claim me as a dependent.

If you meet all of the above conditions, enter the year effective and "EXEMPT" here . . . ▶ **7** 19 ____

8 Are you a full-time student? (**Note:** *Full-time students are not automatically exempt.*) . . . . **8** ☐ Yes ☐ No

Under penalties of perjury, I certify that I am entitled to the number of withholding allowances claimed on this certificate or entitled to claim exempt status.

Employee's signature ▶ _____ Date ▶ _____ , 19 ____

9 Employer's name and address (Employer: Complete 9 and 11 only if sending to the IRS)	10 Office code (optional)	11 Employer identification number

---

FIGURE 10–6 Form W-4: Employee's Withholding Allowance Certificate.

Health insurance. Available; may require some co-payment and may not be provided if employee is covered by insurance with spouse's employment.

■ **Disability** insurance. Will cover a percentage of the salary if the employee is unable to work because of a disabling condition.

■ Life insurance. Usually for a set amount such as equal to a year's salary.

■ **Profit sharing**. A form of pension plan to employees who meet certain requirements such as: at least twenty-one years old, work a minimum of 1000 hours in a year, employed for at least a year to establish eligibility. Each plan will have its own requirements. For example an amount equal to a certain percentage of the employee's salary is deposited annually into the plan by the employer. This amount accumulates interest and grows tax free until it is withdrawn. The employee is normally responsible for the taxes due. There is usually a period of time, five years for example, before an employee becomes **vested** in the plan. This means the person must be employed at least five years before being eligible to receive the money in the account should employment be terminated. This type of benefit can add up to a nice sum. As an example, a person earns $10 per hour, $20,800 per year. If 10% of the salary ($2080) is placed into the plan for ten years, it would be valued at $20,800 plus the interest earned. Even if there were no increase in salary and therefore no increase in annual contributions, with an interest rate of only 5%, the amount would be approximately $23,000 at the end of ten years—a very impressive fringe benefit.

Another benefit, which is often overlooked, is the medical care you may receive as an employee. Depending on the type of practice in which you work, you may realize a considerable amount of complimentary health care. It is also of benefit to be a physician's employee when you need referral to another physician or medical specialist.

Medical practices that offer a good benefit package in addition to a competitive salary usually have a much more stable staff. This, in turn, results in reduced expense and maintenance of a high level of productivity because training time for new employees is not needed.

Complete Chapter 10, Unit 3 in the workbook to help you meet the objectives at the beginning of this unit and therefore achieve competency of this subject matter.

UNIT 4

General Management Duties

■ OBJECTIVES

Upon completion of the unit, meet the following terminal performance objectives by verifying knowledge of the facts and principles presented through oral and written communication at a level deemed competent.

1. Discuss refunds to patients.
2. Explain why no-shows are a concern.
3. Discuss a method to ensure inventory supplies.
4. Identify office equipment requiring frequent attention.
5. Describe a manager's responsibility to the employees.
6. Describe a manager's responsibility to the physicians.
7. List general facility responsibilities.
8. Spell and define, using the glossary at the back of the text, all the words to know in this unit.

■ WORDS TO KNOW

calibration	inventory
delegation	maintenance
expenditure	management
extensive	negligent
fiscal	reimbursement

Many duties performed in a medical office can be categorized under the broad classification of general **management** duties. These are activities that coordinate and maintain the functions within an office. This unit identifies a wide range of miscellaneous duties to acquaint you with those "behind the scenes" activities needed to efficiently operate a successful medical practice.

DAILY AND MONTHLY ACCOUNT RECORDS

Medical offices use a variety of bookkeeping and accounting systems. Regardless of the system used, some method will be needed to maintain a sense for **fiscal** status. It is essential to identify expenditures and income totals to ensure the practice is earning sufficient income to meet office expenses, taxes, insurance premiums and benefits payments and to provide an income for the physician. In addition, it is necessary to build assets for equipment purchases, investments, and perhaps hiring additional employees when needed.

In a medical practice, a percentage of patients may be **negligent** in paying for services. This can represent a sizeable amount of lost income. If it is allowed to continue or increase in percentage, it can present a serious problem and must be dealt with by the manager. Because of this fact, many physicians now require payment when services are delivered. In long-term care situations, such as with obstetrical patients, a standard fee to cover the anticipated form of delivery is established and the patient makes periodic payments prior to the delivery.

It is necessary to keep a record of accounts receivable. You can do this with a record page that allows you to begin the month with the amount carried over from the preceding month. Then each day you list charges and receipts and increase or decrease your total accounts receivable balance depending on whether your receipts or charges were greater. A trial balance, or total of all outstanding accounts, should be calculated each month. The total should agree with the accounts receivable balance.

The accounts payable records include all invoices for purchases, the checkbook, and the disbursement journal. All **expenditures** must be carefully entered in the disbursement journal. Office expenses must be separated from the physician's personal expenses. Office expenses are tax deductible but not all personal expenses are.

In an office where a computer is used for accounting transactions, you will receive instructions before being expected to perform the work. Every system has special features not found in other systems.

Many offices send their billing and invoices to a computerized accounting service through a telephone-linked terminal. Still other offices prepare all accounting records in a batch and take them to an accounting service computer center to be processed.

When a personal accountant is employed, the records will be maintained and a report provided to the medical practice each month, which indicates the expenditures, balances, and accounts receivable.

In addition to those already mentioned, the 1099 forms issued by third party payers, which indicate the total amount paid directly to the physician during the year, must be saved and given to the accountant for inclusion with the tax forms.

MISSED APPOINTMENTS

Another related area that a manager may need to address is missed appointments. If a patient does not show, no payment is received for that scheduled time of the day. In addition, another patient who needed to schedule an appointment was either scheduled at another time or referred if necessary. As an example, say there is one no-show for an average charge of $32. If this occurs three days in a week for forty-eight weeks during a year, $4608 income is lost. A policy of calling to remind patients may be established or a fee assessed for additional missed appointments after the patient has been notified in writing.

OFFICE POLICY MANUAL

The office manager would be responsible for developing and maintaining the policy and procedure manual for the office. There should be regular staff meetings to allow input from employees and exchange of ideas. This can help greatly in maintaining office harmony. To have a successful meeting, it is necessary to have an agenda or order of business so that you will be organized and know in advance what topics will be covered. If you are making decisions that will affect office operation, you should be sure a written record in the form of minutes is kept so that you will have a reference for any necessary changes in the policy and procedure manual. The office manager should be familiar with basic parliamentary procedures.

PATIENT INFORMATION BROCHURE

The office manager may be asked to compose a patient information brochure to be distributed to new and/or existing patients. This should be a brief explanation of office policies.

A brief history of the physician(s) education and practice interests should be included as well as office hours, appointments, telephone calls, after hours calls, accepted insurance plans, payment policies, and hospital affiliation(s).

This brochure should be printed on a good quality paper. If the practice has a logo, this could be placed on the cover of the brochure. This can be as simple as a single sheet neatly folded or as complex as a booklet. An added touch would be a picture of the physician(s) and a map showing the office location. A brochure can be sent to a new patient as confirmation of an appointment or given to the patient at their initial appointment. The brochure will need to be updated as physicians or services are added or deleted from the practice.

PATIENT REFUNDS

Managers usually assume the responsibility of verifying overpayment to a patient's account before approving **reimbursement** to the patient. This situation occurs when both the patient and the insurance company pay the physician or an error in the amount due is made.

EQUIPMENT MAINTENANCE AND SUPPLY INVENTORY

The manager or the medical assistant is expected to keep track of equipment **maintenance** and maintain an **inventory** of clinical and administrative supplies. An office that has been in operation for several years will have an established list of companies that supply its needs. You should not change to another company without consulting the physician. You should be alert to the best quality for the best price, however. You will be a valuable member of the health care team if you are able to control costs without sacrificing the quality of the products and supplies you use. New medical assistants will usually have to prove their capability to handle routine office affairs before being entrusted with maintaining an inventory.

The best method for organizing office supplies is to prepare a separate inventory card for each item used. These should be reviewed and updated in a systematic manner. Some high usage items may require a daily update, whereas a weekly update is sufficient for others. The inventory card should indicate the supplier's name, address, phone number, and the cost of the item. A file should be maintained of the maintenance contracts on equipment along with the names and phone numbers of service personnel to be called.

Good housekeeping rules must be followed in storage of supplies. The storage areas should be clean and dry. All medications should be stored in a cool, dark area to avoid deterioration. Narcotics should always be in a locked cabinet. Some laboratory supplies must be refrigerated. Supplies should be stored near the area where they will be used.

It is not possible to give quality care to patients with faulty office equipment. You must be aware of daily, weekly, or monthly maintenance that must be carried out to keep equipment in good working order. Always go through a troubleshooting checklist to see if you can correct a problem before requesting outside help. Maintenance personnel charge for plugging in a machine just as they do for repair service.

Autoclaves require regular cleaning to work effectively in sterilization procedures. Typewriters should be covered when not in use. The **calibration** of aneroid sphygmomanometers should be checked periodically. The mercury level of mercury manometers should be checked to ensure an accurate blood pressure reading (see Chapter 13, Unit 3). Electrocardiograph machines must be maintained. Light sources on sigmoidoscopy, otoscope, and ophthalmoscope should be checked and replaced when necessary. There should always be a supply of batteries and light bulbs to be used in maintenance of equipment.

A part of office maintenance that cannot be overlooked is linen supplies. Some offices use gowns, towels, pillow cases, and sheets, which must be sent to a laundry. If disposable items are used, there must be an adequate supply at all times.

RESPONSIBILITY FOR DECISION-MAKING

In large practices, clinics, and corporations, it is advisable to divide the decision-making responsibilities among the physicians according to their area of interest or expertise. When decisions need to be made, the manager has to confer with only that physician or two instead of the total partnership. An example of division of responsibility is:

- Employment/personnel concerns
- Purchasing and office facility concerns
- Lab and radiology
- Fees, investments, and other financial matters

Decisions made by designated physicians are then usually discussed at the general meeting.

RESPONSIBILITIES TO EMPLOYEES

The manager in large practices often has the following responsibilities related to the support staff employees.

- Interview, hire, and terminate employees in concert with physicians if desired.
- Supervise or personally train employees. This applies to new personnel as well as updating current staff.
- Conduct staff meetings to inform, discuss, and exchange information.
- Make out work schedules.
- Arrange vacations and coverage if needed. Work in the position if necessary.
- Conduct performance evaluations, establishing probationary periods as deemed necessary.
- Consult physicians concerning salary increases and benefit changes.

RESPONSIBILITY FOR THE FACILITY

The physical structure of the office must be observed and maintained. The manager assumes responsibility for:

- Maintenance of office services such as cleaning and laundry
- Subscriptions to magazines and health-related literature
- Monitoring and paying utilities
- Suggesting improvements: repairs, decorating, organization of rooms

RESPONSIBILITIES TO PHYSICIANS

Physicians also need to be kept informed and aware of conditions affecting the practice. The manager has a great deal of obligation to the physicians. Some areas the manager must consider are:

- Assist in creating or updating business policies to increase efficiency
- Attend meetings pertaining to office management such as those sponsored by the medical association and other professional organizations
- Update physicians on Medicare, health plans, and insurance company policy changes, fee schedules, and reimbursement rates (for example, changes in ICD or CPT codes or descriptors or the reduction in Medicare coverage affecting reimbursement when accepting consignment). Approximately 85% of a physician's income is from third party payers, either directly or indirectly. It is critical that physicians learn to code their services correctly to obtain the full amount allowed for their care.
- Order CPT and ICD books annually. Review for deleted numbers.
- Hold physician meetings to discuss practice concerns.

MANAGER'S REWARDS

The role of office manager can be as limited or **extensive** as the physician(s) feel comfortable in the **delegation** of authority. A trusted employee who performs well in the role of office manager becomes a tremendous asset to the practice. This role in large medical offices carries a great amount of authority and responsibility, but the rewards are worthwhile both financially and personally. It is a challenge you should look forward to accepting should the opportunity arise.

Complete Chapter 10, Unit 4 in the workbook to help you meet the objectives at the beginning of this unit and therefore achieve competency of this subject matter.

Medical-Legal Ethical Highlights

Throughout this chapter you should be mindful of all medical-legal/ethical implications. Listed below are a few important reminders.

1. Keep accurate and complete records.
2. Secure important papers and documents in safe or fireproof storage.
3. Keep records private and confidential.
4. Stay abreast of current changes in tax laws and interest rates.

Ms. Right . . .

is organized and efficient in completing information on patients' records. She is mindful in storing important documents in a fireproof storage for safekeeping. She respects the privacy of patients and never leaves charts or records out where other patients can read them. When bulletins are received, she carefully reads them and notes important changes in tax laws and interest rates.

Employment outlook: Continuous.

Mrs. Wrong . . .

is careless in leaving charts and other important documents out in full view of other patients. She leaves charts and other information out wherever she pleases and has a difficult time finding things. She ignores bulletins concerning tax laws and interest rates because she doesn't like to read. She is negligent in recording important information on patients' charts because she is so disorganized.

Employment outlook: Termination.

REFERENCES

American Medical Association. "The Business Side of Medical Practice."

Diehl, Marcia, and Fordney, Marilyn. *Medical Typing and Transcribing Techniques and Procedures,* 3d Ed. Philadelphia: W. B. Saunders, 1991.

Douglas, Lloyd V., James T. Blanford, and Ruth I. Anderson. *Teaching Business Subjects,* 3d Ed. Englewood Cliffs, NJ: Prentice Hall, 1973.

Ehrlich, Ann, M.A. *The Role of Computers in Medical Practice Management.* Champaign, IL: Colwell Systems, Inc., 1981.

Frew, Mary, and Frew, David. *Comprehensive Medical Assisting: Administrative and Clinical Procedures,* 3d Ed. Philadelphia: F.A. Davis, 1995.

King, Colleen, RN. Office Manager, Northwest Family Physicians. Interview, October 1991.

Kinn, Mary E. and Derge, Eleanor. *The Medical Assistant: Administrative and Clinical,* 7th Ed. Philadelphia: W. B. Saunders, 1993.

Simmers, Louise. *Diversified Health Occupations,* 4th Ed. Albany: Delmar, 1997.

Appendix

CONVERTING MEASUREMENTS

LENGTH	Centimeters	Inches	Feet
1 centimeter	1.000	0.394	0.0328
1 inch	2.54	1.000	0.0833
1 foot	30.48	12.000	1.000
1 yard	91.4	36.00	3.00
1 meter	100.00	39.40	3.28

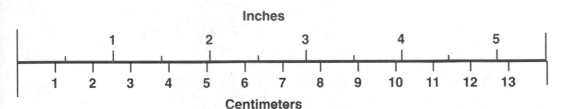

Comparison of Centimeters and Inches

VOLUMES	Cubic Centimeters	Fluid Drams	Fluid Ounces	Quarts	Liters
1 cubic centimeter	1.00	0.270	0.033	0.0010	0.0010
1 fluid dram	3.70	1.00	0.125	0.0039	0.0037
1 cubic inch	16.39	4.43	0.554	0.0173	0.0163
1 fluid ounce	29.6	8.00	1.000	0.0312	0.0296
1 quart	946.0	255.0	32.00	1.000	0.946
1 liter	1000.0	270.0	33.80	1.056	1.000

WEIGHTS	Grains	Grams	Apothecary Ounces	Pounds
1 grain (gr)	1.000	0.064	0.002	0.0001
1 gram (gm)	15.43	1.000	0.032	0.0022
1 apothecary ounce	480.00	31.1	1.000	0.0685
1 pound	7000.00	454.0	14.58	1.000
1 kilogram	15432.0	1000.00	32.15	2.205

RULES FOR CONVERTING ONE SYSTEM TO ANOTHER

Volumes

Grains to grams—divide by 15
Drams to cubic centimeters—multiply by 4
Ounces to cubic centimeters—multiply by 30
Minims to cubic millimeters—multiply by 63
Minims to cubic centimeters—multiply by 0.06
Cubic millimeters to minims—divide by 63
Cubic centimeters to minims—multiply by 16
Cubic centimeters to fluid ounces—divide by 30
Liters to pints—divide by 2.1

Weights

Milligrams to grains—multiply by 0.0154
Grams to grains—multiply by 15
Grams to drams—multiply by 0.257
Grams to ounces—multiply by 0.0311

Temperature

Multiply centigrade (Celsius) degrees by $\frac{9}{5}$ and add 32 to convert Fahrenheit to Celsius
Subtract 32 from the Fahrenheit degrees and multiply by $\frac{5}{9}$ to convert Celsius to Fahrenheit

COMMON HOUSEHOLD MEASURES AND WEIGHTS

1 teaspoon	= 4-5 cc. or 1 dram
3 teaspoons	= 1 tablespoon
1 dessert spoon	= 8 cc. or 2 drams
1 tablespoon	= 15 cc. or 3 drams
4 tablespoons	= 1 wine glass or $\frac{1}{2}$ gill
16 tablespoons (liq)	= 1 cup
12 tablespoons (dry)	= 1 cup
1 cup	= 8 fluid ounces or $\frac{1}{2}$ pint
1 tumbler or glass	= 8 fluid ounces or 240 cc.
1 wine glass	= 2 fluid ounces, 60 cc.
16 fluid ounces	= 1 pound
4 gills	= 1 pound
1 pint	= 1 pound

Medical Symbols and Abbreviations

m̲	minim	s̄s	one half
℥	dram	s̄	without
℥	ounce	c̄	with
O	pint	−	minus, negative, alkaline reaction
#	pound, number	+	plus, excess, acid reaction, positive
℞	recipe, prescription	×	multiply
'	foot, minute	÷	divide
"	inch, second	=	equals
a̅a̅	equal parts	>	greater than
°	degree	<	less than
%	percent	∞	infinity
♂	male	↑	increase
♀	female	↓	decrease

Abbreviations

a, aa	of each
a.c.	before meals
ad lib	as desired
A & P	anterior and posterior
aq	aqueous, water
BE, ba.en.	barium enema
blf	black female
bib	drink
b.i.d. BID	twice a day
bm, BM	bowel movement
blm	black male
BP, B/P	blood pressure
BUN	blood urea nitrogen
c̄	with
C	centigrade
Ca	calcium
cap	capsule
CBC	complete blood count
cc	cubic centimeter
CCU	coronary care unit
CHF	congestive heart failure
cm	cubic centimeter
CNS	central nervous system

Abbreviations (*continued*)

CO$_2$	carbon dioxide
comp	compound
COPD	chronic obstructive pulmonary disease
CPR	cardiopulmonary resuscitation
CSF	cerebrospinal fluid
CVA	cerebrovascular accident
cysto	cystoscopy
D & C	dilatation and curettage
Dil, dil	dilute
DOA	dead on arrival
DPT	diphtheria, pertussis, tetanus
dr.	dram
dx, Dx	diagnosis
ECG	electrocardiogram
EEG	electroencephalogram
EENT	eye, ears, nose, throat
EKG	electrocardiogram
elix	elixir
ER	emergency room
et	and
expl lap	exploratory laporatomy
ext.	extract
F	fahrenheit
F	female
FBS	fasting blood sugar
fl	fluid
fl. dr.	fluid dram
fl. oz.	fluid ounce
Fx	fracture
GB	gallbladder
GI	gastrointestinal
Gm	gram
GP	general practitioner
gr	grain
gtt Gtt gtts	drop, drops
GU	genitourinary
GYN	gynecology
H, h	hour
HCL	hydrochloric acid
Hgb	hemoglobin
h.s.	hour of sleep, bedtime
Hx	history
hypo	hypodermic, under
ICU	intensive care unit
I & D	incision and drainage
IM	intramuscular
inj	injection
I & O	intake and output
IPPB	intermittent positive pressure breathing
IT	inhalation therapy
IUD	intrauterine device
IV	intravenous
IVP	intravenous pyelogram

k	potassium
KUB	kidney, ureter, and bladder
L, lb	pound
lat	lateral
liq	liquid
LLQ	left lower quadrant
LMP	last menstrual period
LUQ	left upper quadrant
m	minim
M	male
mm	millimeter
MS	multiple sclerosis
NB	newborn
no.	number
noxt.	at night
NPO	nothing by mouth
N & V	nausea and vomiting
O	pint
OB	obstetrics
OD	overdose
O.D.	right eye
OP	outpatient
OR	operating room
os	mouth
O.S.	left eye
O.U.	both eyes
oz	ounce
Path	pathology
PBI	protein bound iodine
p.c.	after meals
Peds	pediatrics
per	through, by
PID	pelvic inflammatory disease
PKU	phenylketonuria
PO, p.o.	by mouth
prn	as desired, needed
pro time	prothrombin time
Psych	psychiatry
pt	patient, pint
pulv	powder
Px	physical examination
q	every
qd	every day
q 4 h	every 4 hours
qh	every hour
q.i.d., QID	four times a day
qns	quantity not sufficient
qs	quantity sufficient
qt	quart
R	right
Ra	radium
RBC	red blood cells
REM	rapid eye movement

Abbreviations (*continued*)

rep	let it be repeated
R/O	rule out
ROM	range of motion
ROS	review of systems
Rx	prescription, take
s̄	without
sig	instructions, directions
SOB	short of breath
sol	solution
solv	dissolve
s.o.s.	distress signal
sp. gr.	specific gravity
ss	half
stat	immediately
subq	subcutaneous
syr.	syrup
T	temperature
T & A	tonsilectomy and adenoidectomy
tab	tablet
TIA	transient ischemic attack
t.i.d.	three times a day
tinct.	tincture
TPR	temperature, pulse, respiration
TUR	transurethral resection
UA	urinalysis
ung.	ointment
URI	upper respiratory infection
UTI	urinary tract infection
VD	venereal disease
vin	wine
VS	vital signs
WBC	white blood cells
WF	white female
WM	white male
WNL	within normal limits
wt. Wt.	weight

MEDICAL TERMINOLOGY DERIVATIVES

and—et
arm—brachium; brachion (Gr)
artery—arteria
attachment—adhaesio

back—dorsum
backbone—spina
backward—retro
belly—venter
bend—flexus
bile—billis; chole (Gr)
bladder—vesica
blind—obscurus
blister—pustulo
blood—sanguis; haima, aima (Gr)
blood vessel—vena

body—corpus; soma (Gr)
bone—os; osteon (Gr)
bony—osseus
bowels—intestina, viscera
brain—cerebrum
breach—ruptura
breast—mamma; mastos (Gr)
buttock—gloutos (Gr)

cartilage—cartilago; chondros (Gr)
chest—thorax
choke—strangulo
confinement—puerperium
corn—callus, clavus
cornea—cornu; keras (Gr)
cough—tussio
cramp—spasmus

dead—mortuus
deadly—lethalis
dental—dentalis
digestive—pepticus
disease—morbus
dose—potio

ear—auris
egg—ovum
entrails—viscera
erotic—amatorius
exhalation—exhalatio
expell—expello
expire—expiro
external—externus
extract—extractum
eye—oculus; ophthalmos (Gr)
eyeball—pupula
eyelid—palpebra

face—facies
fat—adeps; lipos (Gr)
feel—tactus
fever—febris
finger—digitus
flesh—carnis
foot—pedis; pous (Gr)
forearm—brachium
forehead—frons

gall—bilis
gravel—calculus
gum—gingiva
gut—intestinum

hair—capillus
half—dimidius
hand—manus; cheir (Gr)
harelip—labrum fissum
head—caput; kephale (Gr)
healer—medicus
health—sanitas
hear—audio

Medical Terminology Derivatives (*continued*)

heart—cor; kardia (Gr)
heat—calor
heel—calx, talus
hysterics—hysteria

illness—morbus
infant—infas, puerilis
infectious—contagiosus
infirm—debilis
injection—injectio
intellect—intellectus
internal—intestinus
intestine—intestinum; enteron (Gr)
itch—scabies
itching—pruritis

jaw—maxilla
joint—artus; anthron (Gr)

kidney—ren; nephros (Gr)
knee—genu
kneecap—patella

lacerate—lacero
larynx—guttur
lateral—lateralis
leg—tibia
limb—membrum
listen—ausculto
liver—jecur, hepar (Gr)
loin—lapara
looseness—laxitas
lukewarm—tepidus
lung—pulmo, pneumon (Gr)

mad—insanus
male—masculinus
malignant—malignus
maternity—conditio matris
milk—lac
moist—humidus
month—mensis
monthly—menstruus
mouth—os; stoma (Gr)

nail—unguis
navel—umbilicus; omphalos (Gr)
neck—cervis; trachelos (Gr)
nerve—nervus; neuron (Gr)
nipple—papilla
no, none—nullus
nose—nasus; rhis (Gr)
nostril—naris
nourishment—alimentus

ointment—unguentum
orifice—foramen
pain—dolor
patient—patiens
pectoral—pectoralis

pimple—pustula
poison—venenum
powder—pulvis
pregnant—gravida
pubic bone—os pubis
pupil—pupilla

quinsy—angina

rash—exanthema
recover—convalesco
redness—rubor
rib—costa
ringing—tinnitus
rupture—hernia

saliva—sputum
scab—scabies
scalp—pericranium
scaly—squamosus
sciatica—ischias
seed—semen
senile—senilis
sheath—vagina
shin—tibia
short—brevis
shoulder—humerus; omos (Gr)
shoulderblade—scapula
shudder—tremor
side—latus
skin—cutis; derma (Gr)
skull—cranium; kranion (Gr)
sleep—somnus
smell—odoratus
socket—cavum
solution—dilutum
sore—ulcus
spinal—dorsalis, spinalis
spine—spina
spittle—sputum
sprain—luxatio
stomach—stomachus; gaster (Gr)
stone—calculus
sugar—saccharum
swallow—glutio

tail—cauda
taste—gustatus
tear—lacrima
teeth—dentes
testicle—testis; orchis (Gr)
thigh—femur
throat—fauces; pharygx (Gr)
throb—palpito
tongue—lingua; glossa (Gr)
twin—geminus

urine—urina

vagina—vagina; kolpos (Gr)
vein—vena; phleps (Gr)

Medical Terminology Derivatives (*continued*)
vertebra—vertevra; spondylos (Gr)
vessel—vas

wash—lavo
water—aqua
wax—cera
weary—lassus
wet—humidus
windpipe—arteria aspera
woman—femina
womb—uterus; hystera (Gr)
worm—vermis
wrist—carpus; karpos (Gr)

yolk—luteum

PREFIXES AND SUFFIXES

a- an-	without, negative
ab- abs-	away from
ad-	toward
adeno-	gland
aero-	air
-aesthesia	sensation
-algia	pain
ambi-	both
angio-	blood vessel
ano-	anus
ante-	before
anti-	against
arterio-	artery
arthro-	joint
auto-	self
bi-	two, twice
brady-	slow
broncho-	bronchial
cardio-	heart
cata-	down
-cele	tumor, cysts
cent-	hundred
-centesis	puncture
cephal-	head
chole-	gall
chromo-	color
-cide	causing death
circum-	around
-cise	cut
co- com- con-	together
colo-	colon
colpo-	vagina
contra-	against
costo-	rib
cranio-	skull
cysto-	bag, bladder
-cyte -cyto	cell
dacry-	tears
de-	from, down
deca-	ten
deci-	tenth
demi-	half

dent-	teeth
derma-	skin
di-	double
dia	through, between
diplo-	double
dis-	negative, apart
dys-	difficult, painful
ecto-	out, on the outside
-ectomy	cutting out
-emesis	vomiting
-emia	blood
en-	in, into
encephalo-	brain
endo-	within
entero-	intestine
epi-	above, over
-esthesia	sensation
ex- exo-	out
extra-	on the outside
fibro-	connective tissue
fore-	before, in front of
-form	form
-fuge	to drive away
galact- galacto-	milk
gastro-	stomach
-gene -genic	origin, formation
glosso-	tongue
gluco- glyco-	sugar, sweet
-gram	a tracing, record
-graph	machine
-graphy	the process
gyne-	woman
hema- hemato- hemo-	blood
hemi-	half
hepa- hepato-	liver
herni-	rupture
histo-	tissue
homo-	same, similar
hydra- hydro-	water
hyper-	above, increased, over
hypo-	below, under, decreased
hyster-	uterus
-iasis	condition of
ictero-	jaundice
idio-	peculiar to the individual
ileo-	ileum
in-	in, into, not
infra-	beneath
inter-	between
intra- intro-	within
-ism	condition, theory
-itis	inflammation of
ize	to treat by special method
karyo-	nucleus, nut
kata- kath-	down
kera-	horn, indicates hardness
-kinesis	motion
lact-	milk
laparo-	abdomen
-lepsy	seizure, convulsion
leuco- leuko-	white

Prefixes and Suffixes (*continued*)

lipo-	fat	-penia	too few, lack
lith-	a stone	per-	through, excessive
-logia -logy	science of, study of	peri-	around
-lysis	disintegration	pharyng-	throat
macro-	large, long	phelebo-	vein
mal-	bad, poor	-phobia	fear
-mania	insanity	-phylaxis	protection
mast-	breast	-plasty	operate to revise
med- medi-	middle	-plegia	a stroke, paralysis
mega-	large, great	-pnea	breathing
-megalia -megaly	large, great, extreme	pneumo-	air, lungs
melan-	black	poly-	many, much
men-	month	post-	after
meso-	middle	pre-	before
meta-	beyond, over, between, change, transportation	pro-	before, in behalf of
-meter	measure	procto-	rectum
metro- metra-	uterus	proto-	first
micro-	small	pseudo-	false
mio-	smaller, less	psych-	the mind
mono-	single, one	pyelo-	kidney, pelvis
multi-	many	pyo-	pus
my- myo-	muscle	pyro-	heat
myel- myelo-	marrow	re-	back, again
narco-	sleep	reni- reno-	kidney
naso-	nose	retro-	backward, behind
necro-	dead	-rhage -rhagia	hemorrhage, flow
neo-	new	-rhaphy	a suturing, stitching
nephr- nephro-	kidney	-rhea	flow
neu- neuro-	nerve	rhino-	nose
niter- nitro-	nitrogen	sacchar-	sugar
non- not-	no	sacro-	sacrum
nucleo-	a nucleus	salpingo-	a tube, fallopian tube
o-	ovum, an egg	sarco-	flesh
ob-	against	sclero-	hard, sclera
oculo-	eye	-sclerosis	dryness, hardness
-ode -oid	form, shape	-scopy	to see
odont-	a tooth	semi-	half
oligo-	few	septi-	poison, infection
-ology	study of	stomato-	mouth
-oma	a tumor	-stomy	to furnish with a mouth
oophor-	ovary	sub-	under
ophthalmo-	eye	super- supra-	above
-opia	vision	syn-	with, together
orchid-	testicle	tele-	distant, far
-orrhaphy	to repair a defect	tetra-	four
ortho-	straight	-therapy	treatment
os-	mouth, bone	-thermy	heat
-osis	disease, condition of	thio-	sulfur
oste- osteo-	bone	thoraco-	chest
-ostomy	to make a mouth, opening	thrombo-	clot
oto-	ear	thyro-	thyroid gland
-otomy	incision, surgical cutting	trans-	across
oxy-	sharp, acid	tri-	three
pachy-	thick	uni-	one
pan-	all, entire	-uria	urine
para-	alongside of	urino- uro-	urine, urinary organs
path- -pathy	disease, suffering	vaso-	vessel
ped- (Greek)	child	venter- ventro-	abdomen
ped- (Latin)	foot	xanth-	yellow

Glossary

abandonment—to desert, to give up entirely.

abbess—a mother superior; a woman who is the head of an abbey of nuns.

abbreviation—a shortened form.

abdomen—the cavity in the body between the diaphragm and the pelvis.

abdominal—pertaining to the abdomen.

abdominopelvic—pertaining to the anterior body cavity below the diaphragm.

abduct—to move away from the midline.

ablation—a surgical procedure utilizing a resectoscope inserted into the uterus through the cervix.

abnormality—person, thing, or condition that is not normal.

abortion—the termination of pregnancy before the stage of viability; spontaneous or induced.

abrasion—an injury caused by rubbing or scraping off the skin.

abrupt—sudden; blunt, curt.

absolute—free as to condition, unlimited in power.

absorb—to suck or swallow up, to drink in.

abstract—a summary of the principal parts of a larger work.

absurd—contrary to sense or reason.

accelerator—increasing action or function.

accessible—capable of being reached.

accommodation—the process of the lens changing shape to permit close vision.

accountant—one who keeps, audits, and inspects the financial records of individuals or businesses.

account history—the past financial record.

accreditation—the assignment of credentials; approval given for meeting established standards.

accumulated—to pile up; collect; gather.

accuracy—correctness, exactness.

accurate—correct, exact, without error

accurate and precise testing (APT)—refers to a standard for performing laboratory procedures to ensure reliability of results.

acetylcholine—a hormone released at the parasympathetic and skeletal nerve endings.

Achilles tendon—a tendon attaching the gastrocnemius muscle of the leg to the heel.

acidosis—a disturbance of the acid-base balance of the body.

acne—a skin condition characterized by inflammation of sebaceous glands and producing pimples.

acquaintance—the state of knowing a person or subject.

acquire—to gain by one's own efforts or actions; to get.

acquisition—to acquire; to get by one's own efforts.

acromegaly—a chronic condition characterized by enlargement of bones of the extremities and some bones of the head; thickening of facial soft tissues.

acronym—a word formed from the initial letters of each major word in a term.

action potential—the temporary electrical charge within a cell.

activate—to make active or more active.

acupuncture—involves the insertion of needles at various points in the body to treat disease or relieve pain.

acute—sharp, severe. Having a rapid onset, severe symptoms and a short course; not chronic.

adaptability—the act of or the result of adjusting to a new circumstance or change.

addiction—the state of being governed or controlled by a habit, as with alcohol or drugs.

adduct—to draw together toward the midline.

adenitis—inflammation of lymph nodes or a gland.

adequate—equal to the requirement or occasion, sufficient.

adhere—to stick fast, become firmly attached; to be devoted to.

adjective—a word added to (modifying) a noun to quantify or limit it.

adjustments—changes to fit or bring into harmony.

administer—to manage; to conduct, as in business.

administrative—duties that manage or direct activities; in medical assisting, refers to tasks other than clinical in nature; front office duties.

admissions clerk—a person who processes information and forms for a patient who will be entering the health facility.

adrenal—pertaining to the adrenal glands which sit atop each kidney.

adrenaline—an internal secretion derived from the adrenal glands; can be commercially prepared from animal glands; acts as a stimulant.

adrenocorticotrophic hormone (ACTH)—a hormone secreted by the anterior lobe of the pituitary gland.

advantageous—beneficial, profitable.

adverb—a word added to (modifying) a verb, an adjective, or another adverb.

advocate—one who pleads for or defends a cause or a person.

aerobe—a microorganism which can live and grow only in the presence of oxygen.

aesthetic—relating to the principles of beauty and taste.

afebrile—without fever.

affiliate—to unite, to join or become connected.

agar—a dried mucilaginous substance, or gelatin, extracted from algae, used as a culture medium.

agent—one that acts or has the power or authority to act for another.

aggressive—pushy, assuming the offensive without cause; forceful.

Al-Anon—a support group for family members of alcoholics.

Al-Ateen—a support for teenagers with an alcoholic parent.

albino—a person who lacks pigment in the skin, hair, and eyes, either partial or total; a person with albinoism.

alcoholic—an individual who uses alcohol to excess.

Alcoholics Anonymous—an organization formed to assist alcoholics to refrain from the use of alcohol.

aldosterone—a mineralocorticoid hormone secreted by the adrenal cortex.

alignment—being in proper position.

alimentary canal—the intestinal tract, from the esophagus to the rectum, and accessory organs.

allege—to state positively but not under oath and without proof; to affirm.

allergic rhinitis—inflammation of the nose due to an allergy.

allergist—a physician specializing in the care of patients with allergies.

allergy—an altered or acquired state of sensitivity; abnormal reaction of the body to substances normally harmless.

allosteric—a protein found in erythrocytes that transports oxygen in the blood; hemoglobin.

alopecia—the loss of hair; baldness.

alpha search—look by alphabetical order.

alveoli—microscopic air sacs in the lung.

amber—orange/yellowish color.

amblyopia—lazy eye; a condition characterized by the inward turning of the affected eye.

ambulate—to walk, not be confined to bed.

amenity—pleasantness, pleasant ways, civilities.

amenorrhea—absence of menses; without menstruation

American Society for Clinical Laboratory Science (ASCLS)

amniotic—pertaining to the amniotic fluid within the amniotic membrane surrounding the fetus.

amphetamine—a central nervous system stimulant, often referred to as an upper.

amplifier—a device on an electrocardiograph which enlarges the EKG impulses.

ampule—a small glass container that can be sealed and its contents sterilized.

amputate—to cut off, remove a part.

anaerobe—a microorganism having the ability to live without oxygen.

anal—pertaining to the anus or outer rectal opening.

analysis—the examination of anything to determine its makeup; a description of the process or the examination, point by point.

analytical—characterized by a method of analysis, a statement of point-by-point examination.

anaphylaxis—a hypersensitive reaction of the body to a foreign protein or a drug; the term implies symptoms severe enough to produce serious shock, even death.

anatomical—pertaining to the anatomy or structure of an organism.

anatomy—the study of the physical structure of the body and its organs.

anchor—the attachment of a skeletal muscle; the wrapping at the start of a gauze or elastic bandage.

anemia—a deficiency of red blood cells, hemoglobin, or both.

aneroid—operating without a fluid; when used in reference to a sphygmomanometer, measuring by a dial instead of a mercury column.

anesthesia—without sensation, with or without loss of consciousness.

anesthesiology—the study of anesthesia.

anesthetic—an agent which produces insensibility to pain or touch, either generally or locally.

aneurysm—a widening, external dilation due to the pressure of blood on weakened arterial walls.

angina—pain and oppression radiating from the heart to the shoulder and left arm; a feeling of suffocation.

angiography—a radiological study of an artery using a radiopaque medium.

angle—the inclination of two straight lines which meet in a point.

annotate—to provide with explanatory notes.

annotating—to provide critical or explanatory notes.

annuity—a sum of money to be received yearly, either in a lump sum or by installments.

anorexia—loss of appetite; with anorexia nervosa, loss of appetite for food not explainable by disease, which may be a part of psychosis.

antagonize—to annoy; to arouse opposition.

antecubital—the inner surface of the arm at the elbow.

anterior—before or in front of.

antibody—a protein substance carried by cells to counteract the effect of an antigen.

antibody-mediated—humoral immunity; when antibodies and complement work together to destroy antigens.

anticipation—expect, forsee.

anticoagulant—a substance that prohibits the coagulation of blood.

antigen—any immunizing agent which, when introduced into the body, may produce antibodies.

antihistamine—a class of drugs used to counteract allergic reactions or cold symptoms.

antiseptic—an agent which will prevent the growth or arrest the development of microorganisms.

antitoxin—a protein that defends the body against toxins.

anuria—the absence of urine.

anus—the external opening of the anal canal.

anxiety—a condition of mental uneasiness arising from fear or apprehension.

aorta—the main trunk of the arterial system of the body.

apex—the point, tip, or summit of anything; in reference to the heart, the point of maximum impulse of the heart against the chest wall.

apical—referring to the apex.

apnea—the absence of breathing.

aponeurosis—extension of connective tissue beyond a muscle in round or flattened tendons; a means of insertion or origin of a flat muscle.

apostrophe—a punctuation mark showing the absence of a letter or letters; possession.

apothecary—one who dispenses drugs and medicines.

appearance—outward show.

appendectomy—the excision of the appendix.

appendicitis—inflammation of the appendix.

appendicular—pertaining to the limbs or things that append (attach) to other parts.

applicable—capable of being applied, suitable.

appointment—an engagement; a meeting at a particular time.

apprehension—anticipation of something feared, dread; a mental conception.

apprenticeship—a training or learning period; study under the guidance of a skilled, experienced worker.

apprise—to inform.

appropriate—correct, suitable.

aqueous humor—a watery, transparent liquid which circulates between the anterior and posterior chambers of the eye.

arachnoid—a delicate, lacelike membrane covering the central nervous system.

arbitrary—depending on will or whim, self-willed; depending on choice or discretion.

ardently—eagerly, passionately, intensely.

areola—a ringlike coloration about the nipple of the breast.

arrhythmia—without rhythm; irregularity.

arteriography—a radiological study of an artery using a radiopaque medium.

arterioles—small blood vessels connecting arteries with capillaries.

arteriosclerosis—a degeneration and hardening of the walls of arteries.

artery—a blood vessel carrying blood away from the heart, usually filled with oxygenated blood.

arthritis—inflammation of a joint.

articulate—to join together, as in a joint.

artifact—something extraneous to what is being looked for. Activity which causes interference on EKGs.

ascending—referring to that portion of the colon which ascends from the lower right quadrant to the upper right quadrant of the abdomen.

ascertain—to make certain.

ASCLS—see American Society for Clinical Laboratory Science.

asepsis—a condition free of organisms.

aseptic technique—means of performing tasks without contamination by organisms.

asphyxiation—suffocation, loss of consciousness as the result of too little oxygen and too much carbon dioxide.

aspirate—to remove by suction.

assault—physical harm; a violent attack.

assess—to determine, to appraise the condition or state.

asset—anything owned that has exchange value, all the entries on a balance sheet that shows the property or resources of a person or business.

associate—to connect in thought; to join in friendship or partnership; a degree granted by a junior college at the end of a two-year course.

asthma—an allergic reaction to a substance resulting in wheezing, shortness of breath, and difficulty in breathing.

astigmatism—blurring of the vision due to an abnormal curvature of the cornea.

asymmetry—lack of same size, shape, and position of parts or organs on opposite sides.

atelectasis—lack of air in the lungs due to the collapse of the alveoli of the lungs.

atherosclerosis—fatty degeneration of the walls of the arteries.

atmosphere—any surrounding influence.

atrial depolarization—the excitement and contraction caused by the SA node at the beginning of the cardiac cycle.

atrioventricular—see **A-V node.**

atrium—cardiac auricle; the upper chamber of the heart.

atrophy—wasting away of a muscle.

attenuated—diluted; to reduce virulence of a pathogenic organism.

attitude—state of thought or feeling.

attribute—quality or characteristic; to give credit for.

audible—loud enough to be heard.

audiometry—testing of the hearing sense.

auditory—pertaining to the sense of hearing; the external canal of the ear.

aural—the ear; temperature measurement using tympanic infrared scanner.

augmented—refers to leads 4, 5, and 6 of the standard 12-lead EKG tracing; these leads are of different voltage.

auscultate—to listen for sounds produced by the body.

authorization—the giving of authority.

autoimmune—a condition wherein the person's antibodies react against their own normal tissues.

autologous—given by oneself.

automation—behavior in an automatic or mechanical fashion.

autonomic—spontaneous; the part of the nervous system concerned with reflex control of bodily functions.

autonomous—self-governing.

autotrophs—microorganisms that feed on inorganic matter.

A-V node—atrioventricular node; the beginning of the Bundle of His in the right auricle/atrium; nerve fibers responsible for the contraction of the ventricles.

axial—pertaining to the spinal column, skull, and rib cage of the skeleton.

axilla—the underarm area, armpit.

axillary—referring to the underarm area.

axon—an extension from a nerve cell.

BSA—see **body surface area.**

bacteria—unicellular microorganism concerned with the fermentation and putrefaction of matter; disease-causing agent.

balance—to bring into or keep in equilibrium; to have equal weight and power.

bankruptcy—the state of being bankrupt, being legally declared unable to pay debts.

barbiturate—a sedative or hypnotic drug, also known as a downer.

barrier—to prevent access; bar passage.

barter—to give one thing in exchange for another.

Bartholin's glands—two small mucous glands, situated one on each side of the vaginal opening at the base of the labia minora.

baseline—the initial information on which additional data is based.

basophil—a granulated white blood cell.

battery—any illegal beating of another person.

benefits—anything that promotes or enhances wellbeing.

benign—non-malignant; not cancerous.

benign hypertrophy—nonmalignant enlargement.

beriberi—a disease resulting from lack of vitamin B, thiamine.

biceps—the muscle of the upper arm which flexes the forearm.

biconvex—the curving out on both sides.

bicuspid—heart valve between the left atrium and left ventricle, also known as the mitral valve.

biennially—happening once in two years.

bile—a secretion of the liver; a greenish-yellow fluid with a bitter taste.

bimanual—two-handed; with both hands.

bimonthly—occurring once in two months.

binge—a spree; to overindulge such as with alcohol or food.

binocular—pertaining to the use of both eyes; possessing two eyepieces as with a microscope.

biochemistry—a science concerned with the chemistry of plants and animals.

biohazardous—any material that has been in contact with body fluid and is potentially capable of transmitting disease.

biopsy—excision of a small piece of tissue for microscopic examination.

bizarre—odd, unusual, strikingly out of the ordinary.

bladder—a membranous sac or receptacle for a secretion; the gallbladder, urinary bladder.

blood pressure—the amount of force exerted by the heart on the blood as it pumps the blood through the arteries.

body mechanics—the use of appropriate body positioning when moving and lifting objects in order to avoid injury.

body surface area (BSA)—refers to the total surface of the human body.

bolus—a mass of masticated food which is ready to be swallowed.

bookkeeper—one who records the accounts and transactions of a business.

booster—a subsequent injection of immunizing substance to increase or renew immunity.

bowel—refers to intestines.

Bowman's capsule—part of the renal corpuscle; surrounds the glomerulus of the nephron.

brachial—refers to the brachial artery in the arm; the artery used in measuring blood pressure.

bradycardia—slow heart rate.

braille—printing for the blind, using a system of raised dots.

brain scan—a diagnostic test using a scanner to measure radioisotopes within the brain.

breach—violation of a law, contract, or other agreement.

brochure—a small pamphlet or booklet providing information.

bronchi—the primary divisions of the trachea.

bronchiole—small terminal branches of the bronchi which lack cartilage.

bronchitis—inflammation of the mucous membranes of the bronchial tree.

bruit—an adventitious sound of venous or arterial origin heard on auscultation; usually refers to the sound produced by the mixing of arterial and venous blood at dialysis shunts.

buccal—the mouth; oral cavity.

bulbourethral gland—two small glands, one on each side of the prostate gland, terminating in the urethra by way of a duct.

bulimia—a condition characterized by alternating periods of overeating followed by forced vomiting and the use of laxatives to remove food from the body.

bundle—a number of things bound together.

bunion—a bursa with a callus formation.

bursa—a sac or pouch in connective tissue chiefly around joints.

CAT scan—see **computerized axial tomography.**

CLIA—see **Clinical Laboratory Improvement Amendments (1988).**

COPD—see **chronic obstructive pulmonary disease.**

caduceus—the wand of Hermes or Mercury; used as a symbol of the medical profession.

calculate—to compute.

calculi—commonly called stones; usually composed of mineral salts.

calibrations—a set of graduated markings to indicate values.

callus—in fractures, refers to the formation of new osseous material around the fracture site.

calorie—a unit for measuring the heat value of food.

calyces—two or more calyx.

calyx—the cuplike division of the kidney pelvis.

cancellation—to strike out by crossing with lines; marking a postage stamp, check, etc. to delete an appointment or event.

cancellous—a latticework structure, as the spongy tissue of bone.

cancer—a malignant tumor or growth; specifically the hyperplasia of cells with infiltration and destruction of tissue.

cannula—a tube or sheath enclosing a trocar (triangular bore needle); after insertion the trocar is removed.

capillary—a microscopic blood vessel connecting arterioles and venules.

caption—heading, title, or subtitle.

carbohydrate—an organic combination of carbon, hydrogen, and oxygen as a sugar, a starch, or as cellulose.

carbon dioxide—a gas found in the air, exhaled by all animals; the chemical formula is CO_2.

carbon monoxide—a colorless, odorless, poisonous gas caused by the incomplete combustion of carbon.

carboxyhemoglobin—combined carbon monoxide and hemoglobin in red blood cells.

carbuncle—a staphylococcal infection following furunculosis, characterized by a deep abscess of several follicles with multiple draining points.

carcinoembryonic antigen—a tumor marker which can be detected in the blood when tested.

carcinogenesis—the malignant transformation of a cell.

carcinogenic—cancer causing agents.

carcinoma—a malignant tumor from epithelial tissue.

cardiac—pertaining to the heart.

cardiac sphincter—the muscle which encircles the esophagus where it enters the stomach.

cardinal signs—principal signs: temperature, pulse, respiration, and blood pressure.

cardiologist—a physician specializing in the care of patients with diseases of the heart.

cardiology—the study of the heart and its diseases.

cardiovascular—pertaining to the heart and blood vessels.

carotid—pertaining to the carotid artery.

carpal tunnel syndrome—the symptoms associated with the entrapment of the median nerve within the carpal bones and the transverse ligament at the wrist.

carpals—bones of the wrist.

carrel—a small, partitioned space.

carrier—one who carries, transports; with insurance, it's the company who provides the policy.

cartilage—a strong, tough, elastic tissue forming part of the skeletal system; precalcified bone in infants and young children.

cataract—an opacity of the lens of the eye resulting in blindness.

catarrhal—pertaining to inflammation of mucous membranes; causing severe spells of coughing with little or no expectoration.

catastrophic—of great consequence; disastrous.

categorize—to arrange by class or kind; to place like things together.

catheterize—to insert a catheter into a cavity (for example, urinary bladder to remove urine) to remove body fluid.

caudal—pertaining to any taillike structure.

caustic—capable of burning; an agent that will destroy living tissue.

cauterize—to burn with an electrical cautery or chemical substance.

cautery—an iron or caustic used to burn tissue.

cavities—a hollow space, such as within the body or organs.

cecum—the beginning of the ascending portion of the large intestine which forms a blind pouch at the junction with the small intestine.

celiac disease—dilatation of the small and large intestines.

cell-mediated—direct cellular response to antigens.

cell membrane—the structure which surrounds and encloses a cell.

central—situated at or related to a center.

centrifuge—a machine for the separation of heavier materials from lighter ones through the use of centrifugal force.

centriole—an organelle within the cell.

cerebellum—lower or back brain below the posterior portion of the cerebrum.

cerebral—pertaining to the cerebrum of the brain.

cerebrospinal—referring to the brain and spinal cord.

cerebrospinal fluid—the liquid that circulates within the meninges of the spinal cord and ventricles and meninges of the brain.

cerebrovascular accident—a stroke; hemorrhage in the brain.

cerebrum—the largest part of the brain. It is divided into two hemispheres with four lobes in each hemisphere.

certificate—a written declaration of some fact.

certificate of waiver—refers to a list of basic laboratory tests that may be performed in the physician's office, by non-laboratory personnel.

certification—written declaration.

certified—holding a certificate; being certificated; guaranteed in writing.

certified ophthalmic technician—a person trained and certified in diagnostic testing procedures and limited examination of the eye.

cerumen—waxlike brown secretion found in the external auditory canal.

cervical—pertaining to the neck portion of the spinal column; also to the entrance into the uterus.

cervix—the entrance into the uterus.

cesarean—surgical removal of an infant from the uterus.

cessation—ceasing or discontinuing.

chaos—a state of complete confusion; disorder.

charting—the recording of observations, subjective and objective findings, diagnostic procedures, treatments, and other pertinent data in the patient file.

chemical—a simple or compound substance used in chemical processes.

chemotherapy—the use of chemical agents in the

treatment of disease, usually associated with cancer therapy.

Cheyne-Stokes—a breathing pattern characterized by alternating periods of apnea and hyperventilation.

chiropractic—a system of healing based upon the theory that disease results from a lack of normal nerve function; treatment by scientific manipulation and specific adjustment of body structures such as the spinal column.

chiropractor—a health care provider who utilizes chiropractic methods to treat patients.

chlamydia—a sexually transmitted disease caused by a bacteria that lives as an intracellular parasite.

chloroform—a liquid compound that yields a gas which dulls pain and causes unconsciousness.

cholecystectomy—surgical removal of the gallbladder.

cholelithiasis—stones in the gallbladder.

cholenergic—nerve fibers capable of secreting acetylcholine.

cholera—an acute, specific, infectious disease characterized by diarrhea, painful cramps of muscles, and a tendency to collapse.

chorionic gonadotropin—a hormone detectable in the urine of a pregnant female soon after conception.

choroid—the vascular coat of the eye between the sclera and the retina.

chromosome—structures within the cell's nucleus which store hereditary information.

chronic—continuing a long time, returning; not acute.

chronic obstructive pulmonary disease (COPD)—a syndrome characterized by chronic bronchitis, asthma, and emphysema, or any combination of these conditions, resulting in dyspnea, frequent respiratory infections, and thoracic deformities from attempting to breathe.

chronological—the arrangement of events, dates, etc., in order of occurrence.

chyme—the mixture of partially digested food and digestive secretions found in the stomach and small intestines during digestion of a meal.

cilia—hairlike projections from epithelial cells as in the bronchi.

circulatory—refers to the circulatory system. The process of blood flowing through the vessels to all the cells of the body.

circumcision—surgical removal of the foreskin of the penis.

cirrhosis—an interstitial inflammation with hardening of the tissues of an organ, especially the liver.

civil—pertaining to the rights of private individuals; legal proceedings concerning rights that are not criminal.

clarity—clearness, absence of cloudiness.

classified—arranged in a group or classification according to some system.

clause—part of a sentence with a subject and a predicate.

claustrophobia—an abnormal fear of being in enclosed or confined places.

clavicle—the collar bone, articulating with the sternum and scapula.

clinical—based on observation; in medical assisting, pertains to duties considered "back office"; not administrative in nature.

Clinical Laboratory Improvement Amendments (CLIA)—legislation dealing with the operation of a clinical laboratory.

clitoris—an erectile organ located at the anterior junction of the labia minora.

clone—an exact copy.

coagulate—to lessen the fluidity of a liquid substance; to clot or curdle.

coccyx—the tailbone; the last four bones of the spine.

cochlea—the snail-shaped portion of the inner ear.

coercion—to force or compel; to restrain or constrain by force.

coitus—sexual intercourse between a man and a woman.

colitis—inflammation of the colon.

collaborate—to work together.

colleague—an associate at work, usually one of similar status.

colon—the large intestine.

colorimeter—an instrument used for measuring the amount of pigments and determining the amount of hemoglobin in the blood.

colostomy—incision of the colon for the purpose of making a more or less permanent opening.

colposcopy—a diagnostic examination to visualize the cervix through a colposcope.

coma—an abnormal deep stupor from which a person cannot be aroused by external stimuli.

comminuted—a crushed bone fracture with many fragments.

commonality—people in general; a body corporate or its membership.

common bile duct—a duct carrying bile from the hepatic and cystic ducts to the duodenum.

communication—the act of communicating; information given; a means of giving information.

compatible—able to be mixed or taken together without destructive changes (as in blood typing and cross-matching); matching; not opposed to.

compensate—to make amends; be equivalent to.

compensation—anything given as an equivalent or to make amends; pay.

competent—fit, able, capable.

complement—a group of about twenty inactive enzyme proteins present in the blood.

complexity—the state of being complicated.

compliance—consent; conformity to formal or official requirements.

complicated—not simple, involved; having many parts; not easy to solve.

compose—to form by putting together, creating.

compound—not simple, composed of two or more parts; with fractures, refers to bone fragments piercing the skin externally.

comprehensive—covering all areas; inclusive.

compression—to exert force against, press.

computer—a mechanical, electric or electronic device that stores numerical or other information and provides logical answers at high speed to questions bearing on that information.

computerized—to store in a computer; to put in a form a

computer can use; to bring computers into use to control an operation.

computerized axial tomography (CAT)—a series of X-ray views of the body used to construct a three-dimensional picture.

conceal—to hide, to keep secret, to withhold, as information.

conceive—to become pregnant; the uniting of the sperm and ovum.

conception—the union of the sperm of a male and the egg of a female; fertilization.

concise—condensed, short.

condenser—part of a microscope substage that regulates the amount of light directed on a specimen.

confidentiality—to be held in confidence; a secret.

confinement—restriction within certain limits.

confirm—to verify or ratify.

confirmation—making firm or sure; convincing proof.

conflict—a clash of opinions or interests; a fight or struggle; an inner moral struggle; to come into opposition.

confront—to stand face to face with.

congestive heart failure—a complex condition of inadequate heart action with retention of tissue fluids; may be either right or left side failure, or both.

congratulations—to express pleasure; a recognition of accomplishment.

conjunction—meeting; a word that connects.

conjunctiva—a mucous membrane which lines the eyelids and covers the anterior sclera of the eyeball.

connective—that which connects or binds together; one of the five main tissues of the body.

connotation—something implied or suggested.

consciousness—awareness, full knowledge of what is in one's own mind.

consecutive—following in order, successive.

consecutively—a series of things that follow each other.

conserve—to keep from damage or loss; to maintain.

constipation—a sluggish action of the bowel; usually refers to an excessively firm, hard stool which is difficult to expel, or lack of a bowel movement over a period of time.

constrict—to narrow; to become smaller due to contraction of a sphincter muscle.

contact dermatitis—inflammation and irritation of the skin due to contact with an irritating substance.

contagious—catching; able to be transmitted by contact.

contaminate—to place in contact with microorganisms.

contemporary—happening or existing at the same time; a person living at the same time as another.

content—the matter dealt with in a field of study; matter contained.

context—the part of a written or spoken statement that surrounds a particular word or passage and can clarify its meaning.

contraception—against conception.

contract—to draw together, reduce in size, or shorten.

contractions—the muscle action of the uterus during labor.

contracture—permanent shortening or contraction of a muscle.

contradiction—the act of contradicting; to deny; to assert to the contrary of.

contrast—to show difference; in radiology, refers to a radiopaque medium used to outline body organs.

contributory—giving a share; helping toward a result.

controversial—open to dispute; relating to discussion of opposing views.

conventional—growing out of custom; not spontaneous.

convey—to impart, as an idea; to transfer.

convulsion—attack of involuntary muscular contractions often accompanied with unconsciousness.

cooperate—to work together.

coordination—a state of harmonious adjustment or function.

cornea—the transparent extension of the sclera that lies in front of the pupil of the eye.

coronal plane—a line drawn through the side of the body from head to toe, making front and back section.

coronary—referring to the arteries surrounding the heart muscle; also refers to a "heart attack" which involves the coronary arteries.

corpus luteum—the yellow body that develops in the ruptured graafian follicle after the ovum has been discharged.

cortex—the outer portion of the kidney.

corticosteroids—hormones used to treat inflammation.

COT—see certified ophthalmic technician.

countershock—(in cardiology) a high intensity, short duration, electric shock applied to the area of the heart, resulting in total cardiac depolarization.

courteous—polite, considerate, and respectful in manner and action.

CPT—see current procedural terminology.

cramp—a spasmodic, painful, contraction of a muscle or muscles.

cranial—pertaining to the cranium or skull.

cranium—the skull; the eight bones of the head enclosing the brain; generally applied to the 28 bones of the head and face.

crenated—notched or scalloped, as the crenated condition of blood corpuscles.

cretinism—a congenital condition due to the lack of the hormone thyroxin.

criminal—of, involving, or having the nature of a crime.

crisis—the turning point of a disease; a very critical period. An emergency situation.

criterion—a standard of criticism or judgment (plural: criteria).

critique—a critical examination of a thing or situation, to determine its nature, worth, or conformity to standards.

Crohn's disease—an inflammation of the GI tract with debilitating symptoms.

cross-match—a blood test used to assure compatibility of the donor to the recipient when transfusing blood.

crutch—a staff with a cross-piece at the top to place under the arm of a lame person.

cryosurgery—the use of a substance at subfreezing temperature to destroy and/or remove tissue.

cryptorchidism—failure of the testicles to descend into the scrotum.

CTD—see cumulative trauma disorder.

CTS—see carpal tunnel syndrome.

cultivate—to form and refine; to improve.

cummulative trauma disorder (CTD)—an injury resulting from repetitive movement of a body part.

currency—any form of money.

current—happening now; of the present time; the latest information.

current procedural terminology (CPT)—a numerical listing of procedures performed in medical practice; a standardized identification of procedures.

curriculum—a course of study at a school or university.

Cushing's syndrome—a disorder resulting from the hypersecretion of glucocorticoids from the adrenal cortex.

customarily—by custom, the usual course of action under similar circumstances.

cyanosis—a bluish discoloration of the skin due to lack of oxygen.

cyst—a bladder; any sac containing fluid.

cystic—pertaining to a cyst; of disease, refers to a condition with multiple cysts.

cystic fibrosis—a disease condition of fibrous tumors which have undergone cystic degeneration, accumulating fluid in the interspaces; also known as fibrocystic disease.

cystitis—inflammation of the urinary bladder.

cystoscope—an instrument for examining the interior of the urinary bladder.

cytology—the study of cell life and cell formation.

cytoplasm—cellular matter, not including the nucleus of a cell.

cytotechnologist—a laboratory specialist who prepares and examines tissue cells to study cell formation.

cytotoxic—capable of destroying cells.

DACUM—an acronym for "design a curriculum."

D & C—see dilatation and curettage.

DEA—see Drug Enforcement Administration.

data—facts from which conclusions can be inferred.

debilitated—weaken; impaired the strength of.

debridement—to clean up or remove, as is done with damaged tissue around a wound.

decline stage—becoming less intense, subsiding. A period of time when the symptoms of disease start to disappear.

dedicated—committed to; set apart for a special use.

deductions—to deduct or subtract; remove, take away.

defamation—to slander, or to attack the reputation of an individual or group.

defecate—to pass stool or move bowels.

defibrillation—to cause fibrillation to end; restore to normal action.

dehydration—withdrawal of water from the tissues naturally or artificially.

delegation—a person or group of persons officially elected or appointed to represent another or others.

delete—to remove, erase.

delirium tremens—a psychic disorder involving hallucinations, both visual and auditory, found in habitual users of alcohol.

deltoid—the muscle of the shoulder.

demeanor—behavior; bearing.

demography—the study of population statistics concerning births, marriage, death and disease as well as many other indicators.

dendrite—an extension from a nerve cell.

denial—a refusal to believe or accept; disowning.

denote—to indicate, to mean.

dental assistant—a health care worker employed by a dentist to perform management and clinical functions and provide chairside assistance.

dental hygienist—a licensed health care provider who is trained to X-ray and perform prophylactic treatments on teeth.

dentist—a licensed health provider who cares for the teeth, repairing and replacing as needed.

deoxyribonucleic acid—DNA; material within the chromosome that carries the genetic information.

dependable—that which may be relied upon.

depict—to represent by a picture; portray.

depleted—consumed, emptied, exhausted.

deposit—to entrust money to a bank or other institution.

deposition—testimony given under oath.

depressant—a drug which causes a slowing down of bodily function or nerve activity.

depressed—a state of depression, a period of low spirits; referring to a fracture, usually a fracture of the skull where bone fragments are driven (depressed) inward.

deprivation—to be deprived; without; having to do without or unable to use.

dermatitis—an inflammation of the skin, often the result of an irritant.

dermatologist—a physician who specializes in the diseases and disorders of the skin.

dermatology—the study of the skin and its diseases.

dermis—true skin.

descending—refers to the portion of the large intestine from the splenic flexure to the sigmoid.

description—a word picture.

desensitization—the process of making an individual less susceptible to allergens.

design—working plan; layout; sketch.

designate—to point out; indicate; appoint.

detection—find out or discover.

detrimental—harmful, injurious.

devastate—to lay waste, plunder, destroy.

dextrose—a simple sugar, also known as glucose.

diabetes mellitus—a metabolic disease caused by the body's inability to utilize carbohydrates.

diabetic—one afflicted with the condition diabetes.

diagnostic—referring to measures which assist in the recognition of diseases and disorders of the body.

dialysis—removal of the products of urine from the blood by passage of the solutes through a membrane.

diaphanography—a type of transillumination used to examine the breast, using selected wavelengths of light and special imaging equipment.

diaphoresis—profuse sweating.

diaphragm—the muscle of breathing which separates the thorax from the abdomen.

diarrhea—frequent bowel movements, usually liquid or semisolid.

diarthroses—a movable joint; another word for synovial.

diastole—the relaxation phase of the heartbeat; the period of least pressure.

dictation—something dictated; recorded voice communication.

dietician—one who is trained in dietetics, which includes nutrition, and in charge of the diet of an institution.

differential—refers to determining the number of each type of leukocyte in a cubic millimeter of blood.

diffuse—to scatter or spread.

diffusion—a process whereby gas, liquid, or solid molecules distribute themselves evenly through a medium.

digestion—the process by which food is broken down, mechanically and chemically, in the gastrointestinal tract and converted into absorbable forms.

digestive—pertaining to digestion.

digital—pertaining to or resembling a finger or toe, as an examination using a finger or fingers.

dilatation and curettage (D & C)—dilation of the cervix and scraping of the interior lining of the uterus.

dilate—to enlarge, expand in size; to increase the size of an opening.

dimpling—a condition characterized by indentations in the skin.

diphtheria—an acute infectious disease characterized by the formation of a false membrane on any mucous surface, usually in the air passages, interfering with breathing.

diplomate—an advanced status of medical practice.

disability—a legal incapacity.

disaster—an occurrence inflicting widespread destruction and distress.

disciplinary—designed to correct or punish breaches of conduct.

discipline—self-control, conduct, system of rules.

disclose—to uncover, reveal.

discoid—a type of Lupus which is confined to the skin; also called cutaneous.

discreet—wisely cautious, prudent.

discrepancy—inconsistencies; variances.

discretion—the use of judgment, prudence.

disease—sickness, illness, ailment.

dislocate—the displacement of a part; usually refers to a bone temporarily out of its normal position in a joint.

dispense—to distribute; to deal out in portions.

displacement—the transfer of emotions about one person or situation to another person or situation.

disposition—the act or manner of putting in a particular order; arrange.

dissect—to cut into separate parts for examination; to separate.

distal—farthest from the center, from the medial line, or from the trunk.

distend—to become inflated, to stretch out.

distinctive—unmistakable, different from anything else.

distort—to misrepresent; to twist out of usual shape.

diversion—the act of diverting or turning aside.

diverticulitis—inflammation of the diverticula.

diverticulum—a sac or pouch in the walls of a canal or organ, particularly the colon.

divulge—to make public; to make known; reveal.

DNA—see deoxyribonucleic acid.

doctorate—a postgraduate degree conferred following extensive course work, an individual research project, and the writing of a dissertation; a PhD.

doctrine—the principles of any branch of knowledge; a belief held or taught.

documentary—presenting facts without inserting fictional matter.

domestic—not foreign; private.

dominant—strongest; prevailing, the prime or main.

dorsal—pertaining to the back.

dorsalis pedis—a pulse point palpable on the instep of the foot.

douche—an irrigation of the vagina.

downtime—refers to being off-line; computer failure; time when nothing is scheduled.

dribbling—uncontrolled leakage of urine from the bladder.

drill—disciplined repetitive exercises as a means of perfecting a skill or procedure.

droplet—a very small drop.

Drug Enforcement Administration (DEA)—a division of the federal government responsible for the enforcement of laws regulating the distribution and sale of drugs.

duodenum—the first segment of the small intestine.

dura mater—the outer membrane covering the brain and spinal cord.

duration—period of time a thing continues.

dwarfism—a condition caused by inadequate growth hormone during childhood.

dysmenorrhea—painful menstruation.

dyspnea—difficult or labored breathing.

dystrophy—progressive atrophy or weakening of a part, such as the muscles.

dysuria—painful urination; difficulty in urination.

ECG/EKG—see **electrocardiogram.**

echocardiography—ultrahigh-frequency sound waves directed toward the heart to evaluate function and structure of the organ.

echoes—reflections of sound.

ectopic—in an abnormal position; in pregnancy refers to the embryo or fetus being outside the uterus.

eczema—a non-contagious skin disease characterized by dry, red, itchy and scaly skin.

edema—a condition of body tissues containing abnormal amounts of fluid, usually intercellular; may be local or general.

effacement—the thinning out of the cervix during labor.

efficiency—the ratio of energy expended to results produced.

ejaculation—the expulsion of seminal fluid from the male urethra.

ejaculatory duct—the duct from the seminal vesicle to the urethra.

elasticity—ability to return to shape after being stretched.

electrical—charged with electricity; run by electricity.

electrocardiogram (EKG, ECG)—a graphic record of the electric currents generated by the heart; a tracing of the heart action.

electrocardiograph—a machine for obtaining a graphic recording of the electrical activity of the heart.

electrocautery—an apparatus used to cauterize tissue with heat from a current of electricity.

electrocoagulation—coagulation of tissue by means of a high-frequency electric current.

electrode—an instrument with a point or a surface which transmits current to the patient's body.

electroencephalogram—a graphic record of the electric currents generated by the brain; a tracing of brain waves.

electrolyte—a substance, which in solution, conducts an electric current.

electromagnet—a soft iron core that temporarily becomes a magnet when an electric current flows through a coil surrounding it.

electromagnetic radiation—rays produced by the collision of a beam of electrons with a metal target in an X-ray tube.

electromyography—the insertion of needles into selected skeletal muscles for the purpose of recording nerve conduction time in relation to muscle contraction.

electron—a minute particle of matter charged with the smallest known amount of negative electricity; opposite of proton.

electronic—operated by the use of electrons.

elements—substances in their simplest form; the basic building blocks of all matter.

elicit—to draw out, to derive by logical process.

eliminate—to remove, get rid of, exclude; also to pass urine from the bladder or stool from the bowel.

elite—choice, superior, select.

ellipses—a mark or series of marks used in writing or printing to indicate an omission, especially of letters or words.

emaciated—to become abnormally thin; the loss of too much weight.

emancipated minor—no longer under the care, custody, or supervision of a parent or guardian.

embolus—a circulating mass in a blood vessel; foreign material which obstructs a blood vessel.

embryo—the initial eight weeks of development after fertilization.

emergency—an unexpected occurrence or situation demanding immediate action.

emergency medical technician (EMT)—an individual trained to respond in emergency situations and provide appropriate initial medical treatment.

emesis—to vomit.

emetic—medication that induces vomiting.

empathy—sympathetically trying to identify one's feelings with those of another.

emphysema—a chronic lung disease characterized by overdistention of the alveolar sacs and inability to exchange oxygen and carbon dioxide.

empyema—exudate (pus) within the pleural space of the chest cavity.

enact—to make into law.

encompass—to surround, enclose.

encounter—to meet, unexpectedly or by chance.

endocardium—the serous membrane lining of the heart.

endocrine—a gland that secretes directly into the blood stream.

endocrinologist—a physician specializing in the diseases and disorders of the endocrine system.

endocrinology—the study of the endocrine or ductless glands of internal secretion.

endocytosis—a cellular process to bring large molecules of material into the cytoplasm of the cell.

endometrium—the mucous membrane lining of the uterus.

endoplasmic reticulum—an organelle within the cytoplasm of a cell.

endorse—to approve, recommend, or sponsor.

endorsement—the act of endorsing; approving.

endoscope—an instrument consisting of a tube and optical system for observing the inside of an organ or cavity.

enema—the instillation of fluid into the rectum and colon.

engorge—to fill with blood to the point of congestion; to devour or engulf.

enhance—to intensify, improve.

enthusiasm—intense interest; zeal; passion.

entity—a thing having reality.

enucleation—surgical excision of the eyeball.

enumerate—to count separately, name one by one.

enunciate—to speak or pronounce clearly.

envelope—to enclose completely with a cover; a paper container for a letter.

environment—surroundings.

enzyme—a complex chemical substance produced by the body, found primarily in the digestive juices, which acts upon food substances to break them down for absorption.

eosinophil—a white blood cell or cellular structure that stains readily with the acid stain eosin; specifically an eosinophilic leukocyte.

epidemic—affecting many persons at one time.

epidermis—the outer layer of the skin; literally *over the true skin.*

epididymis—a convoluted tube resting on the surface of the testicle, which carries sperm from the testicle to the vas deferens.

epigastric—pertaining to the area of the abdomen over the stomach.

epiglottis—a cartilagenous lid which closes over the larynx when swallowing.

epilepsy—a chronic disease of the nervous system characterized by convulsions and often unconsciousness.

epinephrine—a hormone produced by the adrenal medulla.

epiphysis—a portion of bone not yet ossified; the cartilagenous ends of the long bones which allow for growth.

episiotomy—an incision in the perineum to avoid tearing during childbirth.

epistaxis—nosebleed; hemorrhage from the nose.

epithelial—pertaining to a type of cell or tissue that forms the skin and mucous membranes of the body.

equity—the value of property beyond the total amount owed on it.

equivalent—equal to in value, size, or effect.

erectile—refers to tissue which is capable of erection, usually due to vasocongestion.

ergonomics—the applied science of being concerned with the nature and characteristics of people as they relate to design and activities with the intention of producing more effective results and greater safety.

erythema—diffuse redness over the skin due to capillary congestion and dilation of the superficial capillaries.

erythrocyte—a red blood cell (RBC).

erythropoiesis—the formation of red blood corpuscles.

esophagus—a collapsible tube from the pharynx to the stomach through which passes the food and water the body ingests.

essential—necessary; when referring to blood pressure, indicates an elevation without apparent cause.

estrogen—a female hormone produced by the ovaries.

ether—a colorless liquid used to produce unconsciousness and insensibility to pain.

ethical—right, according to the principles of ethics.

ethics—standards of conduct and moral judgement.

etiquette—conventional rules for correct behavior.

euphoria—a feeling of well-being, elation.

eustachian tube—refers to the tube of the middle ear which connects to the pharynx.

evacuate—to empty, especially the bowels.

evacuation—withdrawal, to remove, to make empty.

evaluation—assessment; judgment concerning the worth, quality, significance, or value of a situation, person, or product.

evoke—to call forth or up; summon; elicit.

excretion—the process of expelling material from the body.

exemplify—to show by example.

exempt—excluded; not liable; freedom from duty or service; privileged.

exemption—freed from or not liable for something to which others are subject.

exfoliate—to scale off dead tissue.

exhale—to breathe out.

exocrine—a gland which secretes substances through a duct into the body.

exocytosis—a cellular process which moves materials within the cell to the outside.

exogenous—originating outside an organ or part.

exophthalmia—abnormal protrusion of the eyeball.

exorcism—the act of expelling an evil spirit.

expectorate—to spit, to expel mucus or phlegm from the throat or lungs.

expedient—suitable means for achieving or attaining a purpose or end. Of immediate advantage, convenient.

expedite—to hasten.

expend—to spend or use, as with money or energy.

expertise—special knowledge or skill.

expiration—the expulsion of air from the lungs in breathing.

explicit—clearly and definitely expressed; unambiguous; leaving no room for questions.

express—to utter; to make known in words or by action.

extensive—having a wide range.

extensor—the muscle of a muscle team which extends a part, allowing the joint to straighten.

externship—a supervised employment experience in a qualified health care facility as part of the educational curriculum.

extinguish—to put out; put an end to.

extinguisher—a device for putting out fire.

extracellular—outside the cell.

extract—a substance distilled or drawn out of another substance.

extremity—refers to the terminal parts of the body—the arms, legs.

exudate—pus; the collection of purulent material in a cavity.

eyewash—a device utilizing water to remove foreign material from the eyes, usually in emergency situations.

facility—a building; in medical situations, a building for the care and treatment of patients.

facsimile—an exact copy.

facultative—able to live under conditions of temperature or oxygen supply which vary; having the capability to adapt to more than one condition, as a facultative anerobe.

fallopian tube—the ovaduct; the passageway for the ova from the ovary to the uterus.

family practice—one which cares for patients of all ages and all conditions not requiring specialization.

fascia—a fibrous membrane covering, supporting, and separating muscles; may also unite the skin with underlying tissue.

fasting—to abstain from food; without food or water.

fatal—causing death.

feasible—possible; practicable.

febrile—pertaining to a fever.

fecal—pertaining to feces.

feces—stool, bowel movement.

fee schedule—listing of allowable charge.

femoral—pertaining to the artery that lies adjacent to the femur.

femur—the thigh bone of the leg.

fenestrated—having a window or opening.

fertilization—impregnation of the ovum by the sperm; conception.

fetal—pertaining to a fetus, pregnancy beyond the third month.

fetus—an embryo after eight weeks of gestation.

fibrillation—the quivering of muscle fibers; ineffective, rapid but weak heart action.

fibroid—a tumor made up of fibrous and muscular tissue.

fibula—a long bone in the leg from the knee to the ankle.

filtration—the movement of solutes and water across a semipermeable membrane as a result of a force such as gravity or blood pressure.

fiscal—of or pertaining to finances in general.

fissure—an ulcer, split, crack, or tear in the tissue.

fistula—an abnormal tubelike passage from a normal cavity or an abscess to a free surface.

flatulence—the existence of flatus or intestinal gas.

flatus—intestinal gas.

flexed—bent, as at a joint.

flexibility—easily bent, compliant, yielding to persuasion.

flexor—the muscle of a muscle team that bends a part.

flextime—refers to the practice of permitting work hours within a range of time.

flora—plant life as distinguished from animal life; plant life occurring or adapted for living in a specific environment, as flora in the intestines.

flu—an abbreviation for the word influenza; a respiratory or intestinal infection.

fluoroscope—a device consisting of a fluorescent screen in conjunction with an X-ray tube to make visible shadows of objects interposed between the screen and the tube.

flush—sudden reddish coloration of the skin.

follicle—a small excretory duct or sac or tubular gland; a hair follicle.

folliculitis—a staphylococcal infection of a hair follicle.

foreign—anything that is not normally found in the location; usually refers to dirt, splinters, etc.

foreskin—loose skin covering the end of the penis.

forge—to imitate, especially to counterfeit, as a signature.

formaldehyde—a colorless, pungent gas used in its liquid form to harden tissue for pathological study, or as a germicide, disinfectant, or preservative, according to the strength of the solution.

fovea centralis—a depression in the posterior surface of the retina which is the place of sharpest vision.

fracture—the sudden breaking of a bone.

fraudulent—characterized by cheating and deceit; obtained by dishonest means.

frequency—the need to void urine often, though usually only a small amount at one time.

friction—resistance of one surface to the motion of another surface rubbing over it.

fringe benefits—benefits included in or added to the salary paid, such as health insurance, retirement fund, etc.

frontal—anterior; the forehead bone; refers to the plane drawn through the side of the body from the head to the foot.

functional—practical, working, useful.

fungus—a vegetable, cellular organism that subsists on organic matter, such as bacteria or mold; a disease condition that causes growth of fungal lesions on the surface of the skin.

furuncle—the medical term for a boil.

GYN—see **gynecology.**

gait—manner of walking.

gallbladder—a small sac suspended beneath the liver which concentrates and stores bile.

galley proof—printed matter in preliminary form, to be corrected.

galvanometer—an instrument that measures current by electromagnetic action.

gamete—a germ cell; any reproductive body.

ganglion—a mass of nerve tissue which receives and sends out nerve impulses.

gangrene—a form of necrosis; the putrefaction of soft tissue.

gastric—pertaining to the stomach.

gastrocnemius—the large muscle in the calf of the leg.

gastroenterologist—a physician specializing in the care of patients with diseases and disorders of the gastrointestinal tract.

gastroenterology—the study of the stomach and intestines and their diseases.

gastrointestinal (GI)—pertaining to the stomach and intestines.

gastroscopy—examination of the stomach with a gastroscope.

gauge—the size of a needle bore; the smaller the number the larger the needle bore.

gene—a substance within the chromosome that dictates heredity.

generate—to produce, as heat, ideas, power.

generic—general; characteristic of a genus or group.

genetic—pertaining to the genes.

genital herpes—fluid-filled lesions on the external genitalia which are contagious upon direct contact.

genitalia—the external sexual organs.

genucubital—pertaining to the elbows and knees; the knee-elbow position.

genupectoral—pertaining to the knees and chest; the knee-chest position.

geriatrics—the study and treatment of the diseases of old age.

gerontologist—a physician specializing in the care of the aged.

gigantism—a condition resulting from the overproduction of growth hormone during childhood.

glance—a quick look or view.

glaucoma—a disease of the eye characterized by increased intraocular pressure.

glomerulonephritis—inflammation of the glomerulus of the nephron of the kidney.

glomerulus—the microscopic cluster of capillaries within the Bowman's capsule of the nephron.

glucohemoglobin—sugar in the blood.

glucose—a colorless or yellow, thick, syrupy liquid obtained by the incomplete hydrolysis of starch; a simple sugar.

gluteus maximus—the large muscle of the buttocks.

glycosuria—sugar in the urine.

goiter—an enlargement of the thyroid gland.

golgi apparatus—an organelle within the cytoplasm of a cell.

gonadotrophic—related to stimulation of the gonads.

gonads—the sex glands, the ovaries in the female and the testicles in the male.

gonorrhea—a venereal disease of the reproductive organs which is highly contagious upon direct contact.

graafian follicle—the vesicle in which ova are matured and which releases them when ripened.

graft—a constructed part.

gram-negative—bacteria which take on a pink color with Gram staining process.

gram-positive—bacteria which take on a purple color with Gram staining process.

greenstick—an incomplete fracture, occurring in children.

grillwork—a bar-like device, usually constructed of heavy metal; an open grating for a door or window.

groin—the depression between the thigh and the trunk of the body; the inguinal region.

gross—exclusive of deductions; total; entire.

gross anatomy—refers to the study of those features that can be observed with the naked eye by inspection and dissection.

guaiac—a solution used to test for the presence of occult blood in the stool.

guarantee—assurance that something will be done as specified; a pledge.

guarantor—a person who makes or gives a guarantee or pledge, often to pay another's debt or obligation in the event of default.

guilds—associations of persons engaged in the same trade or calling for mutual protection.

gynecologist—a physician specializing in the care of diseases and disorders of women, particularly the genital organs.

gynecology (GYN)—the study of diseases of the female, particularly of the organs of reproduction.

HCFA—Health Care Financing Administration.

HHS—Health and Human Services.

HIB/hib—hemophilus influenzae type B.

haemophilus—bacterial strains that grow best in hemoglobin.

hallucinogen—a substance which causes hallucinations.

hamstring—a group of muscles of the posterior thigh.

handicap—to hinder; with (people) those who are physically disabled or mentally retarded.

harassment—continual annoyance; persecution.

hard copy—information printed on a solid surface such as paper instead of displayed on a CRT screen or stored on a disk.

harmonious—having parts combined in a proportionate, orderly, or pleasing arrangement; being peaceable or friendly.

hazardous—dangerous; risky.

health—a state of complete physical and mental or social well-being.

heart block—a condition in which impulses from the S-A node fail to carry over to the A-V node resulting in a slow heart rate and a different rate of contraction between the upper and lower heart chambers.

heartburn—a burning sensation beneath the breastbone, usually associated with indigestion.

hematocrit—an expression of the volume of red blood cells per unit of circulating blood.

hematologist—a physician specializing in the care of patients with disorders and diseases of the blood and blood-forming organs.

hematology—the study of the blood and its diseases.

hematoma—a tumor or swelling which contains blood.

hematuria—blood in the urine.

hemodialysis—a process whereby blood is passed through a thin membrane and exposed to a dialysate solution to remove waste products.

hemoglobin—the combination of a protein and iron pigment in the red blood cells that attracts and carries oxygen in the body.

hemolysis—dissolution; the breaking down of red blood cells.

hemophilia—hereditary condition, transmitted through sex-linked chromosomes of female carriers; affects males only, causing inability to clot blood.

hemorrhage—abnormal discharge of blood either internally or externally from venous, arterial, or capillary vessels.

hemorrhoidectomy—surgical excision of hemorrhoidal tissue.

hemorrhoids—varicose veins of the anal canal.

hemothorax—blood within the pleural space of the chest cavity.

heparin—a substance formed in the liver which inhibits the coagulation of blood.

hepatic—pertaining to the liver.

hepatitis—inflammation of the liver.

hernia—a projection of a part from its normal location.

herniorrhaphy—the surgical repair of a hernia.

Herpes Simplex—the medical term for fever blister, an acute viral infection of the face, mouth or nose.

Herpes Zoster—the medical term for shingles, an acute viral infection of the dorsal root ganglia.

hesitancy—difficulty in starting a urine stream.

heterosexual—sexual attraction toward the opposite sex.

heterotrophs—microorganisms that feed on organic matter.

hiatus—pertains to a herniation of the stomach through an opening or hiatus.

hiccough—(Also hiccup) a result of the spasmodic closing of the epiglottis and spasm of the diaphragm.

hilum—the recessed area of the kidney where the ureter and blood vessels enter.

hinge—a type of joint.

Hippocratic—refers to the oath taken by a doctor bonding him to observe the code of medical ethics contained in the oath by Hippocrates in the 4th century.

histamine—a substance normally present in the body.

histologist—(Histotechnologist) a person engaged in the study of the microscopic structure of tissue.

histoplasmosis—a fungal infection caused by an organism found in bird and bat droppings.

holistic—considering the whole or entire scope of a situation.

Holter monitor—a device that attaches electrodes to a patient's chest for the purpose of obtaining a 24-hour EKG tracing in an accessory tape recorder.

homeostasis—maintenance of a constant or static condition of internal environment.

homosexual—sexual attraction toward the same sex as oneself.

honesty—the state of being truthful, trustworthy; genuine.

horizontal—not vertical; flat and even; level; parallel to the plane of the horizon.

hormone—a chemical substance secreted by an organ or gland.

hostility—unfriendliness, enmity.

hpf—high-power field; refers to microscope lens.

humble—modest, unassuming.

humerus—the long bone of the upper arm.

humoral—antibody-mediated immunity.

hyaline membrane disease—a condition resulting from incomplete development of the respiratory system in premature infants.

hydrocele—the accumulation of fluid in the scrotum.

hydrochloric acid—a digestive juice found in the stomach.

hygiene—the study of health and observance of health rules.

hygienist—one who provides health related services, such as dental procedures.

hymen—a membranous fold partially or completely covering the vaginal opening.

hyperglycemia—increase of blood sugar, as in diabetes.

hyperopia—a defect of vision so that objects can only be seen when they are far away; farsightedness.

hypersensitive—over sensitive; abnormally sensitive to a stimulus of any kind.

hypertension—elevated blood pressure.

hyperthermia—higher than normal temperature.

hyperthyroidism—a condition caused by excessive secretion of the thyroid glands.

hypertonic—having a higher concentration of salt than found in a red blood cell.

hyperventilation—excessive deep and frequent breathing.

hypoallergenic—unlikely to cause an allergic reaction.

hypochondriac—pertaining to the upper outer regions of the abdomen below the thorax; also someone with a morbid fear of disease, resulting in abnormal concern about one's health.

hypogastric—referring to an abdominal area in the middle lower third of the abdomen.

hypoglycemia—deficiency of sugar in the blood.

hypotension—abnormally low blood pressure.

hypothalamus—a structure of the brain between the cerebrum and the midbrain; lies below the thalamus.

hypothermia—below normal body temperature.

hypothyroidism—a condition caused by a marked deficiency of thyroid secretion.

hypotonic—having a lower concentration of salt than found in a red blood cell.

hypoxia—a lack of oxygen.

hysterectomy—surgical removal of the uterus.

hysteroscopy—a procedure utilizing the hysteroscope to view the endometrium of the uterus.

ICD—see International Classification of Diseases.

I & D—see **incision and drainage.**

IVP—see **intravenous pyelography.**

identification—anything by which a person or thing can be identified.

idiopathic—disease without recognizable cause.

ileocecal—the valve between the end of the small intestine and the cecum.

ileostomy—a surgical opening from the ileum onto the abdominal wall.

ileum—the last section of the small intestine.

iliac—the edge or crest of the pelvic bone.

ilium—the hip bone.

illegible—impossible to read.

illicit—improper; unlawful; not sanctioned by custom or law; illegal.

illuminate—to enlighten, throw light on.

imaging—a representation or visual impression produced by a lens, mirror, etc.

immobilize—to keep out of action or circulation; stationary.

immune—protected or exempt from a disease.

immunization—becoming immune or the process of rendering a patient immune.

immunodeficiency—lacking the components necessary to mount an immune response.

immunoglobulin—a large protein molecule which assists in the immune response.

immunological—pertaining to immunology.

immunosuppressed—a condition wherein the immune system has been overpowered and cannot function adequately.

impacted—refers to a fracture where the broken ends are jammed together.

impaction—a collection of hardened feces in the rectum which cannot be expelled.

impending—to be at hand or about to happen.

implant—something implanted into tissue; a graft; artificial part.

implement—a tool or instrument for doing something; to put into effect.

implementation—put into effect.

implication—involvement, bringing into connection.

impotence—inability of a male to obtain or maintain an erection.

impulse—a charge transmitted through certain tissues, especially nerve fibers and muscles, resulting in physiological activity.

inappropriate—not appropriate, out of place.

incinerate—to burn, set afire.

incision—cut.

incision and drainage (I & D)—cutting into for the purpose of providing an exit for material, usually a collection of pus.

inclined—leaning or tending toward.

incomprehensible—beyond belief, not to be grasped by the mind.

incongruous—lacking harmony or agreement.

incontinent—unable to control the bladder or bowel.

increments—becoming greater; amount of increase; gain.

incubation—the interval between exposure to infection and the appearance of the first symptom.

incus—the anvil, the middle bone of the three in the middle ear.

indigent—needy, poor, destitute.

indigestion—difficulty in digesting food.

inevitable—unavoidable, destined to occur.

infarct—infiltration of foreign particles; material in a vessel causing coagulation and interference with circulation.

infectious—capable of producing infection; denoting a disease in the body caused by the presence of germs; tending to spread to others.

inferior—below, under.

infertility—inability to achieve conception.

infirmity—illness, disease.

inflict—to strike, to cause punishment.

influenza—an acute illness characterized by fever, pain, coughing, and general upper respiratory symptoms.

infrared—pertaining to those invisible rays just beyond the red end of the visible spectrum which have a penetrating heating effect.

infusion—to instill; introduction of a substance into a vein.

ingest—to eat.

inguinal—referring to the region where the thigh joins the trunk of the body; the groin.

inguinal canal—a passageway in the groin for the spermatic cord in the male.

inguinal hernia—the presence of small intestine in the inguinal canal.

inhale—to breathe in.

initial—the first; beginning; the first letter of each of a person's names.

initiate—to get something started, begin.

initiative—the action of taking the first step; ability to originate new ideas.

innate—inborn; inherent.

inoculating loop—a laboratory instrument used to transfer organisms from one source to another.

inorganic—not living; occurring in nature independently of living things.

inseminate—to impregnate with semen.

insertion—the place where a muscle is attached to the bone that it moves.

insidious—hidden, not apparent.

insignificant—unimportant; petty; of little or no value.

insomnia—abnormal inability to sleep.

inspect—to examine closely.

inspection—the first part of a physical examination; close observation.

inspiration—to breathe in, inhale.

institute—to originate as a custom.

insufficient—not as much as needed.

insulin—a hormone secreted by the Islands of Langerhans in the pancreas.

insurance—a contract to guarantee compensation for a specified situation.

intact—unbroken, undamaged.

intangible—that which cannot be touched, easily defined or grasped.

integrity—soundness of character; honesty in particular.

integumentary—the skin; a covering.

intellectualization—to employ reasoning to avoid confrontations or stressful situations.

intelligence—the ability to learn or understand.

interaction—to act upon one another.

intercostal—between the ribs.

interference—confusion of desired signals due to undesired signals, as in artifacts on an EKG.

interferon—a lymphokine that helps regulate the activities of macrophages and NK cells.

interjection—a part of speech; an exclamation.

interleukin—a substance which is a messenger between leukocytes.

intermediate—in the middle.

intermittent—stopping and starting again at intervals.

intermuscular—within the muscle.

International Classification of Diseases—ICD; a comprehensive listing of diseases and disorders of the human body.

interneurons—neurons connecting sensory to motor neurons.

internist—a physician specializing in the care of patients with internal diseases.

internship—a period of time following graduation wherein practice of the profession is performed.

interpersonal—between persons.

interpret—to explain, translate; to determine the meaning.

interval—time between events; space.

intervention—taking action to modify, hinder, or change an effect.

intervertebral—between the vertebrae.

intestine—the alimentary canal extending from the pylorus of the stomach to the anus.

intimidate—to make afraid, to frighten.

intimidation—to make afraid; to deter with threats.

intracellular—within the cell.

intradermal—within the skin.

intraocular—within the eyeball.

intrauterine device (IUD)—an object inserted into the uterus to prevent pregnancy.

intravenous—to insert into the vein.

intravenous pyelography (IVP)—the insertion of a radiopaque material into the vein for the purpose of X-raying the kidneys and ureters.

intricate—complicated, complex, elaborately interwoven.

intubation—insertion of a tube into the larynx for entrance of air.

intuition—the immediate knowing or learning of something without the conscious use of reasoning.

inunction—the process of administering drugs through the skin.

invasive—diagnostic methods involving entry into living tissue.

inventory—an itemized list of goods in stock.

involuntary—independent of or even contrary to will or choice.

iodine—a nonmetallic element belonging to the halogen group.

iris—the colored, contractible tissue surrounding the pupil of the eye.

irrational—lacking the power to reason; senseless.

irreparable—damaged beyond possibility of repair.

ischemia—temporary and localized anemia due to obstruction of the circulation to a part.

ischium—posterior and inferior portion of the hip bone.

Ishahara—refers to an eye test to determine color vision.

Islet of Langerhans—clusters of cells in the pancreas.

isotonic—having the same concentration of salt as found in a red blood cell.

issue—to send forth; to put into circulation.

Jaeger—a system for measuring near vision acuity.

jaundice—a yellowish discoloration of the sclera and skin due to the presence of bile pigments in the blood.

jejunum—the middle segment of the small intestine, which measures approximately 8 feet in length.

journal—a record of happenings; a diary.

journalizing—entries on the daily log.

judgment—a decision; ability to make the right decisions.

keloid—an overgrowth of new skin tissue; a scar.

keying—pressing a lever or button, as on a typewriter, that is pressed with the finger to operate the machine.

kidney—a bean-shaped organ that excretes urine and is located retroperitoneally, high in the back of the abdominal cavity.

KUB—kidneys, ureters, and bladder; refers to a radiological study.

kyphosis—a convex curvature of the spine; humpback.

L & A—light and accommodation.

labia majora—the two large folds of adipose tissue lying on each side of the vulva of the female; external genitalia.

labia minora—the two mucocutaneous folds of membrane within the labia majora.

laboratory—a room or building in which scientific tests or experiments are conducted.

laboratory technician—a health care worker who performs specialized chemical, microscopic, and bacteriologic tests of blood, tissue, and body fluids.

laceration—a cut or tear.

lacrimal—pertaining to tears; the glands and ducts which secrete and convey tears.

laminectomy—the removal of a portion of the vertebral posterior arch.

lancet—a sharp, pointed instrument used to pierce the skin to obtain a capillary blood sample.

laryngeal—pertaining to the larynx.

laryngectomy—surgical removal of the larynx or voice box.

larynx—the voice box.

lateral—pertaining to the side.

latissimus dorsi—the large muscle of the back.

laxative—a substance which induces the bowels to empty.

ledger—the principal account book of a business establishment, containing the credits and debits.

legible—easy to read, readable.

Legionnaires disease—an acute bronchopneumonia.

leisure—spare or free time, away from the pressure and responsibilities of work.

lens—a part of the eye which bends or refracts images onto the retina.

lesion—an injury or wound; a circumscribed area of pathologically altered tissue.

lethal—deadly; capable of causing death.

leukemia—a disease characterized by a great excess of white blood cells; it exists in a lymphatic and myelogenous form; it is often fatal, especially in adults.

leukocyte—a white blood cell.

liability—anything to which a person is liable, responsible, legally bound.

liaison—intercommunication between two entities.

license—a legal permit to engage in an activity.

licensed practical nurse (LPN)—an individual trained in basic nursing techniques, to provide direct patient care under the supervision of an RN or physician.

ligament—fibrous tissue which connects bone to bone.

ligation—to tie off; the process of binding or tying.

limbs—refers to the arms and legs.

liter—a unit of measure; 1,000 ml or approximately 1 quart.

liver—the largest gland in the body, located in the upper right quadrant of the abdomen beneath the diaphragm.

lithotomy—an examination position wherein the patient lies upon the back with thighs flexed upon the abdomen and legs flexed upon the thighs.

lithotripsy—destruction of stone; stonecrusher.

LMP—last menstrual period.

longevity—a long duration of life; lasting a long time.

longitudinal fissure—the deep cleft between the two hemispheres of the cerebrum.

lordosis—abnormal anterior curvature of the lumbar spine.

lpf—low-power field; refers to microscope lens.

lubb dupp—sounds made by the heart.

lumbar—pertaining to the back, specifically to the five vertebrae above the sacrum.

lumbar puncture—the insertion of a needle between the vertebrae in the lumbar area for the purpose of withdrawing spinal fluid.

lumen—the space within an artery, vein, or capillary; the space within a tube.

lung—the organ of respiration, located within the thoracic cavity.

lupus erythematosus—a chronic autoimmune disease which causes changes in the immune system.

luteinizing—a hormone effect which causes ovulation and progesterone in the female and sperm production and testosterone in the male.

Lyme Disease—a disease caused by a spirochete which is carried by the deer tick.

lymph—a body fluid formed within the tissue spaces and circulated throughout the body.

lymphatic system—a network of transparent vessels carrying lymph fluid throughout the body.

lymphocyte—a type of white blood cell.

lysosomes—an organelle within the cytoplasm of the cell.

MI—see myocardial infarction.

MRI—see magnetic resonance imaging.

MUGA—see multiple-gated acquisition scan.

macrophage—a phagocytic cell that destroys antigens.

macule—a discolored spot or patch on the skin neither elevated nor depressed.

magnetic—having the properties of a magnet, able to attract.

magnetic resonance imaging (MRI)—a diagnostic test using magnetic waves to visualize internal body structures.

magnify—to make something look larger than it really is.

mailable—a standard for judging written correspondence as satisfactory for sending.

maintenance—to preserve; the act or work of keeping something in proper condition.

malaise—a feeling of discomfort or uneasiness.

malignant—a cancerous growth; tumor.

malinger—to pretend illness to escape dealing with a situation or obligation.

malleus—the largest of the three bones of the middle ear, also called the hammer.

mammary glands—the breasts.

mammograph—an X-ray of the breast.

management—the act, manner, or practice of managing, handling, or controlling something.

mandate—an order of authorative command; instruction.

manifestation—act of disclosing; revelation; display.

manipulation therapy—any treatment or procedure involving the use of the hands; movement of a joint to determine its range of extension and flexion; additional manual skills utilized by osteopathic physicians.

marginal—close to the lower limit of acceptability.

marrow—the soft tissue in the hollow of long bones.

masses—a multitude; a large number of people.

mastectomy—surgical removal of a breast.

matrix—a format for establishing a time schedule for appointments.

maturation—refers to a stage of cellular development.

maturity—a state of full development.

measles—a highly contagious disease characterized by the presence of maculopustular eruptions.

mechanical—pertaining to machinery.

medial—pertaining to the middle or midline.

Medicare—a federal health program for paying certain medical expenses of the aged.

Medigap—refers to situations not covered by Medicare insurance.

medulla—the inner section of the kidney.

medulla oblongata—enlarged portion of the spinal cord; the lower portion of the brain stem.

melanin—a pigment which gives color to the skin, hair, and eyes.

melanocyte—cells which produce the pigment of the skin, melanin.

membrane—a thin, soft, pliable layer of tissue which lines a tube or cavity or covers an organ or structure.

menarche—the first menstrual period.

Meniere's disease—a disorder of the ear characterized by nausea, vomiting, tinnitus, and hearing loss.

meninges—the membranes covering the brain and spinal cord.

meningitis—inflammation of the meninges of the brain and/or spinal cord.

meniscus—a concave level of fluid in a tube or cylinder.

menopause—the permanent cessation of menstruation.

menorrhagia—excessive menstrual flow, hemorrhage.

menstruate—to periodically discharge bloody fluid from the uterus.

mensuration—the process of measuring.

mercury—a liquid metal used in measurement devices such as thermometers and sphygmomanometers; chemical symbol, Hg.

merit—to deserve reward or praise; excellence.

mesentery—a peritoneal fold connecting the intestine to the posterior abdominal wall.

metabolism—the successive transformations to which a substance is subjected from the time it enters the body to the time it or its decomposition products are excreted, and by which nutrition is accomplished and energy and living substance are provided.

metacarpals—pertaining to the five bones of the hand between the wrist and the phalanges.

metastasis—movement of cancer cells from one part of the body to another.

metatarsals—the five bones of the feet between the instep and the phalanges.

methodical—systematic, following a plan or method.

microbial—related to microbes.

microfiche—a sheet of microfilm capable of accommodating and preserving a considerable number of book pages in reduced form.

microorganism—a microscopic living body not perceivable by the naked eye.

microscopic—visible only with a microscope.

microscopic anatomy—an area of study that deals with features that can be seen only with a microscope.

micturation   the passing of urine.

midbrain—that portion of the brain connecting the pons and the cerebellum.

midline—the middle.

migraine—a severe headache with characteristic symptoms.

minute—a measurement of time equal to 60 seconds; very small, tiny.

misalignment—out of alignment; not straight.

misspelled—to spell incorrectly.

mitochondria—an organelle within the cytoplasm of the cell.

mitosis—the division of a cell.

mitral—the valve in the heart between the chambers of the left side, also known as the bicuspid.

mobility   quality of being mobile; easy to move.

modifier—changes; limits the meaning.

modifies—changes the form or quality of; alters slightly.

molten—melted.

monilia—a family of parasitic fungi or molds.

monitor—to oversee or observe.

monoclonal—a laboratory-produced hybrid cell which produces antibodies.

monocular—possessing a single eyepiece as with a microscope.

monocyte—single nucleated cells which leave the blood and enter into tissues to become macrophages.

monotone—a single, unvaried tone; having the same pitch; a tiresome sameness.

mons pubis—a pad of fatty tissue and coarse skin overlying the symphysis pubis in the female.

mores—folkways that, through general observance, develop the force of a law.

morphology—a branch of biology dealing with the form and structure of organisms.

motor—refers to the nerves which permit the body to respond to stimuli.

mouth—the oral cavity; can also refer to the opening to organs.

mucosa—pertaining to mucous membrane.

multi-channel—refers to the capability of ECG equipment of processing impulses from multiple leads.

multi-skilled—having more than one skill area for employment.

multiple-gated acquisition scan (MUGA)—a diagnostic test to evaluate the condition of the myocardium of the heart.

mumps—an acute contagious disease characterized by inflammation of the parotid gland and other salivary glands.

murmur—a soft blowing or rasping sound heard on auscultation of the heart.

muscle—a type of tissue composed of contractile cells or fibers which effect movement of the body.

muscle team—a pair of skeletal muscles, one which flexes and one which extends the joint.

muscle tone—a state of muscle contraction in which a portion of the fibers are contracted while others are at rest.

muscular—pertaining to muscles.

musculoskeletal—pertaining to the muscular and skeletal systems.

mutation—a change in an inheritable characteristic; cellular change due to an influence.

myelin—a fatlike substance forming the principal component of the myelin sheath of nerve fibers.

myelography—an X-ray examination of the spinal cord following an injection of a radiopaque material.

myocardial infarction (MI)—blockage of a coronary artery which interrupts the flow of blood to the heart muscle.

myocardium—the muscle layer of the heart.

myometrium—the muscular structure of the uterus.

myopia—a defect in vision so that objects can only be seen when very near; nearsightedness.

myxedema—a condition resulting from the hypofunction of the thyroid gland.

narcolepsy—overwhelming attacks of sleep which the victim cannot inhibit; sleeping sickness.

narcotic—a drug capable of producing sleep and relieving pain or inducing unconsciousness and even death, depending upon the dosage.

nasal—pertaining to the nose.

nausea—an inclination to vomit.

negate—to deny the existence or truth of.

negligent—guilty of neglect; lacking in due care or concern; act of carelessness.

negotiable—capable of being discussed and terms arranged.

neoadjuvant—new attachment process; giving chemotherapy prior to surgery to shrink the tumor before removal.

neonate—a newborn infant.

neoplastic—new abnormal tissue formation; cancer related.

nephrologist—a physician specializing in the diseases and disorders of the kidney.

nephrology—the study of the kidney and its diseases.

nephron—the structural and functional unit of the kidney.

nephrotic syndrome—term applied to renal disease of whatever cause characterized by massive edema, proteinuria, and usually elevation of serum cholesterol and lipids.

nerve—a group of nervous tissues bound together for the purpose of conducting nervous impulses.

nervosa—loss of appetite for food not connected with a disease; part of a psychosis.

net—remaining after all deductions have been made; to clear as profit.

neurilemma—a thin membranous sheath enveloping a nerve fiber.

neurologist—a physician specializing in the diseases and disorders of the nervous system.

neurology—the study of the nervous system and its diseases.

neuron—a nerve cell.

neurosurgery—surgical procedures performed on the nervous system.

neutrophil—a granulated white blood cell.

nicotine—a poisonous alkaloid extracted from tobacco leaves.

nit—the egg of a louse or other parasitic insect.

nocturia—having to void at night.

node—a knot, knob, protuberance, or swelling.

nomenclature—a system of technical or scientific names.

nominal—too small to be considered, or a very small amount.

nomogram—representation by graphs, diagrams, or charts of the relationship between numerical variables.

nonchalant—unconcerned, indifferent.

non compos mentis—general legal term for all forms of mental illness.

non-invasive—a diagnostic method not requiring entry into body tissue.

nonpathogen—an organism which does not produce a disease.

nonspecific urethritis—inflammation of the urethra in males, vaginitis or cervicitis in females, due to bacteria or an allergy to substances used by a sexual partner.

norepinephrine—a hormone secreted by adrenal medulla in response to sympathetic stimulation.

normal saline—a solution with the same salt content as that found within a red blood cell.

nuclear—pertaining to the nucleus of an atom.

nuclear medicine—the branch of medicine which utilizes radionuclides in the diagnosis and treatment of disease.

nucleolus—a structure found within the nucleus of the cell

nucleus—the vital body in the protoplasm of a cell.

numeric—denoting a number or system of numbers.

nurse practitioner—an RN with advanced clinical experience and education in a special branch of practice.

nurture—to care for, train, or educate.

nutrition—refers to edible material, food, things that nourish.

nutritionist—a member of the health care team who studies and applies the principles and science of nutrition.

OSHA—Occupational Safety and Health Act.

OTC—see **over the counter.**

objective—the end toward which action is directed; of a disease symptom, perceptible to persons other than the one affected; on a microscope, a lens or series of lenses.

obligate—to bind legally or morally.

obliterate—to blot out; leaving no trace; destroy.

observant—quick to notice, watchful.

obsolete—out of use, discarded, no longer useful.

obstetrician—a physician who specializes in the care and treatment of women during pregnancy and childbirth.

obstetrics—the branch of medicine dealing with women during pregnancy, childbirth, and postpartum.

obturator—anything that obstructs or closes a cavity or opening; refers to that internal portion of an examining instrument which facilitates the introduction of the instrument into the body and is then withdrawn permitting visualization of the internal area.

occipital—pertaining to the back part of the head, the posterior lobe of the cerebrum.

occlude—to close up, obstruct.

occult—obscure, hidden.

occulta—obscure; hidden.

occupational medicine—diagnosing and treating disease or conditions arising from occupational circumstances.

occupational therapist—a health care worker involved in the use of purposeful activity with individuals who are limited by physical injury or illness, psychosocial dysfunction, developmental or learning diabilities, poverty and cultural differences, or the aging process to maximize independence, prevent disability, and maintain health.

occupational therapy assistant—OTA; a person trained to assist an occupational therapist.

O.D.—oculus dexter, or right eye.

office manager—(Business Office Manager) an individual responsible for the overall operation of the medical office.

ointment—a salve; a fatty, soft substance having antiseptic or healing properties.

olfactory—pertaining to the sense of smell.

oliguria—scanty production of urine.

oncogenes—a gene in a tumor cell.

oncology—the branch of medicine dealing with tumors, usually malignant.

ophthalmologist—a physician specializing in the diseases and disorders of the eye.

ophthalmology—the study of the eye and its diseases.

opportunistic—seizing the opportunity; taking advantage of the situation.

opposition—action against, resistance.

optic—pertaining to the eye or sight.

optic disc—the blind spot where the optic nerve exits from the retina of the eye.

optometrist—a person who measures the eye's refractive power and prescribes correction of visual defects when needed.

oral—pertaining to the mouth.

orbital—refers to the cavity within the skull where the eye is located.

organ—a part of the body constructed of many types of tissue to perform a function.

organ of Corti—terminal acoustic apparatus in the cochlea of the inner ear.

organelles—functional structures within the cytoplasm of a cell.

organic—pertaining to or derived from animal or vegetable forms of life.

origin—the beginning or source of anything; of muscles, the anchor.

orthopedics—the branch of medicine dealing with the structure and function of bones and muscles.

orthopedist—a physician who corrects deformities and treats diseases and disorders of the bones, joints, and spine.

orthopnea—respiratory condition in which breathing is possible only in an erect sitting or standing position.

orthostatic—standing; concerning an erect position.

O.S.—oculus sinister, or left eye; also a mouth or opening.

oscilloscope—an instrument that displays a visual representation of electric variations on the fluorescent screen of a cathode ray tube.

osmosis—the process of diffusion of water or another solvent through a selected permeable membrane.

osseous—bonelike, concerning bones.

osteopathy—any bone disease; also refers to a school of medicine based on the belief that the bony fragment of the body largely determines the structural relations of its tissues.

osteoporosis—a condition resulting from a decrease in the amount of calcium stored in the bone.

OTA—see occupational therapy assistant.

otitis—inflammation of the ear; can be referenced to the external, middle, or internal ear.

otorhinolaryngologist—a physician specializing in diseases and disorders of the ear, nose, and throat.

otorhinolaryngology—the study of the ear, nose, and larynx and their diseases.

otosclerosis—condition characterized by progressive deafness due to the fixation of the stapes of the middle ear.

O.U.—oculus uterque, or each eye.

ovary—the female gonad which produces hormones causing the secondary sex characteristics to develop and be maintained.

over the counter (OTC)—referring to accessible, nonprescription drugs.

ovulation—the periodic ripening and rupture of a mature graafian follicle and the discharge of the ovum.

ovum—an egg, the female gamete or reproductive cell.

oxalate—a salt of oxalic acid.

oxygen—a colorless, odorless, tasteless gas found in the air; chemical symbol, O_2.

oxygenate—combine or supply with oxygen.

PDR—*Physician's Desk Reference.*

PKU—see **phenylketonuria.**

POL—physician's office laboratory.

PS—see **postscript.**

pacemaker—the S-A node of the heart; also refers to an artificial device which initiates heartbeat.

pallor—lack of color, paleness.

palpate—to feel; to examine by touch.

pancreas—an organ which secretes insulin and pancreatic digestive juice.

pancreatitis—inflammation of the pancreas.

pandemic—epidemic over a large region; epidemic in many regions.

pantomime—motions or gestures used for expressive communication.

Papanicolaou (Pap) smear—a test to detect cancer cells in the mucus of an organ.

papillae—small protuberances or elevations, such as the taste buds of the tongue.

papillary muscles—muscular attachments to the undersides of the heart valves from the walls of the ventricles, which open the valves during the relaxation phase of the heartbeat.

parabasal—beside, near, an accessory to the base or lower part.

paralytic ileus—paralysis of the intestinal wall with symptoms of acute obstruction.

paramedic—health care providers who provide emergency and supportive medical care. Have additional training beyond EMT status.

parameter—quantity to which an arbitrary value may be given as a convenience in expressing performance or for use in calculations.

parasite—an organism that lives in or on another organism without rendering it any service in return.

parasympathetic—a division of the autonomic nervous system.

parathyroid—small endocrine glands located close to the thyroid gland.

parenteral—other than by mouth.

parietal—a central portion of the cerebrum located on each side of the brain.

paroxysmal—a sudden attack of a disease; fit of acute pain, passion, coughing, or laughter.

patella—the kneecap.

pathogen—any microorganism or substance capable of producing a disease.

pathological—a condition due to a disease.

pathologist—a physician specializing in the interpretation and diagnosis of changes caused by disease in tissues and body fluids.

pathology—the study of the nature and cause of disease.

pathophysiology—the study of mechanisms by which disease occurs, the responses of the body to the disease process, and the effects of both on normal function.

patience—calm in waiting, endurance without complaint.

patient care technician—PCT; a health care worker who utilizes both nursing and medical assisting skills to provide patient care in a hospital setting.

payee—a person to whom money is paid.

PCT—see patient care technician.

pectoralis major—the principal muscle of the chest wall.

pediatrician—a physician specializing in the diseases and disorders of children.

pediatrics—the branch of medicine dealing with the care of children and their diseases.

pediculosis—the scientific name for lice.

peer—equal; usually refers to someone of similar standing or status.

pelvic—pertaining to the pelvis.

penis—the male external sex organ.

peptic—pertaining to digestion; can also refer to an ulcer of the upper digestive tract.

per capita—for each person.

perceive—to become aware of through the senses; to understand.

percentage—rate or proportion of each hundred.

perception—awareness through the senses; the receipt of impressions; consciousness.

percussion—tapping the body lightly but sharply to determine the position, size, and consistency of an underlying structure.

perfusion—passing of a fluid through spaces; the act of pouring over or through.

pericarditis—inflammation of the pericardium, the covering of the heart.

pericardium—the membranous sac that covers the heart.

perineum—the region between the vagina and anus of the female and the scrotum and anus of the male.

periodic—occurring, appearing, or done again and again, at regular intervals.

periosteum—the fibrous membrane covering the bone except at the articulating surfaces.

peripheral—pertaining to a portion of the nervous system; an item attached to a computer system.

peristalsis—a progressive, wavelike muscular movement which occurs involuntarily in the urinary and digestive system.

peritoneal—pertaining to the peritoneum.

peritoneum—the membrane which lines the abdominal cavity and covers the abdominal organs.

permeable—capable of being penetrated; allowing entrance.

pernicious anemia—a severe anemia characterized by progressive decrease in the production of red blood cells.

perplexing—troubling with doubt, puzzling.

persecute—treat badly; do harm to again and again; pursue to injure.

perserverance—the act of continuing steadfastly, especially in the face of discouragement.

personality—the personal or individual qualities that make one person different from another.

perspective—a view of things, or facts, in which they are in the right relations.

pertinent—having to do with what is being considered; relevant or to the point.

pertussis—an acute infectious disease characterized by a paroxysmal cough, ending in a whooping inspiration.

petechiae—small, purplish, hemorrhagic spots on the skin.

petition—a written plea in which specific court action is sought.

petty—small, having little value, mean, narrow-minded.

pH—a measure of acidity or alkalinity.

phagocyte—a white blood cell that engulfs and destroys antigens.

phagocytosis—ingestion and digestion of bacteria and particles by phagocytes.

phalanges—bones of the fingers and toes.

phalanx—any one of the bones of the fingers or toes.

phantom limb—an illusion following amputation of a limb that the limb still exists.

pharmaceutical—concerning drugs or pharmacy.

pharmacist—a licensed health care provider who prepares and dispenses drugs.

pharmacology—the study and practice of compounding and dispensing medical preparations.

pharmacy technician—PT; an assistant to a pharmacist who prepares and in some situations administers medication.

pharynx—the throat; that portion of the alimentary canal between the mouth and the esophagus.

phenylalanine—an amino acid of a protein.

phenylketonuria (PKU)—a genetic disorder resulting from the body's failure to oxidize an amino acid, perhaps because of a defective enzyme.

phimosis—a narrowing of the opening of the foreskin of the penis.

phlebitis—inflammation of a vein.

phlebotomist—a health care worker who specializes in obtaining blood samples.

photocopy—a photographic reproduction of written matter made by a special device.

photophobia—sensitive to light; avoiding light.

physical—pertaining to the body; also used for the examination of the body.

physical medicine—the branch of medicine dealing with the treatment of disorders and diseases with mechanical devices, as in physical therapy.

physical therapist—one who is licensed to assist in the examination, testing, and treatment of physically disabled or handicapped people through the use of special exercise, application of heat or cold, use of sonar, and other techniques.

physician—a medical doctor; one skilled in the practice of medicine.

physician's assistant—a person trained in certain aspects of the practice of medicine to provide assistance to the physician.

physician's office laboratory—a designated room in the physician's office where laboratory procedures and tests are performed by qualified persons.

physiology—the study of the function of the cells, tissues, and organs of the body.

pia mater—innermost of the three meninges of the brain and spinal cord.

pigment—any coloring matter.

pineal body—a small endocrine gland attached to the posterior part of the third ventricle of the brain.

pinocytosis—the process whereby a cell engulfs large amounts of liquid.

pitch—the frequency of vibrations of sound which enable one to classify sound on a scale from high to low.

pitfall—trap or hidden danger.

pituitary—a small endocrine gland attached to the base of the brain; the "master" gland.

PKU (phenylketonuria)—a genetic disorder resulting from the body's failure to oxidize an amino acid, perhaps because of a defective enzyme.

placenta—the structure through which the fetus obtains nourishment during pregnancy; the afterbirth.

plague—a deadly epidemic or pestilence.

planes—a flat or relatively smooth surface; points of reference by which positions or parts of the body are indicated.

plasma—the liquid part of the lymph and blood.

platelet—a type of cell found in the blood which is required for clotting.

pleura—a serous membrane which covers the lungs and lines the thoracic cavity.

pleurisy—inflammation of the pleura.

plexuses—a network of nerves.

plight—unfavorable situation or distressed condition.

pneumoconiosis—a respiratory condition due to inhalation of dust particles from mining or stone cutting.

pneumoencephalography—an X-ray examination of ventricles and subarachnoid spaces of brain following withdrawal of cerebrospinal fluid and injection of air or gas via a lumbar puncture.

pneumonia—inflammation of the lung caused primarily by microbes, chemical irritants, vegetable dust, or allergy.

pneumothorax—a collection of air or gas in the pleural cavity which displaces lung tissue.

podiatrist—(Chiropodist) a person trained to diagnose and treat diseases and disorders of the feet.

podiatry—the branch of medicine dealing with disorders of the feet.

POL—see physician's office laboratory.

polio—(Poliomyelitis) an acute, infectious, systemic disease which causes inflammation of the grey matter of the spinal cord.

polling—pertains to obtaining an unauthorized FAX transmission.

polycystic disease—a condition of multiple cysts.

polycythemia—an excess of red blood cells.

polyp—a tumor with a pedicle, especially on mucous membranes such as in the nose, rectum, or intestines.

polyuria—excessive secretion and discharge of urine.

pons—a portion of the brain stem connecting the medulla

oblongata and cerebellum with upper portions of the brain.

popliteal—pertains to the area back of the knee.

portal—pertaining to the portal circulation of blood from impaired internal organs to the liver for processing before entering the inferior vena cava.

positive—strongly affirmative.

post—to transfer charges from the day sheet to patient account records.

posterior—toward the rear or back or toward the caudal end.

postmark—a dated cancellation of a stamp by the post office which also identifies the place of posting.

postoperative (post-op)—after or following a surgical procedure.

postpartum—the period following delivery of a baby.

postscript (PS)—an addition to a letter written after the writer's name has been signed.

posture—the position and carriage of the body as a whole.

potential—possible; ability to develop into actuality.

Power of Attorney—a legal document authorizing a person to act as another's attorney, legal representative, or agent.

PPMP—see provider-performed microscopy procedures.

practitioner—one who practices the profession of medicine.

precancerous—a state just prior to the development of cancer.

precautions—care beforehand; a preventive measure.

precise—exact; definite; very accurate.

precision—exactness, accuracy.

precordial—pertaining to that area of the chest wall over the heart for the placement of EKG chest leads.

pregnancy—the condition of being with child.

preliminary—coming before, leading up to.

premium—the amount paid or payable. For example, an insurance policy premium.

preoperative (pre-op)—the preparatory period preceding surgery.

presbycusis—impairment of acute hearing in old age.

presbyopia—a defect of vision in advancing age involving loss of accommodation.

prescribe—to lay down as a rule or direction; to order, advise, the use of.

prescription—a written direction for the preparation of a medicine.

prevention—the act of keeping something from coming to pass; to hinder.

preventive—tending to prevent or hinder. Something used to prevent disease.

primary—occurring first in time, development, or sequence; earliest.

prioritize—to arrange in order of importance.

priority—preference; state of being first in time, place or mark.

process—to treat or prepare by some method.

processor—performing a whole sequence of actions or operations.

proclivity—an inclination or predisposition toward something.

procrastination—intentionally delaying action of something that should be done; to postpone.

proctology—the study of the rectum and anus and their diseases.

proctoscope—an instrument for the inspection of the rectum.

proctoscopy—instrumental inspection of the rectum.

procure—to get or obtain.

procurement—to obtain; acquire.

professional—conforming to the technical or ethical standards of a profession.

professionalism—professional status, methods, character, or standards.

proficiency testing—PT; the measurement of acquired knowledge and skills; a means of assessing the competency of someone or of something.

proficient—well advanced in an art, occupation, skill, or branch of knowledge; unusually knowledgeable.

profit sharing—a system by which employees receive a share of the profits of a business enterprise.

progesterone—a hormone secreted by the graafian follicle following the expulsion of the ovum.

programmed—arranged; planned; a sequence of actions performed by a computer.

progress notes—record of the continuing progress and treatment of a patient.

project—to produce and send forth with clarity and distinctness.

prolapse—dropping of an internal part of the body; usually refers to uterus or rectum.

prominent—conspicuous, outstanding.

prompt—to urge to action, to inspire.

prone—a position, lying horizontal with the face down.

pronoun—a word used instead of a noun, to indicate without naming.

proofread—reading of printed proofs to discover and correct errors.

proprietary—privately owned and managed and run as a profit-making organization.

proprietorship—the amount by which assets exceed liabilities.

prostaglandins—a group of chemical substances secreted by mast cells or basophils that constricts smooth muscles in some organs.

prostate—a gland of the male reproductive system which surrounds the proximal portion of the urethra.

prostatectomy—excision of part or all of the prostate gland.

prosthesis—an artificial replacement of a missing body part.

pro tem—acting as (a temporary position); for the time being.

prothrombin—chemical substance existing in circulating blood which aids in the clotting process.

protozoan—a single-cell animal.

provider-performed microscopy procedures (PPMP)—refers to microscopic procedures done in the POL.

provisions—the act of providing; something provided for the future; a stipulation.

proximal—nearest the point of attachment.

pruritus—severe itching.

pruritus ani—itching about the anus.

psoriasis—a chronic inflammatory disease characterized by scaly patches.

psychedelics—hallucinogenic drugs.

psychiatrist—a physician specializing in the diseases and disorders of the mind, including neuroses and psychoses.

psychiatry—the branch of medicine dealing with the diagnosis, treatment, and prevention of mental illness.

psychological—of the mind; mental.

psychologist—a person specializing in the study of the structure and function of the brain and related mental processes.

psychology—the study of mental processes, both normal and abnormal, and their effects upon behavior.

psychoneuroimmunology—a science studying the connection between the brain, behavior, and immunity.

psychopathic—concerning or characterized by a mental disorder.

psychosis—mental disturbance of such magnitude that there is personality disintegration and loss of contact with reality.

psychosomatic—pertaining to interrelationships between the mind or emotions and body.

psychotherapy—the treatment of disease by hypnosis, psychoanalysis, and similar means.

PT—see Pharmacy technician or proficiency testing.

ptosis—a drooping or dropping of an organ or part, for example the eyelid or the kidney.

puberty—the period of life at which one becomes functionally capable of reproduction.

pubic—pertaining to the middle section of the lower third of the abdomen, also referred to as the hypogastric.

pulmonary—concerning or involving the lungs.

pulmonary edema—the presence of interstitial fluid in the lung tissue.

pulmonary embolism—a blockage in the pulmonary artery or one of its branches.

pulse—throbbing caused by the regular alternating contraction and expansion of an artery.

pulse deficit—the difference between the pulse rate measured radially and apically.

pulse pressure—difference between the systolic and diastolic measurements.

punctual—prompt; being on time.

punctuation—standardized marks in written matter to clarify meaning.

puncture—a hole made by something pointed.

pupil—the contractible opening in the center of the iris for the transmission of light.

purge—to empty; to cleanse of impurities; clear.

purkinje—network of fibers found in the cardiac muscle which carries the electrical impulses resulting in the contraction of the ventricles.

pustule—small elevation of the skin filled with lymph or pus.

pyelonephritis—inflammation of the kidney, pelvis, and nephrons.

pyloric—pertaining to the opening between the stomach and the duodenum.

pyrogen—capable of producing fever.

QNS—quantity not sufficient.

quackery—the pretense to knowledge or skill in medicine.

quad-based—refers to a cane with four "feet".

quadrant—one of four regions, as of the abdomen, divided for identification purposes.

quadriceps femoris—a large muscle on the anterior surface of the thigh which is composed of four separate muscles.

quality assurance (QA)—inclusive policies, procedures, and practices as standards for reliable laboratory results that includes documentation, calibration, and maintenance of all equipment, quality control, proficiency testing, and training.

quality control (QC)—inclusive laboratory procedures as standards to provide reliable performance of equipment, including test control samples, documentation, and analyzing statistics for diagnostic tests.

R/O—rule out.

ROM—see **range of motion.**

radial—referring to the radial artery or pulse taken in the radial artery.

radiation—the emission and diffusion of rays; a product of X-ray and radium.

radioactive—capable of emitting radiant energy.

radiograph—a record produced on a photographic plate, film, or paper by the action of X-ray or radium.

radiologic technologist—(X-ray technician) a person with specialized training in the techniques to prepare X-ray films to visualize the tissues and organs of the body.

radiologist—one who diagnoses and treats disease by the use of radiant energy.

radiology—the study of radiation and its uses.

radionuclides—a type of atom utilized in nuclear medicine for the diagnosis and treatment of disease.

radiopaque—impenetrable to the X-ray or other forms of radiation.

radius—a long bone of the forearm.

râles—an unusual sound heard in the bronchi on examination of respirations.

ramification—a subdivision or consequence.

random—by chance; without plan.

range of motion (ROM)—refers to the degree of movement of the body's joints and extremities.

rapport—relationship characterized by harmony and cooperation.

rationalization—to explain on rational grounds, to devise plausible explanations for one's acts.

Raynaud's phenomenon—a symptom of Lupus characterized by fingers which turn white or blue in the cold.

reactivity—rate of nuclear disintegration in a reactor.

reagent—a substance involved in a chemical reaction.

realm—kingdom or empire, as used in text.

reason rule—refers to the purpose or reason for doing a test or procedure, an insurance company criteria for reimbursement.

reception—the fact or manner of being received; a social gathering.

receptionist—one employed to greet telephone callers, visitors, patients, or clients.

receptor—peripheral nerve ending of a sensory nerve that responds to stimuli.

recessive—tending to recede; apparently suppressed in crossbred offspring in preference for a characteristic from the other parent; an organism having one or more recessive characteristics.

recipient—one who receives.

reciprocity—mutual exchange, especially the exchange of special privilege.

reconcile—process to bring checkbook and bank statement into agreement.

rectal—referring to the rectum.

rectocele—the protrusion of the posterior vaginal wall with anterior wall of rectum through the vagina.

rectum—the lower part of the large intestine between the sigmoid and the anal canal.

recumbent—lying down.

recurrent—returning at intervals.

reduce—to restore the ends of a fractured bone to their usual relationship.

redundant—extra, not needed, repetitive.

reference—a source of information or authority.

reflex—an involuntary response to a stimulus.

reflux—a return or backward flow.

refractive—the degree to which a transparent body deflects a ray of light from a straight path.

regimen—regulation of diet, sleep, exercise, and manner of living to improve or maintain health.

register—a formal or official recording of items, names, or actions.

registry—a list of persons qualified in a particular area of expertise.

regulate—control or direction.

Regulations in the POL—standards set for QA and QC in the physician's office laboratory to ensure reliable diagnostic tests.

regulatory—to control according to a rule; to adjust so as to make work accurately.

rehabilitate—to put back in good condition; to restore.

reimburse—to pay back or compensate for money spent, or losses or damages incurred.

reiterate—to say or do again.

rejuvenate—to make young again; to give youthful qualities to.

reliable—dependable, can be relied upon.

reluctant—marked by unwillingness.

rely—to depend on, to trust.

remedy—anything that relieves or cures a disease.

remission—a period that is disease- and symptom-free.

remote—from a distance; far removed in time and place; indirect.

renal—pertaining to the kidney.

renal failure—loss of function of the kidneys' nephrons.

renal threshold—the concentration at which a substance in the blood normally not excreted by the kidney begins to appear in the urine.

render—to present or to deliver, as a service or statement.

renovate—restore; to make new again.

repolarization—reestablishment of a polarized state in a muscle or nerve fiber following contraction or conduction of a nerve impulse.

repression—to force painful ideas or impulses into the subconscious.

reproductive—concerning reproduction.

reputable—having a good reputation; well thought of.

res ipsa loquitur—the thing speaks for itself.

residency—physician training period in a specialty field of medicine.

residual—pertaining to that which is left as a residue.

residual barium—barium remaining in the intestinal tract following evacuation at the completion of X-ray studies.

resistance—opposition, ability to oppose.

resonance—(1) quality of the sound heard on percussion of the chest; (2) the intensification and prolongation of a sound by reflection or by vibration of a nearby object.

resource—a source of support or supply.

respectful—showing respect; honoring; treat with consideration.

respiration—the taking in of oxygen and its utilization in the tissues and the giving off of carbon dioxide.

respiratory—pertaining to respiration.

respiratory therapy technician—a person trained to perform procedures of treatment which maintain or improve the ventilatory function of the respiratory tract.

respite—a temporary cessation of something that is painful or tiring; to delay, postpone.

respondeat superior—let the master answer.

retardation—slowing, delay, lag; slow in development, mental or physical.

retention—inability to void urine which is present in the bladder.

reticuloendothelial—pertaining to that group of cells which appear to aid in the making of new blood cells and the disintegration of old ones.

retina—the innermost layer of the eye which receives the image formed by the lens.

retinopathy—a degeneration of the retina due to a decrease in blood supply.

retraction—a shortening; the act of drawing backward or state of being drawn back.

retroflexed—refers to the body of the uterus being bent backward.

retrograde—refers to an X-ray procedure in which a radiopaque material is instilled by catheter into the bladder, ureters, and kidneys.

retroperitoneal—behind the peritoneum; posterior to the peritoneal lining of the abdominal cavity.

retroverted—refers to the entire uterus being tilted backward.

retrovirus—one with RNA genetic material.

revalidation—the renewing or reconfirmation of credentials.

revoke—to cancel, withdraw, take back.

Rh factor—an antigenic substance in human blood similar to the A and B factors which determine blood groups; apparently present only in red blood cells.

rhinitis—inflammation of the nasal mucosa.

rhinoplasty—plastic surgery of the nose.

rhythm—a measured time or movement; regularity of occurrence.

ribosome—an organelle within the cytoplasm of the cell.

rickets—a disease of the bones primarily due to the deficiency of Vitamin D.

risk—chance; hazard; chance of loss or injury; degree of probability of loss.

roentgen—refers to X-rays.

Role Delineation Study—Occupational analysis study conducted by AAMA and the National Board of Medical Examination in 1997 which identifies the most up-to-date entry-level areas of competence of the medical assisting profession.

rotate—to move around; to turn on an axis.

rubella—(German measles) a mild contagious viral disease which may cause severe damage to an unborn child.

rubeola—(Measles) an acute, highly contagious disease marked by a typical cutaneous eruption.

S-A node—see **sinoatrial node.**

sacrum—five fused vertebrae which lie between the coccyx and the lumbar vertebrae of the spinal column.

safety—freedom from danger or loss.

sagittal—refers to a plane which is made by dividing the body down the center creating a right and left side.

saliva—a digestive secretion of the salivary glands which empties into the stomach.

salivary glands—three pairs of glands that secrete the saliva which begins the digestion of food, primarily the breakdown of starch or complex carbohydrates.

salpingectomy—surgical removal of the fallopian tube or tubes.

salpingo-oophorectomy—surgical excision of the ovary and fallopian tube.

salve—an ointment.

sarcoma—malignant tumors of the connective, muscle, or bone tissue.

sartorius—a long narrow muscle of the thigh; the longest muscle of the body.

scan—to look over quickly but thoroughly.

scapula—the shoulder blade.

schedule—to arrange a timetable; to place in a list of things to be done.

sciatica—inflammation and pain along the sciatic nerve felt at back of thigh running down the inside of the leg.

scientific—based upon or using the principles and methods of science; systematic; exact.

sclera—the white or sclerotic outer coat of the eye.

scoliosis—lateral curvature of the spine.

screening—a preliminary or indicating procedure.

script—manuscript; type designed to look like handwriting.

scrotum—the double pouch containing the testes and part of the spermatic cord.

scurvy—a disease due to lack of fresh fruits, vegetables, and vitamin C in the diet.

sebaceous—an oily, fatty matter; glands secreting such matter.

sebum—oily secretion of the sebaceous glands of the skin.

secondary—one step removed from the first; not primary.

secretary—one employed to conduct correspondence; a person responsible for records and correspondence.

secretion—separation of certain materials from the blood by the activity of a gland.

sector—a section or division.

security—freedom from fear or anxiety.

sedentary—pertaining to sitting; inactivity.

sedimentation—formation or depositing of sediment; of blood, refers to the speed at which erythrocytes settle when an anticoagulant is added to blood.

segment—a part or section of an organ or a body.

seizures—a sudden attack of pain, or disease or of certain symptoms.

self-control—control of ones emotions, desires.

semen—the mixture of secretions from the various glands and organs of the reproductive system of the male, which is expelled at orgasm.

semicircular canals—structures located in the inner ear.

semilunar—the valves of the heart located between the ventricles and the pulmonary artery and aorta.

senility—feebleness of body or mind caused by old age.

sensitivity—abnormal susceptibility to a substance.

sensorineural deafness—a loss of hearing due to transmission failure of the nerves within the inner ear or the auditory nerve.

sensory—refers to the nerves which receive and transmit stimuli from the sense organs.

septum—a membranous wall dividing two cavities, as within the heart or the nose.

sequence—order of succession.

sequentially—arranged in sequence; in an order.

series—a group; a set of things in the same class coming one after another.

serrated—notched, toothed.

sharps—any object which can cut, prick, stab, or scrape the skin.

sheath—a covering structure of connective tissue such as the membrane covering a muscle.

shock—a condition in which the pulse becomes rapid and weak, the blood pressure drops, and the patient is pale and clammy.

sickle cell anemia—a blood disorder in which the red blood cells are shaped like sickles.

sigmoid—an s-shaped section of the large intestine between the descending colon and the rectum.

sigmoidoscopy—an inspection of the sigmoid with an instrument.

signature—a signing of one's own name.

simple—referring to a bone fracture, one without involvement of the skin surface.

simultaneous—occurring at the same time.

sinoatrial (S-A) node—the source of the nerve impulse which initiates the heartbeat; the pacemaker.

sinusitis—inflammation of the sinuses.

skeletal—pertaining to the skeleton or bony structure; also to the muscles attached to the skeleton to permit movement.

skip—a person who owes money but cannot be located.

sling—a hanging support for an injured arm.

slough—to cast off, as dead tissue.

smooth—a type of involuntary muscle tissue found in internal organs.

snap locks—metal locking devices.

Snellen chart—the chart of alphabetic letters used to evaluate distant vision.

sole—only.

solicit—to ask for.

somatic—pertaining to the body as distinguished from the mind; physical.

sonar—a device that transmits high-frequency sound waves in water and registers the vibrations reflected back from an object.

sonogram—record obtained by ultrasound.

sophisticated—not simple or natural; very refined; highly complex or developed in form, technique, etc.

spasm—an involuntary sudden movement or convulsive muscular contraction.

spastic colon—spasmodic contractions of the large intestine.

specificity—something specially suited for a given use or purpose; a remedy regarded as a certain cure for a particular disease.

specified—named particularly; mentioned in detail.

specimen—a sample; a representative piece of the whole.

sperm—the male gamete or sex cell.

spermatozoon—a sperm cell.

sphincter—a circular muscle constricting an opening.

sphygmomanometer—a device that measures blood pressure; also called manometer.

spina bifida—a disorder characterized by a defect in the spinal vertebrae with or without protrusion of the spinal cord and meninges.

spinal—pertaining to the spinal column, canal, or cord.

spinal fusion—the surgical implanting of a bone fragment between the processes of two or more spinal vertebrae to render them immobile.

spiral—having a circular fashion.

spirometer—an apparatus which measures the volume of inhaled and exhaled air.

spleen—an oval, vascular, ductless gland below the diaphragm, in the upper left quadrant of the abdomen.

splinter—a thin sharp piece of wood.

spontaneous—involuntary; produced by itself; unforced.

spores—hard capsules formed by certain bacteria which allow them to resist prolonged exposure to heat.

sports medicine—the branch of medicine dealing with the care of athletes to prevent and treat sports-related injuries.

sprain—the forcible twisting of a joint with partial rupture or other injury of its attachments.

sputum—substance ejected from the mouth containing saliva and mucus; usually refers to material coughed up from the bronchi.

stabilize—to make steady; firmly fixed; constant.

standardization—process of bringing into conformity with a standard; pertaining to EKG, a mark made at the beginning of each lead to establish a standard of reference.

stapes—one of the three bones of the middle ear.

stasis ulcer—an open lesion due to stagnant or inadequate blood supply to an area.

STAT (statim)—immediately.

stationery—writing materials, especially paper and envelopes.

stature—height.

statutory—legally enacted; deriving authority from law.

stenosis—narrowing or constriction of a passage or opening.

sterile—without any organisms.

sternocleidomastoid—a muscle of the chest arising from the sternum and inner part of clavicle.

sternum—the breastbone.

stethoscope—an instrument used in auscultation to convey to the ear the sounds produced by the body.

stimulant—a substance which temporarily increases activity.

stipulations—terms of an agreement.

stomach—a dilated, saclike, distensible portion of the alimentary canal below the esophagus and before the small intestine.

stool—bowel movement, feces.

strabismus—an eye disorder caused by imbalance of the ocular muscles.

strain—injury to muscles from tension due to overuse or misuse.

stratagem—a trick or deception.

stress—to put pressure on; emphasize; urgency; tension, strained exertion. Topical; causing strain or injury to the skin.

striated—a type of muscle tissue marked with stripes or striae.

stricture—the narrowing of an opening, tube, or canal, such as the urethra or esophagus.

stylus—a pen; the EKG writer.

subarachnoid—the space between the pia mater and the arachnoid containing cerebrospinal fluid.

subcutaneous—beneath the skin.

subdural—beneath the dural mater; the space between the arachnoid and the dura mater.

subjective—relating to the person who is thinking, saying, or doing something; personal; of a disease symptom, felt by the individual but not perceptible to others.

sublimation—to express certain impulses, especially sexual, in constructive, socially acceptable forms.

sublingual—under the tongue.

subpoena duces tecum—court process initiated by party in litigation, compelling production of specific documents and other items, and material in relevance to facts in issue in appending judicial proceedings.

subsequent—coming after, following.

substantial—considerable, large.

suction—withdrawal by pressure; a sucking action.

sudden infant death syndrome (SIDS)—the sudden, unexplainable death of an infant.

superficial—on the surface.

superior—above or higher than.

supernatant—floating on the surface.

supine—lying horizontally on the back.

supplement—something added; an additional or extra section.

support—to hold up; to bear part of the weight of.

suppository—a medicated conical or cylindrical shaped material which is inserted into the rectum or vagina.

suppression—the shutdown of kidney function; the absence of urine excretion.

suppression—in psychology it is the deliberate exclusion of an idea, desire, or feeling from consciousness.

suppressor—one that holds back or stops an action.

suprapubic—above the pubic arch.

surfactant—a fatty molecule on the respiratory membranes.

surgeon—a physician with advanced training in operative procedures.

surgery—the branch of medicine dealing with manual and operative procedures for correction of deformities and defects and repair of injuries.

surrogate—a substitute; in place of another.

susceptible—having little resistance to a disease or foreign protein.

suture—to unite parts by stitching them together.

symmetry—the state in which one part exactly corresponds to another in size, shape, and position.

sympathetic—a portion of the autonomic nervous system.

symphysis pubis—the junction of the pubic bones on the midline in front.

symptom—any perceptible change in the body or its functions which indicates disease or the phase of a disease.

synapse—the minute space between the axon of one neuron and the dendrite of another.

syncope—fainting, a transient form of unconsciousness.

syndrome—the combination of symptoms with a disease or disorder.

synergism—something stimulating the action of another so that the effect of both is greater than the sum of the individual effects.

synovial—a movable joint; also called diarthroses.

syphilis—a communicable venereal disease spread by sexual contact.

system—a group of organs working together to perform a function of the body.

systematic—by a system or plan.

systole—the contraction phase of the heart; the greatest amount of blood pressure.

tachycardia—abnormal rapidity of heart action.

tact—delicate perception of the right things to say and do without offending.

tar—a sticky, brown or black carcinogenic substance.

tarsals—pertaining to the seven bones of the instep of the foot.

taut—tightly drawn; tense.

technical—relating to some particular art, science, or trade; also, requiring special skill or technique.

technologist—one skilled in technology; able to apply the technical methods in a particular field of industry or art.

technology—the practice of any or all of the applied sciences that have practical value and/or industrial use.

teleconference—a meeting held over phone lines incorporating video equipment.

temperature—degree of heat of a living body; degree of hotness or coldness of a substance; usually refers to an elevation of body heat.

temporal—relating to the temporal bone on the skull.

tendon—fibrous connective tissue serving to attach muscles to bones.

tendonitis—inflammation of the tendon.

tentative—experimental, provisional, temporary.

terminal—final, end; a terminal illness, refers to a condition which cannot be reversed.

termination—ending.

testes—the male gonads of the scrotum which produce sperm.

testosterone—a male hormone secreted by the testes which causes and maintains male secondary sex characteristics.

tetanus—an acute infectious disease due to the toxins of the bacillus tetani.

tetany—intermittent tonic spasms resulting from inadequate parathyroid hormone.

thalamus—a portion of the brain lying between the cerebrum and the midbrain.

theories—beliefs not yet tested in practice; the general principles on which a science is based.

therapeutic—having medicinal or healing properties; pertaining to results obtained from treatment.

therapist—one who practices the curative and preventive treatment of disease or an abnormal condition.

thermal—characterized by heat; heat activated.

thermography—a technique for sensing and recording on film, hot and cold areas of the body by means of an infrared detector that reacts to blood flow.

thermometer—an instrument used to measure temperature.

thesaurus—a treasury of words, quotations, knowledge; a collection of words with their synonyms and antonyms.

third party—(Insurance) someone other than the patient, spouse, or parent who is responsible for paying all or part of the patient's medical costs.

thoracic—pertaining to the thorax or chest.

thorax—the chest; the body cavity enclosed by the ribs and containing the heart and lungs.

thready—term used to describe a weak pulse which may feel like a thread under the skin surface.

thrombophlebitis—inflammation of a vein associated with the formation of a blood clot.

thrombosis—the formation of a blood clot or thrombus.

thymus—an unpaired organ located in the mediastinal cavity anterior to and above the heart.

thyroid—an endocrine gland located anteriorly at the base of the neck.

thyroidectomy—the surgical removal of the thyroid gland.

tibia—a long bone in the leg from the knee to the ankle.

tibialis anterior—a muscle of the leg.

tinnitus—a ringing or tinkling sound in the ear which is heard only by the person affected.

tissue—a collection of similar cells and fibers forming a structure in the body.

tolerance—the difference between the maximum and

minimum; the amount of variation allowed from a standard.

tongue—the muscular organ of the mouth which assists in the production of speech, contains the taste buds, and provides the ability to swallow.

tonometer—instrument for measuring intraocular tension or pressure.

topical—pertaining to a specific area; local.

tort—any wrongful act, damage or injury done willfully, negligently.

torticollis—stiff neck caused by spasmotic contraction of neck muscles drawing the head to one side with the chin pointing to the other; can be congenital or acquired.

total quality management (TQM)—refers to a management style that uses QA and QC to maintain quality of performance throughout the total process, not just to assure the end result is satisfactory or corrected.

tourniquet—any constrictor used on an extremity to produce pressure on an artery and control bleeding; also used to distend veins for the withdrawal of blood or the insertion of a needle to instill intravenous injections.

toxin—poisonous substance or compound of vegetable, animal, or bacterial origin.

toxoid—a toxin treated so as to destroy its toxicity, but still capable of inducing formation of antibodies on injection.

TQM—see total quality management.

trace—the production of a sketch by means of a stylus passing over the paper as in electrocardiography.

trachea—a cartilaginous tube between the larynx and the main bronchus of the respiratory tree.

tracheostomy—a surgically made opening in the trachea through which a person will breathe.

traction—the process of pulling; with fractures, traction is applied in a straight line to stretch the contracted muscles and permit realignment of the bone fragments.

trait—a feature; a distinguishing feature of character or mind.

transactions—dealings accomplished.

transcript—a copy made directly from an original record, especially an official copy of a student's educational record.

transcription—writing over from one book or medium into another; typing in full in ordinary letters.

transdermal—through the skin.

transducer—a device that transforms power from one system to another in the same or different form.

transfusion—injection of the blood of one person into the blood vessels of another.

transient ischemic attack (TIA)—temporary interruption of blood flow in the brain due to small clots closing off blood vessels.

transillumination—inspection of a cavity or organ by passing a light through its walls.

transition—passing from one condition, place, or activity to another.

transmitted—sent from one person, thing, or place to another.

transpose—putting one in place of another, the accidental misplacing of words or letters.

transurethral—literally means through the urethra; refers to the removal of the prostate by going through the urethral wall.

transverse—lying across; the segment of large intestine which lies across the abdomen; a line drawn horizontally across the body or a structure.

trapezius—the large muscle of the back and neck.

traumatic—caused by or relating to an injury.

traumatize—to cause trauma or injury.

treadmill—an apparatus with a movable platform which permits walking or running in place.

Trendelenburg—a position with the head lower than the feet.

trephining—cutting out a circular section.

trial balance—bookkeeping strategy to confirm accuracy in debits and credits in ledger.

triangular—having three angles and three sides.

triceps—the posterior muscles of the arm which work as a team with the biceps; the triceps straighten the elbow.

trichomoniasis—infestation with parasitic protozoa; usually refers to vaginal involvement.

tricuspid—a valve in the right side of the heart, between the chambers; literally means three cusps or leaflets.

trimester—divided into three sections; the third segment or period.

trivial—of little value, insignificant.

truncated—to cut the top or end off; to lop; with insurance.

tuberculosis—an infectious disease caused by the tubercle bacillus; pulmonary tuberculosis is a specific inflammatory disease of the lungs which destroys lung tissue.

tumor—a swelling or enlargement; a neoplasm; often used to indicate a malignant growth.

turbidity—flaky or granular particles suspended in a clear liquid giving it a cloudy appearance; usually refers to cloudy urine.

tympanic membrane—the eardrum.

typhoid—an acute infectious disease acquired by ingesting contaminated food or water.

Tzanck smear—examination of tissue from the lower surface of a lesion in vesicular disease to determine the cell type.

URI—see **upper respiratory infection.**

UTI—see **urinary tract infection.**

ulcer—an open lesion on the skin or mucous membrane of the body characterized by loss of tissue and the formation of a secretion.

ulceration—suppuration of the skin or mucous membrane; an open lesion.

ulna—a long bone in the forearm from the elbow to the wrist.

ultimately—in the end, finally.

ultrasonic scanning—a process of scanning the body with sound waves to produce a picture on a screen of underlying internal structures.

umbilical—pertaining to the umbilicus or navel of the abdomen.

unemployed—the state of being without work.

unique—one of a kind, unmatched.

unit clerk—a secretarial position on the health care team of a patient care facility.

universal—relating to the universe; general or common to all.

unobtrusive—not forced upon others; not thrust forward or pushed out.

unproductive—not productive; no accomplishment.

unstructured—without specific arrangement.

upper respiratory infection (URI)—inflammatory process involving the nose and throat, may include the sinuses; refers to symptoms associated with the common cold.

uremia—a condition in which products normally found in the urine are found in the blood.

ureter—a tube carrying urine from the kidney to the urinary bladder.

urethra—a membranous canal for the external discharge of urine from the bladder.

urgency—the sudden need to expel urine or stool.

urinalysis—an analysis of the urine; a test performed on urine to determine its characteristics.

urinary meatus—the opening through which urine passes from the body.

urinary tract infection (UTI)—infection occurring within the kidneys, ureters, and/or urinary bladder.

urination—the act of urinating or voiding of urine.

urine—fluid secreted from the blood by the kidneys, stored in the bladder, and discharged from the body by voiding.

urology—the study of the urine and diseases of the urinogenital organs.

urticaria—an inflammatory condition characterized by the eruption of wheals which are associated with severe itching; commonly called hives.

uterus—a muscular, hollow, pear-shaped organ of the female reproductive tract in which a fertilized ovum develops into a baby.

utilization—to put to profitable use.

utilize—to use or make use of.

vaccination—inoculation with modified harmless viruses or other microorganisms to produce immunity, a preventative against diseases.

vaccine—any substance for prevention of a disease.

vagina—a musculomembranous tube which forms the passageway from the uterus to the exterior.

vaginitis—inflammation of the vagina.

vagus—the tenth cranial nerve which has both motor and sensory function, affecting the heart and stomach as well as other organs.

valve—any one of various structures for temporarily closing an opening or passageway, or for allowing movement of fluid in one direction only.

varices—enlarged, twisted veins.

varicose—pertaining to varices; distended, swollen veins, most commonly found in the legs.

vas deferens—the excretory duct of the testes.

vasectomy—the cutting out of a portion of the vas deferens.

vein—a blood vessel carrying blood toward the heart after receiving it from a venule.

vena cava—one of two large veins which empty into the right atrium of the heart.

venipuncture—the puncture of a vein; the insertion of a needle into a vein for the purpose of obtaining a blood sample or instilling a substance.

venous—pertaining to a vein.

ventilatory—that which ventilates, lets in fresh air.

ventral—pertaining to the anterior or front side of the body.

ventricle—one of the two lower chambers of the heart; also used in reference to cavities within the brain.

venule—a minute vein; a blood vessel which connects a capillary with a vein.

verb—the part of speech which expresses an action.

verify—to prove to be true; to support by facts.

veritable—actual, genuine.

vermiform appendix—the appendix; a small tube attached to the cecum.

verrucae—warts; small, circumscribed elevations of the skin formed by hypertrophy of the papillae.

vertebrae—the bones in the spinal column.

vertex—the top of the head, the crown.

vesicle—a small sac or bladder containing fluid; a small, blisterlike elevation on the skin containing serous fluid.

vested—settled; complete; absolute; continuous.

viable—capable of living.

vial—a small glass tube or bottle containing medication or a chemical.

video display terminal—the computer monitor.

villi—tiny projections from a surface; the villi of the small intestine which absorb nutrients during the process of digestion.

villous adenoma—a type of polyp which is invasive and malignant.

virulent—full of poison; deadly; malignant.

virus—a very simple, frequently pathogenic, microorganism capable of replicating within living cells.

visceral—pertaining to viscera, the internal organs, especially the abdomen.

vital—essential; pertaining to the preservation of life (the vital signs).

vital capacity—the total volume of air exchanged from forced inspiration and forced expiration.

vitreous humor—the substance which fills the vitreous body of the eye behind the lens.

void—to pass urine from the urinary bladder; to make ineffective or invalid.

volatile—easily changed into a gas or tending to change into a vapor; usually considered potentially dangerous.

voltage—a measure of electromotive force.

volume—the amount of space occupied by an object as measured in cubic units.

voluntary—under one's control, done by one's own choice.

vomit—to expel the contents of the stomach through the mouth.

voucher—a document that serves as proof that terms of a transaction have been met.

vulnerable—liable to injury or hurt; capable of being wounded.

vulva—the female external genitalia, including the clitoris, the labia minora, and the labia majora.

waiver—to give up; forgo; waiving of a right or claim.

warrant—to justify, to give definite assurance as to the value of; to authorize.

wart—see **verrucae.**

watermark—a mark imprinted on paper that is visible when it is held to the light, usually a sign of quality.

wheals—more or less round and evanescent elevations of the skin, white in center with a pale red edge, accompanied by itching.

wheelchair—a chair fitted with wheels by which a person can propel themself.

whorl—a type of fingerprint in which the central papillary ridges turn through at least one complete circle.

withdrawal—a removal of something that has been deposited.

womb—nonmedical name for the uterus.

work-in—to make time or space for.

writer—the person who writes; the author.

xiphoid—a process which forms the tip of the sternum.

x-linked—connected to the cell's sex chromosome; a characteristic of the sex chromosome.

Z-Tract—a method of injecting medication intramuscularly.

zygote—a cell produced by the union of an ovum and a sperm.

Index

Page numbers followed by *f* indicate figures.
Page numbers followed by *t* indicate tables.